# FEEDING

*Our*

# CHILDREN

A COMPREHENSIVE GUIDE *for* HAVING A HEALTHY, THRIVING CHILD
DURING THEIR FIRST THOUSAND DAYS *and Beyond*

## THOMAS FLASS, MD, MS

# FEEDING OUR CHILDREN

Published by Aware Families LLC

ISBN: 979-8-985-3711-2-3
Digital edition
eISBN-979-8-985-3711-1-6

The information in this book is for educational purposes only. It is not meant to diagnose or treat any medical condition or disease, and is not a substitute for medical care. No physician-patient relationship is stated or implied. Medical concerns must be discussed with a qualified medical provider. Following nutritional advice contained in this book is at the readers own discretion and should always be discussed with the reader's or their child's primary health care provider. Use of any information contained within implies the readers acceptance of this disclaimer.

The publisher and the author have made every effort to ensure that the information presented in this book was accurate at the time of publication. However, while this publication is designed to provide accurate information in regard to the subject matter contained within, the publisher and author assume no responsibility for errors, inaccuracies, omissions, or any other inconsistencies in this text and hereby disclaim any liability to any party for any loss, damage, or disruption caused by errors or omissions, whether such errors or omissions result from negligence, accident, or any other cause.

The publisher and the author make no guarantees concerning any level of success you may experience by following the advice contained in this book. The reader accepts the risk that results will differ for each individual.

# TABLE OF CONTENTS

Preface ........................................................................ v

Chapter 1: Laying the Foundation for a Healthy Life .......................... 1

Chapter 2: The First Thousand Days ......................................... 12

Chapter 3: The Microbiome and Its Role in Human Health .............. 23

Chapter 4: Negative Impacts on the Microbiome ........................... 34

Chapter 5: Being the Best Stewards of Our Children's Microbiome ... 44

Chapter 6: Nutrition Advice for the Expecting Mother ................... 55

Chapter 7: Minimizing Exposure to Toxins and Pollutants .............. 114

Chapter 8: Breastfeeding ................................................... 138

Chapter 9: Infant Formula Feeding ........................................ 162

Chapter 10: Baby's First Foods ............................................ 178

Chapter 11: Feeding Our Toddlers and Young Children .................... 207

Chapter 12: Common Nutrient Deficiencies in Children ................. 245

Chapter 13: Food Allergies and Intolerances ............................. 274

Chapter 14: Celiac Disease and Gluten Sensitivity ...................... 302

Chapter 15: Constipation—The Straight Poop ........................... 315

Chapter 16: Pediatric Feeding Disorders, Feeding Tactics,
and Strategies ............................................................. 326

Chapter 17: Metabolic Health and the Dangers of Sugar ................ 342

Chapter 18: Metabolic Health: The Recovery ............................ 363

Chapter 19: Diet and the Child's Brain ................................... 393

Closing Thoughts........................................................... 421

Glossary ................................................................... 423

## WITH LOVE

To my girls, who wondered what daddy was doing in his office the past few years... you are the inspiration for this book.

To my wife, for giving me the grace and the space to finish this quest; you are the glue that holds our family together.

## ACKNOWLEDGMENTS

To Wolfram and Roberta at Serotonin Press, whose initial edits gave shape to this book.

To Miriam and Michael who took it the rest of the way home.

To all the researchers and healthcare providers who work to improve the health and lives of our children.

*Thank you*

# PREFACE

What if I were to tell you that what you feed your children in the first few years of their lives will impact their health, not only now, but decades into the future? What if you had evidence that feeding your children the Standard American Diet was impairing school performance, eroding their health, and programming their bodies for a life of chronic disease?

We are discovering that diet and chemical exposures in those first few critical years of a child's life may determine whether they will thrive physically and academically or are more likely to have learning difficulties and develop diseases like type 2 diabetes, which can knock ten years off of their lives. Modern science is also providing evidence that what a pregnant mother eats affects not only her child's health but also the health of her future grandchildren and great grandchildren!

It's time we step back and take a good look at what we are feeding ourselves and our children. Once aware of the potential dangers lurking in our food, will we deviate from the easy path of the Standard American Diet and start making positive changes for our children's benefit if not for our own? I am hoping that for you, the answer is yes.

The purpose of this book is not to scare you ... well, ok maybe a little. A little fear can be a good thing if it motivates us to make a positive change. Deep down we all want to do the best thing for our kids. I am hopeful that armed with the knowledge of the dangers that exist in our food supply and environment, we will try to do the right thing and protect our children. This is our job as parents, as well as the medical providers who care for them. My main purpose in writing this book is to inform and empower parents to make better choices for their children's health.

In the thirty years since I began studying nutrition, authorities in this field have published enough conflicting and contradictory information to erode much of your trust, make your head spin, and tie your bowels in a knot. I would like to apologize for this confusion and offer some explanation. Science and medicine are constantly evolving as new findings emerge, but new information is often rejected by doctors and academics who are trapped in the past and view new information as a threat, not a gift. Because of this resistance, new, accurate, and useful information often takes twenty years or more to make it from "the bench" (research labs) to "the bedside" (accepted medical practice). Given the current health of our nation and the world, we don't have twenty years to wait.

Another unfortunate fact is that groups looking to protect their bottom lines or promote their own hidden agendas corrupt some of the research and information they spread. Whenever a headline about some new study hits the media, the savvy reader needs to ask who funded the study and what they may gain by the results. Distortion of research for financial gain is not conspiracy theory; it is unfortunately the way of the modern world.

I am not trying to sell you anything other than my belief that what you feed your children is the single most important choice you can make for the health they will experience throughout their lives. At the time of writing this book, I do not have any financial ties to the food or nutritional supplement industry, and I have no agenda other than to provide objective, evidence-based, and contemporary information to help improve the health of your child.

We have been systematically misled and misinformed about what is healthy and acceptable for our kids. What we don't know can hurt us. **Ignorance is *not* bliss, ignorance is dangerous.** Nutrition has significant power to hurt or heal depending on the choices we make as individuals and as a society. I want to help you make good choices for your child.

To the best of my ability, the information I present in this book is evidence-based and backed up with research published in peer-reviewed scientific and medical journals. I provide references to these validated sources to support my recommendations, equipping you with the science that demonstrates your dietary choices matter. Where the science is new or controversial, I will use the "Hot Topic" sections to offer my professional opinion as a pediatric gastroenterologist and nutrition expert even if it differs with currently established practice. But beyond this, I am in this journey with you. My wife and I used the information provided in this book while raising our two amazing children to make informed food choices and give them the best start possible.

While the material presented in this book is at the forefront of medicine and nutrition, it may not yet be mainstream and may go against present guidelines and recommendations that are obsolete. Beliefs and established "truths" change very slowly and with much resistance.

> *"All truth passes through three stages—first it is ridiculed, then it is violently protested, then it is accepted as self-evident."*
>
> Arthur Schopenhauer, German philosopher.

A surprisingly low percentage of medical schools (29% by recent assessment) include *any* nutrition education in their curriculum. Those that do usually only give a cursory overview of the basics and don't emphasize the increasingly recognized role that nutrition plays in health, much less the physiologic and pharmacologic effects of food. Since most disease is directly impacted by nutrition and lifestyle, nutritional science should be featured as one of the core elements of all medical school curriculums, but this is currently not the case.

I am very fortunate that my road to medical school involved getting an undergraduate degree from Cornell University and a master's degree from Colorado State University, both in human nutrition. I also worked for a number of years in nutrition, health, and wellness prior to medical school. The more I learned about diet and nutrition, the more I realized how very little consideration it was given in the practice of modern medicine.

However, I did not go into nutrition with the conscious intent of becoming a doctor. It wasn't until a defining moment in my life while working on a master's thesis that a research colleague changed the course of my life. During a conversation about our project involving fish oil and brain development, he turned to me and bluntly stated, "You should really be applying to medical school. Everything you are doing, everything we are talking about, relates directly to medicine." When I started making excuses for why I couldn't do it—too many years had passed since my undergraduate degree, the intimidating MCAT entrance exam—he looked me in the eye and said, "You can be forty and *wish* you were a doctor, or you can be forty and *be* a doctor. It's your choice." At that moment I felt my entire life trajectory shift from where I thought I was headed to where I needed to be. I am forever grateful to him for the wakeup call I needed to set me on this path.

I am also grateful that the University of Colorado was willing to take a chance on a non-traditional medical school applicant, and that I was lucky enough to complete my pediatrics and gastroenterology training at Children's Hospital Colorado, one of the top pediatric training programs in the country. Blessed with this education and opportunity, I made it my mission to continuously learn and incorporate evidence-based nutrition into my practice of pediatric gastroenterology and to help other health-care providers incorporate contemporary nutrition science into their own practices. I chose pediatrics because working with younger patients gives me a greater chance to make a difference earlier in the game before bad patterns are fully set, and a lot of the damage is done. Pediatric gastroenterology uses more nutrition in day-to-day medical practice than any other specialty, which is one of the primary reasons I was drawn to this field.

During my medical training and career, I have become extremely interested in the *microbiome,* the collection of microbes that live on and inside our bodies, including probiotic bacteria, and its underappreciated importance in human health. It has become evident to me that many of our kids' health issues likely stem from the fact that the food they eat does not support healthy gut bacteria or proper development of their brains or bodies. Unhealthy foods are programming their bodies for future disease—partially by a process called epigenetics described in the second chapter of this book. These concepts are increasingly backed by evidence, yet still under-valued and seldom incorporated into modern medicine. If parents, healthcare providers, and school administrators better understood the importance of this new research, we would see the health of our children greatly improve.

Becoming a parent, as it has a tendency to do, changes *everything.* Supporting my wife through two pregnancies and breastfeeding and raising my own children has brought my academic, scientific perspective down to a very real, very personal level. How was I going to protect my beautiful little girls from the dangers I knew existed in our food system? How could I best support their growing bodies and brains with what I fed them? Theoretical became practical as I lived the adventure all parents experience.

The following chapters will go in depth on what we are doing wrong and what we are doing right when it comes to *Feeding Our* Children, including

+ The importance of maternal and child nutrition upon the first thousand days of life
+ The impact of nutrition on a child's brain development
+ The vitally important gut bacteria (the microbiome)
+ How diet programs the child's body for health or disease (epigenetics)
+ First foods for babies, and how we have been getting it wrong for decades
+ Common nutritional deficiencies in children
+ The epidemic of feeding disorders and the impact this can have on a child's health
+ How the modern diet fosters metabolic dysfunction and diabetes
+ The link between diet and brain dysfunction and how to maximize brain performance

I'll provide useful, helpful information about how to feed your kids and the scientific reasoning behind nutritional choices that have such a powerful effect on young bodies.

Over the past few years, I have given multiple lectures and grand rounds on nutrition-related topics, including prenatal and infant nutrition, pointing out the abundant research illustrating the importance of nutritional interventions as part of a medical treatment plan. My series of lectures entitled *Feeding Our Children* helped to shape this book. After these lectures, someone in the audience inevitably asks, "Is there a book you would recommend that has all this information in it?" When I've replied, "Not that I have come across," it has often been suggested that I should write one. So here we are.

I will humbly admit that I am just the reporter, the person who likes to connect the dots and piece together the truth of why so many of our children are getting so sick, so young, and to find a way to prevent illness caused by poor nutrition. The real heroes in this story are the physicians and scientists in the trenches, fighting to get honest funding for research, to get published, and get the truth out there. Their voices need to be heard. The other heroes are you—the parents who struggle every day to do their best for their kids, to protect them and keep them healthy. Our children's health is at a crossroads; we have no time to waste. We need to all work together—parents, teachers, physicians, scientists, and community leaders—to prove that what we feed our children matters. Rather than leading us down a road to ruin, our modern diet can be a pillar of health as we fight, reverse, or even eliminate chronic disease.

Thank you for joining me on this journey!

**Thomas Flass, MD, MS**
Kalispell, Montana 2020

Dear Reader;

Please note that this book is heavily referenced with superscripted numbers corresponding to related journal articles. Each chapter is referenced separately for those interested in pursuing more information on the subject matter.

In order to conserve paper and space, the bibliography is posted as a downloadable PDF document available from the author and book websites, and may be updated periodically as new information is published.

www.thomasflass.com
www.feedingourchildren.com

# CHAPTER ONE

# LAYING THE FOUNDATION FOR A HEALTHY LIFE

An epidemic is sweeping our nation, which is set to take the lives of most of the people you know. It is not a virus or plague or bacteria. It is a food-borne illness that can destroy your children's future and rob them of their mental and physical health when they are at their most vulnerable. This epidemic of preventable "diseases of Western civilization" can show itself in many ways, and the pathogen responsible is hiding right under our noses, on our forks.

One of the most concerning ways this epidemic is showing up is with the explosion of diabetes and **pre-diabetes**. **Type 2 diabetes** is a disease, which until recently, has rarely occurred in the pediatric population. (For this reason, it was previously called adult-onset diabetes). Historically the vast majority of cases of diabetes in children were type 1 (juvenile diabetes, a completely different disease than type 2) However, currently more than a quarter of new cases of pediatric diabetes are type 2, not type 1. There has been a 35% increase in type 2 diabetes in children since 2001, and *rates are predicted to increase fourfold by 2050 unless something changes*.[1,2] The rise in cases of type 2 diabetes is unprecedented. Type 2 diabetes has exploded to affect over 30 million Americans and is climbing sharply, destroying people's health and cutting short many lives.[2-4]

Another symptom of the epidemic is the skyrocketing rate of obesity. The majority of adults in the United States are now overweight or obese, and the rate of obesity is predicted to rise from its current rate of 40% to 50%

by the year 2030. (The rate of obesity in the 1970s was 13%, to put things in perspective). One in five children are currently obese. The tsunami of obesity is telling us that something is wrecking our collective **metabolism**. What has happened to our diet and our environment to cause this rapid deterioration?

Equally as concerning are the rising rates of **neurodevelopmental disorders**. Consider the following alarming statistics for children in the United States:

+ Currently, one in six has some type of developmental or learning disability.[5,6]

+ In the past 20 years, the percentage of children diagnosed with ADHD has nearly doubled.[7]

+ Three million children are on ADHD medication, six times the number in 1990.[8]

+ Autism rates went from 1 in 2000 in the 1970s to greater than 1 in 54 today.

What is happening to the brains of our children? These rising rates aren't merely caused by genetics or better testing methods. Increasing evidence implicates environmental causes for these rising rates of neurodevelopmental disorders.

Also of concern are rising rates of many **autoimmune diseases**. Autoimmune diseases are disorders in which the body's immune system attacks and destroys its own tissues. These attacks can include the thyroid gland (Hashimoto's and Grave's disease), the **insulin** producing cells of the pancreas (**type 1 diabetes**), the joints (rheumatoid arthritis), or the gut (**inflammatory bowel disease**), among others, and these diseases are now affecting younger patient populations. Whereas inflammatory bowel disease previously affected mostly teenagers and young adults, pediatric gastroenterologists are now diagnosing alarming numbers of toddlers and young children with this condition, labeled as VEO-IBD (very early onset inflammatory bowel disease). Current research is increasingly focused on the links between diet, the gut bacteria, and autoimmune disease.[9-13]

We need to rethink what we are labeling as "adult" disease or "childhood" disease. *Heart disease and type 2 diabetes are diseases that start in childhood*. The conditions for a heart attack at age 45 began developing in childhood with a poor diet, as did the type 2 diabetes that is diagnosed in our thirties or forties. An overly simplistic response has been to blame our DNA for all that ails us.

However, the rapidly rising rates of chronic diseases illustrate that they are *not* entirely determined by genetics. While certain people may have a predisposition to a certain disease, it is not our genes that have changed in the last four decades; it is our food, our water, and our environment. What is in the environment that threatens our health and the health of our children so significantly? Why are these debilitating health conditions increasingly out of proportion to the population? What can we do to prevent and stop them? This book digs deep into the growing body of evidence pointing the way out of this complex and challenging crisis and the need for immediate change.

I want the best for your children and for mine. Improving our health is going to require some changes in the way we feed ourselves and our children. Too many of us have been misled by social norms or deceptive marketing to think that what we are feeding our children is okay. It is not. Otherwise intelligent, loving parents are unknowingly causing damage to their children by feeding them highly processed food that is void of nutritional value.

Take a look at the average American. Go on, take a *good* look. We are overweight or obese; we are diabetic or on our way; odds are, we will die from a heart attack or cancer. We are stressed, depressed, and our brains are not functioning up to capacity. Is this the way we were meant to live? If you don't want your child to go down this path, you *cannot* feed them like the average American. There is a better way, a way out of this trap.

## THE SIX PILLARS OF HEALTH

Human beings are designed to be healthy given the right environment and the right lifestyle choices. To maintain health and minimize our chance of disease or improve recovery from disease, there are six main fundamental criteria or "pillars" that need to be met. If we pay attention to these pillars, we are generally rewarded with good health. Ignore them, and things start to fall apart. We have deluded ourselves into thinking that we are somehow immune to the forces of nature and of biology. We are not.

## THE SIX PILLARS

**NUTRITION**

**SLEEP**

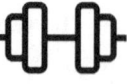

**EXERCISE**

**STRESS MANAGEMENT AND REDUCTION**

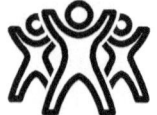

**COMMUNITY AND CONNECTEDNESS**

**SUNLIGHT AND NATURE**

The human body can ignore one or more of these areas for a time, but sooner or later, neglecting these important fundamentals can allow your health or the health of your child to break down. Children are generally more resilient than adults, but they are not invincible. These neglected fundamentals are causing the health issues we are seeing in the modern world. These six pillars are under constant attack. Our diet, sleep, physical fitness, stress levels, and feelings of isolation are not earning us a good report card. Most modern diseases (a.k.a. the diseases of Western civilization) can be traced back to imbalances in one or several of these pillars, all of which are vital to health. It is worth noting that focusing on one area does not make up for being neglectful in several others. For example, lots of exercise cannot make up for a poor diet and lack of sleep. You can't outrun a bad diet! We will explore each of these pillars in more detail.

## 🍎 PILLAR 1: NUTRITION

Because our modern food system gives us such easy access to high-calorie, nutrient-poor food, making healthy choices can be difficult. As a society we have been misinformed and misled about what constitutes a healthy diet. For decades we were told by our government and the media to avoid fat, leading to a high **carbohydrate** (high sugar) diet with disastrous consequences. We have been encouraged by the traditional Food Guide Pyramid or MyPlate Food Guide to eat large amounts of processed grains, which metabolize to simple sugar in the body. Currently more than 75% of processed foods have unnecessary, added sugar to improve taste and increase sales.

The resulting American diet is far too reliant on sugars, processed starches, and flours—leading to the obesity and type 2 diabetes epidemics we see today, as well as a host of other maladies, including chronic inflammatory disease. The sad fact is that many people are consuming too many empty and toxic calories, depriving their brains and bodies of the essential nutrients needed to function optimally.

There are very few absolutes in life, especially when it comes to diets, but healthy nutrition follows some basic ground rules that apply over a broad spectrum of dietary preferences.

1. People must prepare and cook a good proportion of their own food from basic, healthy ingredients.
2. Vegetables that are high in fiber and **phytonutrients** should be eaten in abundance.
3. Highly processed foods and sugar are at the root of most modern diseases (heart disease, diabetes, obesity, autoimmune disease) and should be minimized.

A good diet includes mostly whole, real foods and limits concentrated sugar, highly processed and packaged foods, including most "fast" foods. Our industrial food system is laden with food additives, preservatives, and many questionable chemicals and substances. Interestingly (and frighteningly), most of these food additives have never been tested for safety in humans, much less pregnant women or small children. Many of these chemicals have been given a GRAS listing (Generally Recognized As Safe) based on scant research or data, often provided by the manufacturers without any objective oversight. To avoid many of the questionable items in our food supply, shop mostly around the perimeter of the supermarket where you find vegetables, fruit, nuts, meats, poultry, and fish. These whole foods are the true staples of a healthy diet.

# ⓩ PILLAR 2: SLEEP

Sleep issues are another common problem that can be devastating to your child's health. Good sleep is vital to the human body for its restorative and regenerative properties for both body and brain. Poor sleep can lead to depression and anxiety, cognitive and attention issues, gastrointestinal and immune dysfunction, weight gain, and **prediabetes**.[14,15,16]

Poor sleep may be caused by sleep apnea, trouble falling or staying asleep (often a result of stress or anxiety), poor sleep hygiene, or simply failing to make sleep a priority. Many parents are underestimating how much sleep their children really need, especially teens. The American Academy of Pediatrics endorses the following sleep recommendations to promote optimal health:

### TABLE 1.1 SLEEP REQUIREMENTS BY AGE

| Age | Amount of Sleep, including naps (hours) |
| --- | --- |
| 4-12 months | 12 to 16 |
| 1-2 years | 11 to 14 |
| 3-5 years | 10 to 13 |
| 6-12 years | 9 to 12 |
| 13-18 years | 8 to 10 |

The optimal sleep environment is cool, quiet, and dark, *with no TV, computer, or tablet light in the room.* Blue light, emitted from these screens and other electronic devices directly interferes with the brain's ability to get proper sleep by impairing the production of the crucial sleep hormone melatonin.[17] Avoid screen time and turn down bright lights in the home (or use red lights) within a few hours of bedtime. If you or your older child must use a screen for work or school in the evening, consider apps to reduce blue light and/or wearing blue light-blocking glasses. Also, do not let your children sleep next to a smartphone, tablet, or computer as the light and **electromagnetic field (EMF)** radiation they emit can be detrimental to sleep and rest.[18,19]

Caffeine can also impair sleep. Avoid caffeine entirely for younger children and limit excessive amounts in older children, especially later in the day. Teens, who are increasingly consuming high-caffeine coffee and energy drinks, should also be cautioned about the effects of caffeine on sleep.

So called "sleep aids" are generally not the answer for poor quality sleep. In fact, most prescription sleep aids don't help with sleep, but rather render the person unconscious without attaining the important REM and delta wave phases of sleep needed for repair and recovery of the body and brain. According to sleep experts, these prescriptions may worsen sleep problems in the long term.

Sleep disorders in general are under-recognized and underdiagnosed. If your child has sleep issues, work on these sleep hygiene issues and discuss them with their primary healthcare provider. They may advise a trial of melatonin or a sleep study. Melatonin is a hormone naturally produced by the brain to induce sleep. Available over the counter as a supplement, melatonin can help some people get to sleep without being overly sedating. Many people have difficulty falling asleep because they have a hard time getting their brains to "shut off"—a common affliction that I am very familiar with. Sleep-hypnosis and meditation programs can be useful for people with sleep disturbances and over-active minds.

For more information on sleep disorders and the associated health risks, refer to the suggested reading section at the end of the chapter.

## ⫶⫶ PILLAR 3: EXERCISE AND MOVEMENT

The human body was meant to be fit and active. The primary goal of exercise is not simply to burn calories, but to improve your body's overall metabolism. Metabolism refers to the functioning of your body's machinery and which fuel your body uses to keep it running. Exercise helps your body learn to burn fat more efficiently, even at rest, and it increases and tunes up the little powerhouses of our cells called **mitochondria**. Regular exercise helps prevent heart disease, obesity, and diabetes.

Exercise is just as important for the brain as it is for the body! Intense exercise boosts blood flow to the brain and levels of a substance called **BDNF** (brain derived neurotrophic factor), which is basically "miracle grow" for your brain. BDNF is an important factor in helping to maximize academic performance and in preventing age-related cognitive decline.[20,21] There are studies showing that exercise can improve symptoms of ADHD and improve attention and learning.[22]

Exercise is also the best natural antidepressant. Combined with a healthy diet and good sleep, it could decrease the need for a large proportion of psychiatric medications.[23,24] The recent elimination of physical education in many schools needs to be reexamined and reversed. For some kids, schools provide the only physical activity they will regularly get. Protecting kids' brains and bodies cannot be done without regular physical activity, and we need to encourage exercise in any way possible.

## 🪷 PILLAR 4: STRESS MANAGEMENT & REDUCTION

Everyone has stress, even kids. Some short-term stress can be good if it motivates us to achieve our goals. However, excessive and chronic long-term stress and anxiety can destroy health and quality of life. Anxiety disorders are epidemic in our society, both in children and adults. Excessive stress has been shown to shrink the areas of the brain that are involved with learning and memory while simultaneously making the stress centers of the brain grow stronger. Long-term stress interferes with sleep, digestion, and immune function and increases the risk of developing clinical depression and anxiety disorders, cancer, and heart disease.

Stress management is not about eliminating stress, which is impossible. The key is to increase resilience and change the way that we allow life events to affect us. Handling stress is something we should be teaching all of our kids. People who manage stress well have been shown to be happier and healthier than their peers who do not. Stress can be decreased through positive means with sports and exercise, martial arts, a creative outlet like music, and a regular practice of meditation or mindfulness. There is a reason why practices like meditation and mindfulness have been around for thousands of years—they work to improve resilience and decrease the negative effects of stress in a profound way. Hard science backs up the health and brain benefits of mindfulness and meditation, in adults and children.

A good web resource for people with anxiety issues is AnxietyCanada. com, which also has a site for teens. Check out one of the many beginner meditation apps such as Headspace that have exercises developed specifically for kids. If meditation and mindfulness are so "woo-woo," why does Harvard have a whole research program about it, why does Google offer meditation coursework for all its employees, and why are NFL teams teaching mindfulness to their players to improve their performance? Because it works, that's why.

To learn more about the benefits of meditation, read the online articles listed in the suggested reading section.

## PILLAR 5: CONNECTEDNESS AND COMMUNITY

Humans are meant to be social animals, not isolated and alone. Truly "no man is an island," and we need each other for new ideas, for help, for emotional support, and for a sense of belonging. Social isolation breeds ill health, both mentally and physically.[25] People with a strong social network and community live longer and healthier and suffer from fewer stress-related issues. Finding a way to be of service to others and a larger purpose outside ourselves is an important part of being happy and fulfilled. Help your child find a way to get connected and involved—this can be through your church or temple, your school, sports teams, a community center, volunteer organizations, or even through a large extended family.

## PILLAR 6: SUNLIGHT AND NATURE

A sixth pillar that is increasingly recognized as vital to our health is sunlight and nature. Recent research shows how important sunlight exposure is for human health. Not only do we need sunlight on our skin for vitamin D production, but it also sets our sleep/wake cycle, helping us feel more alert during the day and sleep better at night. Fear of skin cancer has led to bad advice for avoiding all sun exposure and excessively using sunscreen. Avoiding *sunburn* is important, but avoiding *sunshine* may actually increase the risk for certain cancers, heart disease, type 2 diabetes, depression, and autoimmune diseases.[26,27] Morning sun exposure is the best, but moderate exposure to midday sun will also benefit you as long as it does not result in sunburn. Respect the sun but do not fear it; it is your friend.

Spending time outdoors in nature is important to health, and studies are starting to back this up.[28–30] Many kids and adults are suffering from a "nature deficiency," leading to increased risk of depression and anxiety as well as other health issues. Interestingly, studies are showing an association between time spent outdoors in greenspace with lower rates of heart disease, diabetes, cancer, and all-cause mortality (death from any cause). The Japanese have long been proponents of taking "forest baths," immersing themselves in nature for mental and physical health benefits.

We should all be taking nature breaks with our children to reduce their risks of chronic disease.

A body out of balance will often send little "wake-up calls"—like fatigue, depression, digestive issues, frequent infections, or just not feeling good—prior to onset of full-blown disease. Periodically making improvements in any weak areas of the six pillars can have huge payoffs in energy, mood, mental performance, and overall health, and can help your child thrive. By supporting these six pillars, parents can help their children reach their full potential to share their gifts with the world.

On to the rest of the story, and a deeper dive into the reasons why *Feeding Our Children* healthy, real food is so important.

# NUTRITION R$_X$

Periodically review the Six Pillars to identify areas of your children's lives and routines that could use a little attention:

**1** What is their sleep routine? Do they have good sleep hygiene? How long are they sleeping, and is it good quality sleep?

**2** What are they eating? Are they eating several servings of vegetables daily? How much sugar is in their diet?

**3** Are they really stressed out? What are they doing to manage stress?

**4** How active are they? What are they doing to keep themselves fit and active?

**5** Do they have a "tribe" or a group in which they feel they fit in?

**6** Have they been out in the sun and out in nature recently?

## RECOMMENDED READING

1.  www.sleepfoundation.org/articles/children-and-sleep.

2.  Matthew Walker, Why We Sleep, (Scribner, 2017).

3.  https://www.apa.org/topics/mindfulness-meditation

4.  https://www.mindfulschools.org/about-mindfulness/research-on-mindfulness/

5.  https://wellness.huhs.harvard.edu/Mindfulness

6.  www.anxietycanada.com

7.  headspace.com/meditation/kids

8.  https://www.waterford.org/resources/mindfulnes-activities-for-kids/

9.  https://www.mindful.org/mindfulness-for-kids/

# CHAPTER TWO

# THE FIRST THOUSAND DAYS

What if I were to tell you that a significant proportion of the health risks your children will face over the course of their lives could be partially pre-determined before they are two years old? How about the fact that the bacteria that live in your children's intestines largely control their immune system, their **metabolism,** and their brain. Crazy? Scary?

The first thousand days of a child's life, from conception through the second year, represents the most influential time for determining their risk for future health or disease, as well as the health and functioning of their brain.[1-3] Evidence supporting this "**First Thousand Days**" concept is increasingly recognized in the medical literature. Will children do well in school or have a learning disability and struggle academically? Will they be predisposed to become obese and have **type 2 diabetes** or early onset heart disease? Will they be prone to attacks of anxiety or depression? Those first thousand days may determine these outcomes.

### FIRST THOUSAND DAYS

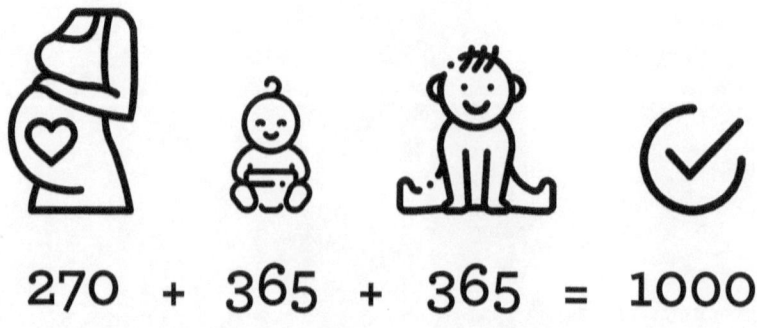

$$270 + 365 + 365 = 1000$$

This chapter is not about giving someone a guilt trip if the first thousand days of their child's life were less than perfect; rather, it is about improving awareness of how we can do better as a society in regard to raising our children. It is about giving every child the best start possible. If the first thousand days were not optimal, all is not lost for that child, but that child may have increased challenges in life and may have to be more vigilant about diet and environment as they get older to maintain good health. Early life programming for "adult" diseases such as heart disease, cancer, and diabetes is a tough concept to grasp, but is gaining traction within the academic medical community. More studies are validating this model of disease development.

The First Thousand Days concept builds upon several major breakthroughs and paradigm shifts in the way we determine risk for disease. The Barker Hypothesis, first published in the 1980s, laid the groundwork for the field of **epigenetics** and the Developmental Origins of Health and Disease (DOHaD) model.[4,5] This hypothesis was based on initial observations that children born during times of starvation were more predisposed to heart disease and **metabolic syndrome (prediabetes)**. Their genetics hadn't changed, but the environment of the child in the womb and during early childhood altered their **gene expression** in ways that resulted in lifelong effects. Additional research has since supported this hypothesis that overnutrition, undernutrition, increased stress, and toxic exposures in the first thousand days influence lifelong risk of certain diseases.[6-16]

In essence, the environment of a child in the first thousand days, starting in the womb on the day of conception, may largely impact future health and functioning. The more diligent we are about what we feed our children and ourselves and the more conscious we are about our environmental exposures, the better start our children have in life. These considerations can have a powerful impact on the first thousand days of a child's life, helping to set the stage for a healthy future and better academic achievement.

Diet during pregnancy, including any nutritional deficiencies or excesses, prenatal drug or **chemical** exposure, and the mother's stress levels all heavily influence the unborn baby. The mode of delivery (C-section or vaginal birth), whether that baby is fed formula or breast milk, the introduction of solid foods and early food choices are all extremely important to the health of the child years into the future.

## MAJOR INFLUENCES ON CHILD'S FIRST THOUSAND DAYS

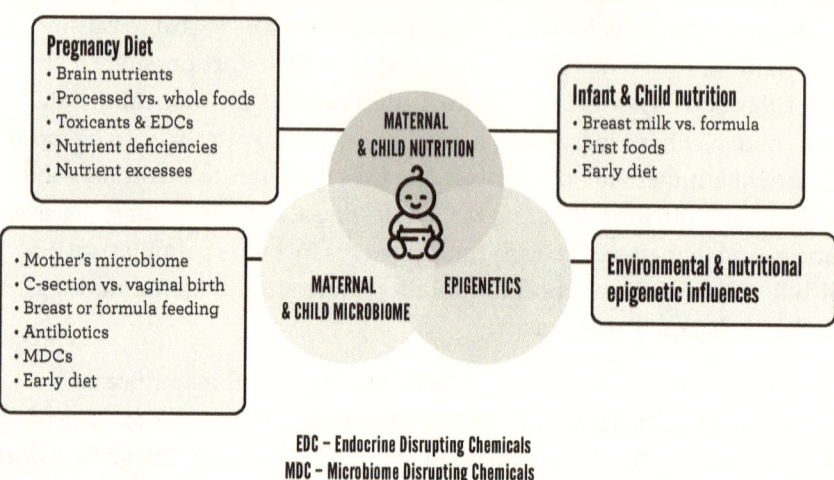

**Pregnancy Diet**
- Brain nutrients
- Processed vs. whole foods
- Toxicants & EDCs
- Nutrient deficiencies
- Nutrient excesses

**MATERNAL & CHILD NUTRITION**

**Infant & Child nutrition**
- Breast milk vs. formula
- First foods
- Early diet

- Mother's microbiome
- C-section vs. vaginal birth
- Breast or formula feeding
- Antibiotics
- MDCs
- Early diet

**MATERNAL & CHILD MICROBIOME**   **EPIGENETICS**

**Environmental & nutritional epigenetic influences**

EDC – Endocrine Disrupting Chemicals
MDC – Microbiome Disrupting Chemicals

*Diagram adapted from Indrio et al. [9]

In the next few chapters, we will explore key areas of research in the fields of **neurodevelopment, epigenetics**, and the **microbiome** to provide a foundational understanding of these topics and how each impacts the first thousand days of our children's life and relates to what we are feeding them.

## CRITICAL WINDOWS OF NEURODEVELOPMENT

The first thousand days of life is the period of the most rapid brain growth (neurodevelopment). During these days, our children's brains are highly susceptible to insults and injuries from nutritional deficiencies, hormone imbalances, or exposure to toxic chemicals.[2,3] If you stop for a moment and think about how in one thousand days we go from an egg and a sperm to a fully functioning human with all the complex biochemistry and brain circuitry, it is nothing short of a miracle. The number of things that have to go *right,* to make sure that the billions of nerves in a baby's brain are communicating correctly and that each organ is formed and functioning, is mind-blowing.

### RAPID BRAIN DEVELOPMENT– PERCENTAGE SIZE OF ADULT BRAIN

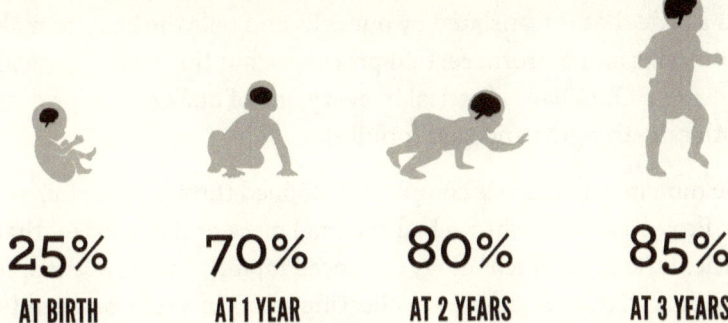

| 25% | 70% | 80% | 85% |
|---|---|---|---|
| **AT BIRTH** | **AT 1 YEAR** | **AT 2 YEARS** | **AT 3 YEARS** |

But when we start messing with mother nature, that's when things go wrong. During this critical window, maternal nutrition during pregnancy and lactation, as well as the early diet of the child heavily impact neurodevelopment.[17] Diet also significantly influences the bacteria that live in the infant's intestines (the microbiome), which recent research is now linking to proper brain growth and function.[18–20] In future chapters, we will delve into specific ways to support and protect our children's brains during the first thousand days extensively, because what the pregnant mother and her baby eat during the first two years of that child's life can have a profound impact on the developing brain of the child.

## GENETICS, EPIGENETICS, AND THE MICROBIOME

Because of recent breakthroughs in the scientific fields of genetics and gene expression, we are starting to look at food ingredients and food additives in a whole new light. The oversimplification that "food is simply calories" to fuel the body is being debunked by this new science.

While we do need calories from food to fuel our bodies, we now know that food provides much more: vitamins and minerals (micronutrients) to help our bodies function, **antioxidants** to protect our bodies, and, importantly, fiber to feed the beneficial bacteria in our gut.

We also know that some "foods" in our modern diet are actually ultra-processed "food-like substances" that foster chronic disease.[21,22] Some of the dangers of the modern diet are being revealed by relatively new areas of research: **Genetics, Epigenetics,** and the **Microbiome.** These may be unfamiliar terms, or perhaps sound like buzzwords found in the media. Let's clarify these important terms before moving ahead.

## What are genetics?

Our genetics, or genome, refer to the DNA we are all born with. DNA contains a code that is translated by our cells and tells the body to make certain proteins and perform certain processes, but this code is individual to each person. Our DNA, identical in every one of our cells, helps determine both our strengths and susceptibilities.

After the human genome was completely mapped through the Human Genome Project, we thought we had the final piece of the puzzle—that we had "cracked the code." Technology advanced rapidly, and now "mapping" our individual DNA is as simple as collecting saliva in a tube and sending it through the mail to be analyzed by one of several companies like 23andMe. These companies send back a report of our ancestry and DNA, telling us if we carry genes that increase our likelihood of developing certain diseases or medical conditions. The hope is that, armed with this information, we can act more proactively to *prevent* disease.

> The ancestry companies compare our DNA to a massive database, which contains information about huge numbers of genetic variations known as single-nucleotide polymorphism (SNPs or "SNiPs") that individualize the coding of our DNA. These SNPs may affect the functioning of certain bodily processes. We know that certain SNPs are associated with increased risks of specific diseases.

But while mapping the human genome has been a monumental achievement, it hasn't told the whole story. Risks based on DNA are not always written in stone, and we have found that there are ways to "change the script" to protect ourselves and our children. These ways are guided by the evolving field of *epigenetics*.

## What are epigenetics?

**Epigenetics** is the study of the influences by which we can either activate or silence our DNA (known as *gene expression*). These influences largely determine whether a gene will be *expressed* (switched on) or *silenced* (switched off) by several biological processes, including those of **methylation** and *acetylation*. It turns out that methylation and acetylation are under significant nutritional control.[1,23]

## EPIGENETICS

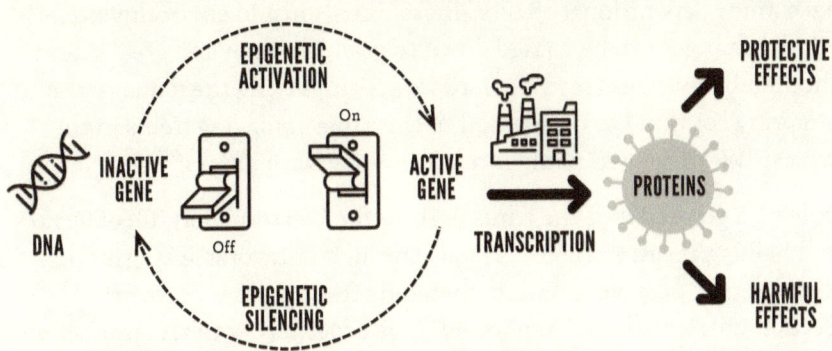

**Activate Protective Genes**
- Healthy microbiome
- Antioxidants & phytonutrients
- SCFA from fiber
- Exercise
- Omega-3 fats
- Breast feeding
- Adequate folate, $B_{12}$, $B_6$, choline
- Vitamin D

**Activate Harmful Genes**
- Smoking
- Stress
- Gestational diabetes
- High sugar diet
- Toxicants & EDC's
- Nutrient deficiencies (iron, zinc, magnesium)
- Inadequate folate, $B_{12}$, choline
- Dysbiosis

Any substance that affects gene expression can be labeled an "**epigenetic modifier.**" A great number of environmental epigenetic modifiers have been discovered: environmental pollutants and **endocrine disrupting chemicals (EDCs)**, emotional and mental stress, exercise, and certain medications, but by far the most important epigenetic modifier currently being studied is diet and its subsequent effects on our microbiome.[9,24]

Why is diet the most important epigenetic modifier? Consider how many times we eat every day. With every meal we are either protecting ourselves by switching off bad genes and turning on good ones, or we are doing the opposite and programming ourselves and our children for the development of disease.

Many diseases, including diabetes, obesity, heart disease and some cancers, are now being linked to poor early-life nutrition and toxic exposures in the first thousand days, which lead to *epigenetic modification*.

A recent finding is that these epigenetic changes to our DNA may even have multi-generational effects. These nutrition and environmentally related changes can be passed down to grandchildren and great grandchildren in a vicious "feed forward" loop, amplifying the damage as our offspring continue to be exposed to the same damaging items in the typical "Western diet" as their parents and grandparents.[25]

Indeed, a good part of the damage from the Western diet, full of sugar and highly processed foods, is likely through unfavorable epigenetic changes that take place both before and after a child is born.[13,26–28] Certain nutrients have been found to be especially powerful protective epigenetic modifiers, including the vitamins $B_{12}$, folate, and choline, as well as the antioxidant nutrients found in fruits and vegetables, which will be explored in later chapters.[9,24,29]

In the following chapters, we will discuss how diet is affecting our children's epigenetics and thereby impacting the risk of certain disorders and diseases. A key message here is that our children's genes are under environmental control, which includes what we feed them. The modern Western diet is programming our kids for a future of heart disease, diabetes, and obesity, in addition to other chronic diseases. Remember that what you eat when you are pregnant and what you feed your children may be turning on "bad" genes and turning off "good ones," programming your children's bodies for disease years in the future.

### What is the microbiome?

The microbiome refers to the collective population of bacteria, viruses, and fungi that reside in or on the human body. It can be used to refer to these organisms in a specific area of the body like the nose or skin, but for our purposes, we will primarily be referring to the intestinal (gut) microbiome.

The human gut microbiome is now being viewed as another organ system, just like our liver, spleen, or kidneys, and a healthy microbiome is vital to children's health.[33] The human gut microbiome contains $10^{14}$ (10 followed by 14 zeros) bacteria, more bacteria than human cells in our own body. This microbial community is now thought to be made up of more than a thousand different species of bacteria, and contains one hundred times as much genetic material as our own body.[34,35] Higher diversity of bacterial species in the gut is associated with improved health; low diversity is associated with poor health and disease.

Several factors, including consumption of highly processed foods and overexposure to antibiotics in our environment, may be decreasing this diversity and altering the microbiome into a state of **dysbiosis**, which contributes to poor health. These gut bacteria have an incredible influence on our health and development as humans and are vital for our children's health across their lifespans.[36]

A child's microbiome "talks to" and significantly influences the rest of the body, including the DNA and the brain. The ability to identify and characterize someone's microbiome and how it is influenced by diet has become a focus of research in the past fifteen years. The science is new, but the evidence of its importance and the effects it has on human health is mounting and changing our medical paradigm.[37]

### What are probiotics?

**Probiotics** are the live microorganisms (mostly bacteria and a few fungi) that provide health benefits when consumed in adequate numbers. This term most commonly refers to probiotic supplements containing certain species of beneficial bacteria such as *Lactobacillus* and *Bifidobacteria,* but it can also refer to bacteria contained within foods like yogurt and sauerkraut (referred to as probiotic foods). We may also use the term **probiotic bacteria** when referring to research about the beneficial effects in the human body of one or several of these species. The most commonly studied probiotic species are listed below. They are often found in probiotic supplements.

+ *Lactobacillus* **species** (*acidophilus, paracasei, rhamnosus, casei, lactis, plantarum, reuteri, salivarius, fermentum, bulgaricus*)
+ *Streptococcus* thermophilus, salivarius
+ *Bifidobacteria* **species** (*infantis, longum, breve, lactis, animalis, bifidum*)
+ *Saccharomyces boulardii* (beneficial yeast)

Keep in mind that *over one thousand species* of bacteria exist in the healthy human intestine. The species listed here represent a small selection that have been studied extensively, but there exists an incredibly complex web of bacterial, viral, and fungal species that make up the microbiome— many with roles yet to be discovered.

### What are prebiotics?

**Prebiotics** are non-digestible substances like soluble fiber in our diet that promote the growth of beneficial (probiotic) bacteria in the body. Prebiotics are the fertilizer for the beneficial bacteria that live in our intestines and support a healthy microbiome.

One of the many unfortunate things about our **Standard American Diet (SAD)** is that it is woefully lacking in fiber, the main fuel for our gut bacteria. Soluble fibers such as inulin, pectins from fruits and vegetables, **oligosaccharides** from human milk and nutritional supplements, and **resistant starches** and other fibers from whole grains are all considered prebiotics that foster the growth of beneficial bacteria.[31]

If we don't feed the good bacteria, they are unable to grow and perform many of their vital functions listed in the next chapter, and harmful microorganisms (unfriendly bacteria, fungi, and viruses) have a better chance of growing in our children's bodies.

### What is dysbiosis?

**Dysbiosis** is the term that refers to a state of imbalance in our intestines with increased numbers of potentially harmful bacteria and too few beneficial bacteria, which can lead to a number of health issues and diseases ranging from **irritable bowel syndrome (IBS)** to **autoimmune diseases and brain disorders**.[32]

### How Does Our Microbiome Develop?

An individual's microbiome starts at birth and continues to develop and evolve during childhood. It is unclear if there is such a thing as a fetal microbiome prior to birth. Some research suggests that amniotic fluid may not be sterile as was previously thought and may contain some bacteria.[38,39,40] For the most part however, a child's intestinal microbiome begins at birth with significant development in the first three years of our children's lives.[36]

During birth, the infant is inoculated (seeded) with bacteria from the mother's vaginal and gut microbiome, or with other non-maternal bacteria if the child has a C-section birth. These bacteria make their way into the baby's mouth, nose, and digestive system, where they become established.

The early microbiome is fed by components in breast milk or formula, namely lactose and prebiotics called oligosaccharides. The most important of these early prebiotics was recently discovered and is called **Human**

**Milk Oligosaccharide (HMO).** It is one of the main components of breast milk that will be described more fully in Chapter 8. HMO helps to fuel the development of the early infant microbiome. The infant can also be further inoculated with beneficial bacteria from mom, contained in her breast milk.

The microbiome then develops with the child, and along the way is shaped and influenced by many factors, including early feeding and weaning choices, environmental factors such as antibiotic and chemical exposures, geographic location, and exposure to nature and animals, as well as ongoing dietary prebiotic fiber or lack thereof. As the child's diet starts to expand, the microbiome expands and changes as well; introducing a wider variety of foods promote bacterial diversity in the intestines. The adult microbiome at some point may become more resistant to change but is still significantly influenced by dietary choices.[41]

The infant and child microbiome, however, is thought to be much more malleable and subject to be changed by the environmental factors listed above. *The first thousand days of that child's life is the most important time for shaping a healthy microbiome that will benefit them for a lifetime.*[35,36,42]

In the next chapter, we will discuss what those intestinal bacteria *do*.

## RECOMMENDED READING

1. Thousand Days non-profit organization: www.Thousanddays.org.

2. The Human Genome Project: www.genome.gov/human-genome-project

3. The Human Microbiome Project: https://commonfund.nih.gov/hmp/overview

# NUTRITION R$_X$

The first thousand days are the most important in a child's life! Protect them and their brain development during this vulnerable period by paying attention to diet, the microbiome and chemical exposures. With our food choices, we are not only feeding the child, but the bacteria that live in their gut.

**1** We can't change a child's genetics but we can change their epigenetics and gene expression! Every meal can turn ON or OFF genes for chronic disease.

**2** Choose healthy, whole foods for yourself and your child to protect them for a lifetime. Make sure you are making food choices that are both turning off harmful genes and feeding the good gut bacteria! Hint- they are usually the same foods!

**3** When pregnant, consume a pregnancy diet with lots of fruits, vegetables, whole grains, and consider probiotic/prebiotic foods (yogurt, kefir, fermented foods like sauerkraut).

**4** Try to avoid unnecessary antibiotics during pregnancy and birth if possible, and discuss treatment options with the PCP, obstetrician, or midwife.

# CHAPTER THREE

# THE MICROBIOME AND ITS ROLE IN HUMAN HEALTH

We humans have co-evolved with our gut bacteria in a symbiotic relation-ship that provides us with multiple health benefits. Advancing research has shown that these intestinal bacteria are not just along for the ride but are essential for our growth, development, and maintenance of health at every stage of the life cycle. They provide functions that our bodies are not capable of performing, and in many ways act to guide and shape the development of our immune system, our nervous system, and our digestive system.

When I started my medical training, little to nothing was taught about the **microbiome**, and **probiotics** were thought to be unscientific quackery only utilized by those on the fringes of medicine. Little or no thought was being given to the long-term effects of multiple rounds of antibiotics in children, C-section births, or the effects of a poor diet on gut bacteria.

Fast forward almost twenty years, and the two hottest areas of medical research are **epigenetics** and the microbiome. Today, thousands of research papers are published each year showing the importance of these concepts to the practice of medicine and especially pediatrics. In fact, almost thirteen thousand research papers on the microbiome were published between 2013 and 2017.[1] Close to ten thousand have been published since then. Obviously, study of the microbiome is a big deal and will eventually change the way medicine is practiced. Unfortunately, things change slowly in the practice of medicine, and outdated dogma dies a slow painful death, even while groundbreaking research discoveries are being made.

## ROLES OF THE HEALTHY MICROBIOME

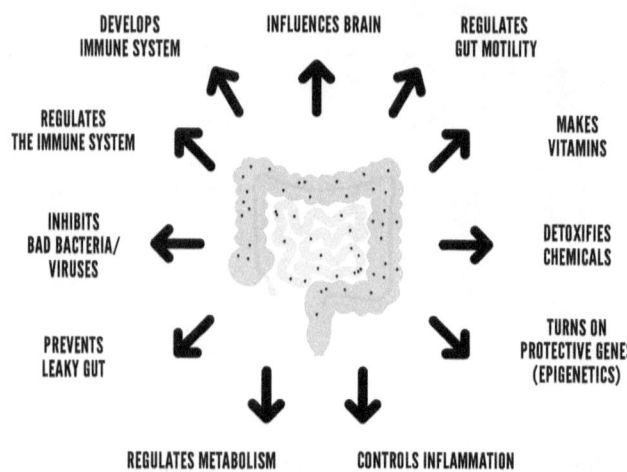

DEVELOPS IMMUNE SYSTEM

INFLUENCES BRAIN

REGULATES GUT MOTILITY

REGULATES THE IMMUNE SYSTEM

MAKES VITAMINS

INHIBITS BAD BACTERIA/ VIRUSES

DETOXIFIES CHEMICALS

PREVENTS LEAKY GUT

TURNS ON PROTECTIVE GENES (EPIGENETICS)

REGULATES METABOLISM

CONTROLS INFLAMMATION

### The microbiome supports our children's immune system

Healthy gut bacteria are vitally important for inhibiting potential invaders. Without healthy gut bacteria, the development and functioning of our body's defense system can be significantly impaired. Infants need early colonization with healthy bacteria to help them establish a properly functioning immune system.[2-11]

Healthy gut bacteria produce chemicals and proteins that kill or ward off harmful bacteria, fungal invaders (yeast), parasites, and viruses in the gut and the vagina of the expecting mother. Probiotic bacteria produce lactic acid and acetic acid to create an unfavorable environment for detrimental bacteria, and they make *bacteriocins,* which are proteins that kill these harmful bacteria. They also stimulate production of defensins (aptly named), which are anti-bacterial molecules in our intestines that also kill viruses and fungi. Simply by having increased numbers of beneficial bacteria in the gut, a healthy microbiome may also suppress dangerous bacteria such as *Clostridioides difficile* (*C. diff*), which can cause a life-threatening intestinal infection.

Not only does a healthy microbiome ward off or kill bad bacteria in the gut, but it can also calm down an overactive immune system and help prevent allergies or **autoimmune disease**. Research shows that our microbiome and certain probiotic bacteria are the "master teachers" of our early immune system. These probiotic bacteria *promote a healthy balanced immune system* in a variety of ways. They stimulate production of secretory Immunoglobulin A (IgA), which is another first line defense protein in our gut, nose, and lungs. This protein's job is to bind up potential invaders and disable them so they can be destroyed by the rest of the immune system. Having a low or ineffective IgA may result in a child being more susceptible to food allergies and respiratory or gastrointestinal infections.

Probiotics "teach" the immune system of the developing infant to recognize friend versus foe. This recognition of non-harmful substances, such as food in the digestive tract, or our body's own tissues and organs, is known as **immune tolerance**. Probiotic bacteria support immune tolerance, in part by increasing numbers of specific white blood cells called T-regulatory cells, whose job it is to tell the immune system when to rest and when to fight.

An overactive immune system and loss of immune tolerance can lead to inflammation, allergies, and autoimmune disease, so this regulation is important. By increasing the activity and number of T-regulatory cells, a healthy microbiome helps to decrease inflammation and the potential for allergies and autoimmune disease. Large studies have suggested that probiotics during pregnancy and infancy in babies born to highly allergic families may help prevent the development of eczema and allergies in the child.[12,13]

Furthermore, it has been shown that probiotic bacteria help to detoxify certain harmful compounds in the gut (like pesticides and heavy metals) and neutralize them before they can do harm to the body. Given these roles, can you start to see why supporting our children's probiotic bacterial population is so important for their immune system and fighting off invaders?

**Probiotic bacteria and a healthy microbiome prevent "leaky gut"**
The barrier separating our digestive system, food particles, and billions of intestinal bacteria from our bloodstream is only one cell layer thick! In health, our bodies only let very select things into the blood from our digestive tract like glucose or fully digested proteins (amino acids). A healthy microbiome helps develop and maintain *tight junctions* between these cells. Tight junctions are the glue that holds our intestinal cells together and prevent unwanted items from crossing into our bloodstream.

## LEAKY GUT

### HEALTHY MICROBIOME AND GUT

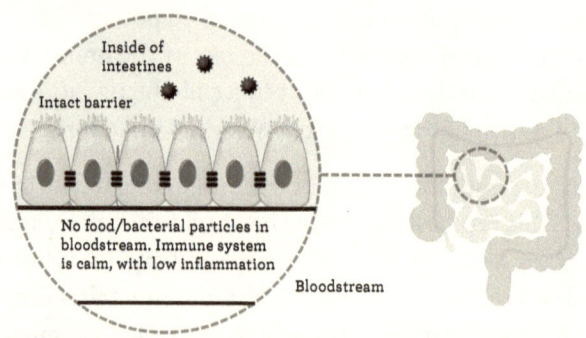

### DYSBIOSIS AND LEAKY GUT

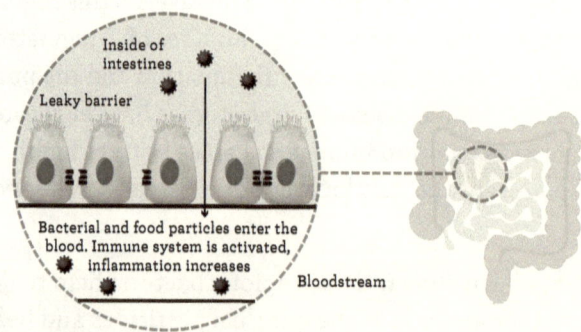

> **Healthy gut versus leaky gut**
>
> Leaky gut allows particles, bacteria into bloodstream where they interact with immune system casuing inflammation and an altered immune response.
>
> Healthy gut only allows very select things into the blood, and the immune system is more regulated with less inflammation.

The body does not like large molecules of food, bacteria, or other foreign particles in the blood. Particles of bacteria or whole bacteria passing unregulated into our bloodstream through a **"leaky gut"** is referred to as **endotoxemia**, which represents a significant challenge to our immune system. Leaky gut is now felt to contribute to a number of inflammatory diseases.[14,15]

If our gut is "leaky," these foreign particles (called antigens) entering our bloodstream from our gut can over-activate our immune system and cause excessive inflammation. This over-activity eventually wears down the immune system and may contribute to autoimmune and cardiovascular disease. It is now suspected that these substances from our gut can also enter our brains—potentially causing cognitive or behavioral issues.[14,16]

It has been shown in medical research that children with autism and people with autoimmune diseases like thyroid issues, **inflammatory bowel disease**, rheumatoid arthritis, **type 1 diabetes**, and multiple sclerosis have a significantly increased incidence of leaky gut compared to healthy people.[17-23] Through cutting edge research, physician-scientist and pediatric gastroenterologist Dr. Alessio Fasano discovered a protein that increases intestinal permeability and causes leaky gut. Production of this protein, named **zonulin**, is stimulated by certain intestinal infections and abnormal gut bacteria, leading to leaky gut. In addition, the wheat protein **gluten** may increase zonulin in susceptible people, even those without celiac disease.[24]

Unfortunately, many physicians are unaware of this process, or they disregard leaky gut as a fringe idea in alternative medicine. The medical literature shows otherwise. The significance of this discovery is revealed in the title of Fasano's 2011 paper, "Zonulin and its regulation of barrier function: the biological door to inflammation, autoimmunity, and cancer."[17] Leaky gut is a very real phenomenon and is backed by current scientific literature and forward-thinking physicians and researchers. *It is an important concept that a diet with too much sugar, saturated fat, processed foods, antibiotics, and chemical additives will damage our microbiome and promote leaky gut.* Protecting against leaky gut by promoting a healthy microbiome is a powerful way to protect our growing children from autoimmune diseases, inflammation, brain disorders, and even future cancer and heart disease. A healthy gut microbiome is their first line defense. [13,16,17,25–29]

### Short Chain Fatty Acids production
**Short Chain Fatty Acids** (SCFA) are substances produced in our large intestines when probiotic bacteria in our microbiome digest soluble fiber from fruits, vegetables, and whole grains. Unlike most fatty acids, which come from dietary fat in our foods, these are made right in our own bodies by beneficial bacteria. These SCFA have multiple beneficial roles in our bodies.[30-32]

SCFA are fuel for the intestinal cells to keep them healthy and functioning and help to prevent leaky gut. They also act directly as anti-inflammatory agents in our intestines and the rest of our body. In fact, past studies have shown that one of these SCFA, called butyrate, when administered into the intestines of patients with ulcerative colitis, successfully helped decrease inflammation.[33,34]

There is evidence that healthy amounts of SCFA in the intestines help prevent colorectal cancer in adults, and may be one of the reasons why a high fiber diet seems to protect against colon cancer.[35,36] Recent research shows that these SCFA have metabolic effects on the entire human body, and may help to regulate our appetite and **metabolism**, protecting against obesity and **type 2 diabetes**.[37-40] These SCFAs are also important immune system regulators and **epigenetic modifiers**, affecting **gene expression**.[41-43]

Studies are showing that SCFA are a potential link between a low fiber diet, **dysbiosis**, and a number of diseases, including obesity, type 2 diabetes, heart disease, autoimmune disease, and even neurological disorders. There is an increasingly recognized role of SCFA effects on the brain as part of the **brain-gut-microbiome axis** described below.[31] It is likely that SCFA production by the microbiome in the infant and child intestine plays a developmental role in their growing brain.[46]

A healthy microbiome, fed by **prebiotics** in breast milk and food, support proper SCFA production, which decreases leaky gut and inflammation, helps regulate appetite and metabolism, and alters gene expression helping to prevent chronic disease in your child.

### What SCFA do in the body

- Provides fuel for intestinal cells
- Prevent leaky gut
- Act as anti-inflammatory agents
- Help prevent colon cancer
- Protect against type 2 diabetes/obesity
- Regulate the immune system
- **Act as epigenetic modifiers**
- Enhance brain development and function

## BRAIN GUT MICROBIOME AXIS

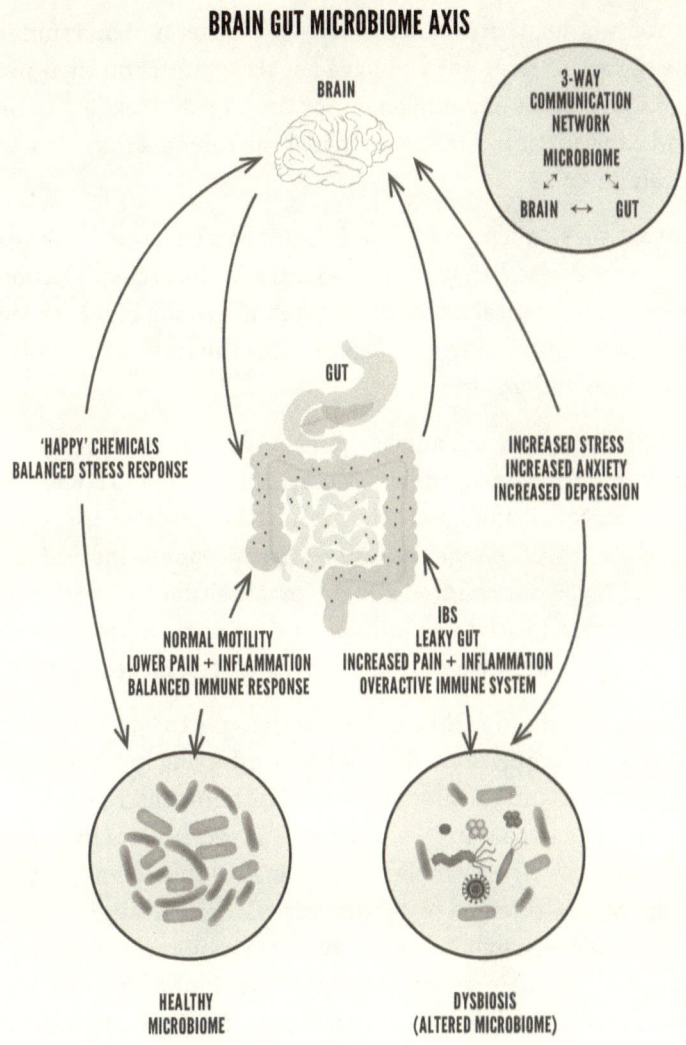

The **brain-gut-microbiome axis (BGM axis)** refers to the complex conversation going on between our gut bacteria, the nerves and immune system of our gut, and our brain. This immense area of research is revealing that *alterations in our children's gut microbiome can have effects on their brain development and function, learning, mood (depression and anxiety), and possibly autism and ADHD.* The interaction of the gut microbiome and the human brain is a fascinating topic that is changing the medical paradigm of neurologic and **neurodevelopmental disorders.**[47-59]

There is mounting evidence that the microbiome and probiotic bacteria help to guide *nerve development* in the brain and in the gastrointestinal

(GI) tract of infants. Disturbances in the gut bacteria of an infant can affect the nerves of their gut and have negative effects on their intestinal motility (contractions and movement of the GI tract) leading to feeding issues and constipation. An altered infant microbiome may also impact brain development.

To think that these microscopic bacteria are somehow controlling our brains, our mood, and behavior may sound a bit like science fiction, but this intricate biochemical dialogue between the brain, digestive tract, and trillions of bacteria residing in the gut is now the focus of a whole new field of research and practice.

Autism, ADHD, depression, anxiety, chronic fatigue syndrome, Parkinson's and Alzheimer's diseases may all be linked in some way to an altered microbiome leading to brain dysfunction and disease. This ground-breaking concept will change the way we practice medicine and disease prevention. Maybe our children's behavioral meltdowns or attention issues can be traced back to an unhappy microbiome asking for more fiber and less sugar. We will dive into this subject a little more in later chapters.

In addition, a disturbed BGM axis is now thought to be a key mechanism leading to **irritable bowel syndrome (IBS)**, affecting more than twenty million Americans and causing frequent abdominal discomfort and constipation or diarrhea. In fact, a panel of world experts in gastrointestinal disorders recently re-labeled "functional GI disorders," including IBS, which are now referred to as **"disorders of gut-brain interaction (DGBI)."** [44] Some researchers also include microbiome in the renamed title (brain-gut-microbiome interactions). Shouldn't this speak volumes to anyone who has doubts about the importance of gut microbiota for our health? [45,47]

## Vitamins
Probiotic bacteria manufacture vitamins right in our intestines! Riboflavin, folate, vitamin $B_{12}$, and vitamin K are all produced by our intestinal bacteria. In addition, probiotic bacteria aid in digestion and help our children get more nutrients out of the food they are eating. [60]

## Constipation
Probiotic bacteria are one of the five things you need for a good "Number Two." ("Number Two" refers to poop, for those not in the know.) Aside from the basic anatomic requirements of a functioning nervous system and an intact GI tract, to have good bowel movements your child needs:

+ A healthy microbiome and good probiotic bacteria in the gut
+ Adequate amounts of soluble and insoluble fiber (especially intact fiber from whole food)
+ Adequate hydration (plenty of water for toddlers and older children, milk or formula for infants)
+ Adequate activity (an inactive child will have an inactive gut)
+ Good bathroom habits (not withholding stool, proper sitting on the toilet with good support)

Probiotic bacteria and pre-biotic fiber increase stool bulk and *promote gastrointestinal motility*, helping prevent constipation. Constipation is one of the main things that brings kids into my office. When I am taking a medical history, I always ask about the mode of birth (C-section or vaginal), early life feeding (formula, breast milk, and early foods) and antibiotic exposure. I see too many children who are set up for dysbiosis (altered intestinal bacteria) because of C-section birth, early antibiotics, and low soluble fiber (due to lack of vegetables) in the diet. This dysbiosis can, in essence, slow down the colon, contributing to constipation.[61,62]

An unhealthy microbiome can be associated with chronic constipation. A multi-species probiotic along with an increase in dietary fiber may be the first things I recommend to get kids' pooping back on track. There is also a known association between difficult-to-treat constipation and an overgrowth of an unfriendly type of methane-producing intestinal bacteria called *methanogens*. It is possible to test for these methane producers with a simple breath test, and treatment of these methanogen bacteria along with restoration of a healthier microbiome may make a significant difference in some people with treatment-resistant chronic constipation.[65-67]

Find a complete discussion about ways to prevent and treat constipation in Chapter 15.

### Epigenetic influence of the microbiome

As stated previously, probiotic bacteria are a major epigenetic influence and "talk" to our DNA via a variety of mechanisms currently being researched. A healthy microbiome may help to "shut off" genes that code for chronic inflammatory diseases, including type 2 diabetes, heart disease, and cancer. As a testament to ancient wisdom, we are rediscovering through science that almost all disease starts in the gut.[68-71]

Going back to the **First Thousand Days** concept, given the increasing knowledge about the importance of the microbiome and epigenetic programming, we start to realize in a different way how important this critical developmental window is for our children. Not only is this the period of the most rapid brain growth, this is also the most sensitive period for epigenetic modification to our children's genes, when certain important genes can be turned on or turned off—potentially for life. This is also the period when the child's microbiome is largely established, carrying with it all the potential risks or benefits of the types of bacteria living in their intestines. A healthy microbiome in the child fosters good health, both mentally and physically. We will go into the importance of the maternal microbiome in the next chapter. However, suffice it to say that the infant's microbiome comes from mom, so it is of vital importance that *she* maintains a healthy population of probiotic bacteria during pregnancy and breastfeeding to pass on to her child. It is the gift that keeps on giving.

## RECOMMENDED READING

1. The Rome Foundation for disorders of gut-brain interaction: https://theromefoundation.org/about/

2. Emeran Mayer, MD, founding director of the UCLA Brain Gut Microbiome Center: www.emeranmayer.com

# NUTRITION Rx

**1** Our intestinal bacteria, referred to as our intestinal microbiome, are vital for human health and development.

**2** Starting at birth, these bacteria shape our children's growth and development.

**3** These bacteria perform a number of roles in the developing child: teaching the immune system, maintaining a healthy, functioning GI tract, guiding brain development, and shaping metabolism.

**4** Many of our modern diseases directly relate to disturbances in the gut microbiome.

# CHAPTER FOUR

# NEGATIVE IMPACTS ON THE MICROBIOME

Many of the health issues your child may face in their lifetime are in part the result of a disturbed and damaged **microbiome**. What can damage their microbiome and how do we prevent or fix it? Below is a list of the *major influences on our children's gut bacteria.*

### FACTORS THAT IMPACT THE MICROBIOME

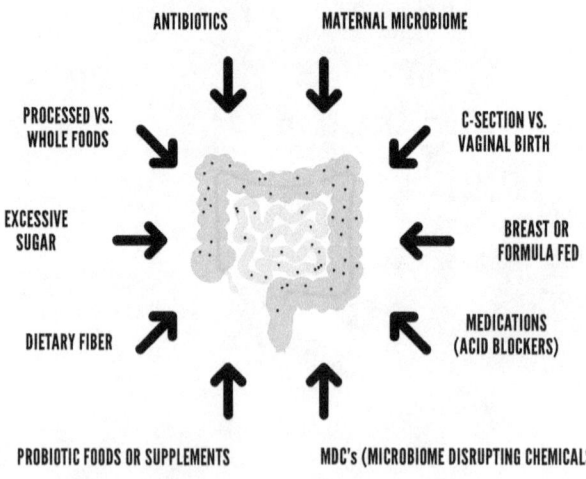

ANTIBIOTICS

MATERNAL MICROBIOME

PROCESSED VS. WHOLE FOODS

C-SECTION VS. VAGINAL BIRTH

EXCESSIVE SUGAR

BREAST OR FORMULA FED

DIETARY FIBER

MEDICATIONS (ACID BLOCKERS)

PROBIOTIC FOODS OR SUPPLEMENTS

MDC's (MICROBIOME DISRUPTING CHEMICALS)

## C-section birth

One third of babies in the U.S. are born by Cesarean section. Some of these are performed to save the baby and mother's lives. Some are elective and may be the mode of delivery chosen by the mom. During an optimal vaginal birth, the infant is "inoculated" with mom's healthy vaginal probiotic bacteria as they pass through the birth canal. These bacteria are nourished by breast milk, and they colonize the intestines of the infant, contributing to a healthy gut and immune system. This is the way mother nature has done it for millions of years.

C-section infants miss out on this important process with potential health implications. C-section infants are more likely to be colonized by the potentially harmful bacteria *Klebsiella*, *Enterobacter*, and *Clostridia*, as well as other skin and hospital bacteria, instead of mom's probiotic bacteria. When these babies are tested later in infancy, studies are finding vaginally born, breastfed infants have more *Bifidobacteria* and *Lactobacillus* (two main species of healthy probiotic bacteria) and fewer potentially harmful bacteria like *Bacteroides*, *C. difficile*, and *E. coli* than infants born by C-section and formula-fed infants. This loss of diversity and fewer probiotic bacteria from C-section births can last well into childhood, carrying with it potential health risks.[1-10, 45-50]

This is NOT a judgement against any mom who has elected to or was required to deliver via C-section, but more of an effort to raise awareness. Knowledge is power. The goal here is to alert parents of the dangers a child may face as a result of a disturbed microbiome and give the means to remedy it. Recent medical literature suggests that *C-section births can carry with them a potential risk to the future health of the child*, even years down the road. While still controversial, large studies are suggesting associations between C-section births and health risks. Women are not being informed of these risks to their children or made aware of the steps they could take to potentially decrease the risks.

For example, in children born by C-section, the risk of allergies and asthma increase by 20% to 30%, **type 1 diabetes** increases by 20%, obesity rates increase by 30% to 60%, while the risk of **inflammatory bowel disease** (Crohn's and Colitis) and celiac disease may or may not be increased. These adverse associations with C-section births are largely thought to be caused by the altered microbiome of the child, the incomplete "teaching" of the newborn immune system, and the downstream epigenetic effects of turning on certain genes coding for these diseases.

What effect does a C-section have on the baby brain? As evidence shows that the gut bacteria may "train the brain" in developing infants, disturbing this balance could have significant brain effects. Current researchers are investigating the impact of C-section versus vaginal birth on the risk of **neurodevelopmental disorders** and effects on later cognitive functioning.[11] Reports on the effects of a C-section birth on the risk of autism and ADHD are mixed, so the jury is still out about these two conditions. However, a large recent **meta-analysis** showed increased risk for autism and ADHD as well as other neuropsychiatric disorders in children born by C-section.[12]

### TABLE 4.1 CHILDHOOD CONDITIONS ASSOCIATED WITH C-SECTION BIRTH (% INCREASED RISK)

| Condition | % increased risk |
| --- | --- |
| Allergic Rhinitis | 15-80% |
| Asthma | 21-83% |
| Celiac Disease | 0-80% |
| Type 1 Diabetes | 19% |
| Gastroenteritis | 31% |
| Obesity | 33%–59% |
| Academic Challenges | 14%–83% |
| ADHD | 17% |
| Autism | 33% |

## HOT TOPIC

Studies are underway looking at various ways to restore a healthy microbiome for C-section babies. A pioneer in this field has been Dr. Maria Gloria Dominguez-Bello at Rutgers University. Her work has focused on the importance of maternal microbiome transfer to the infant. Her research examines the effects that an unhealthy maternal microbiome or an incomplete maternal microbiome transfer plays on the health outcomes of infants.

Dr. Dominguez-Bello and several other researchers at large academic institutions have started research trials of inoculating C-section infants with their mother's own bacteria by using a vaginal swab (a.k.a. vaginal seeding using sterile gauze pads and water to soak up mom's bacteria), which is then applied to the infant's eyes, face, and mouth, simulating what happens in the birth canal. (These mothers are screened for the presence of any bacteria, such as GBS (group B strep), chlamydia or gonorrhea or other infections that could be harmful to the infant).

While ACOG (American College of Gynecology) is currently against widespread use of this practice because of concerns of inadvertently spreading an infection to the infant, the research is ongoing and apparently over 800 subjects have enrolled to date. I am eager to see the outcome of these trials. It does not seem that this practice would be any riskier than what the baby experiences going through the birth canal as long as steps have been taken to ensure a healthy maternal microbiome and rule out dangerous infections. The potential benefits are lifelong, and more research of this type is desperately needed.

I always ask about the mode of delivery when evaluating an infant or young child who comes to me with specific GI complaints. I have seen a trend of children born by C-section coming into my office with complaints of food allergies and sensitivities, chronic constipation, colic, and significant reflux. If there are early issues in a C-section born infant, I may recommend a high quality, multispecies infant-based probiotic (containing at a minimum the **probiotics** *Bifidobacteria infantis* and *Lactobacillus rhamanosus* and *Lactobacillus reuteri* if possible) for these babies to correct their microbiome, oftentimes (but not always) with significant improvement in their symptoms. A small dose of a multi-species infant probiotic mixed with breast milk or formula may "re-inoculate" the baby's gut with healthy bacteria with the hope of preventing future development of disease.

Early studies using probiotics in C-section infants or those given antibiotics at the time of birth have shown a correction of the baby's microbiome to mirror the natural profile of vaginally-born infants, but interestingly, only in those who are breastfed, not formula fed.[16] This observation likely results from the presence of prebiotics (and probiotics) in the breast milk. Dr. Dominguez-Bello feels that "even direct breastfeeding by itself can be highly restorative to the infant microbiome" because of the prebiotics and probiotics contained in healthy mother's milk. Studies are also starting to show improvements in colic and reflux, potentially even eczema and allergies, by using probiotics in babies. It is an exciting new era, but I am in full agreement that ongoing research is needed.

## Premature birth and the NICU

Rates of premature birth in the U.S. and elsewhere continue to rise. Being born prematurely and spending a prolonged period in the Newborn Intensive Care Unit (NICU) is known to significantly alter a baby's microbiome, potentially increasing their risk for serious infections and altered gastrointestinal motility, impaired brain development, and **necrotizing**

**enterocolitis (NEC)**. NEC is a very serious inflammatory condition of the infant's intestines that can be fatal or require surgery to remove large parts of the baby's intestine. As a pediatric gastroenterologist, I have cared for many children who survived NEC but with serious long-term GI consequences. Current research is revealing several things we can do to help prevent some of the serious implications of being born prematurely.

First, prevention. By improving the health, nutrition, and microbiome of the mother (see advice in the pregnancy chapter) we can potentially decrease the risk of premature births and help pass along a healthy microbiome to the baby.)

Secondly, restore the microbiome of the infant who is born early or by C-section.

### HOT TOPIC

Research in this area is ongoing, but multiple studies are showing the safety and benefit of probiotic usage with even the smallest babies in the NICU. Probiotic supplementation (along with breast milk feeding) has been shown to drastically cut down on the rates of NEC and infections and help improve feeding tolerance in these at-risk babies.[19-26] My prediction is that within the next 5 to 10 years, early probiotic and microbiome therapy along with fortified breast milk feeding will be standard of care in the NICU. For now, microbiome therapy is considered experimental. Let's see if this practice will change as the field evolves.

While there have been vocal concerns and resistance to probiotic use by many medical professionals, probiotic supplementation has been shown to be extremely safe. Large trials of probiotics in the NICU have shown no adverse events even among the smallest of babies. In fact, meta-analyses of use of probiotics in the NICU show a reduction in the rates of NEC *by 40%*, as well as a *40% reduction* in life threatening blood infections with *no adverse events* noted. Thousands of babies have been given probiotics with no bad outcomes listed.

Very few medications used in hospitals and given to thousands of people list no side effects or adverse reactions. Use of the proper probiotics could be a potential game changer in premature birth outcomes. If these smallest and most fragile of infants can tolerate probiotic supplementation without any bad effects and with significant health benefits, the chances are that less vulnerable babies may also benefit from their use.

"First, do no harm" is the oath that we take as physicians. Taking steps to promote microbiome restoration in certain circumstances like early antibiotic use, premature or cesarean section delivery are worth considering. There is *evidence of potential harm if we do nothing to reestablish a healthy microbiome* in these babies. If probiotics are safe (and ample studies indicate they are) and may help prevent both immediate and future disease in our children, then we should accelerate research and consider their use now instead of waiting ten years until irrefutable research is available. Supporting evidence is mounting.

I understand the reluctance of many healthcare providers who may be afraid of inadvertently harming their patients. But if you are a healthcare provider, please look at the data (many references are provided in the bibliography of this chapter) for safety profiles and the potential implications of doing nothing. Then make your own educated decision about whether to recommend a probiotic or microbiome restoration.

Do we have *all* the data? No. Do we have enough data showing an acceptable level of safety and suggesting potential major benefits? I say yes. Many medications commonly used in pediatrics have far worse safety profiles, and some that have never been tested or officially approved for use in children. Let's get rid of the double standard.

### Formula feeding
Breast milk is the perfect food to promote proper microbiome development in the infant until foods are added after six months of age, but it can continue to support healthy gut bacteria over the first 1 to 2 years of life for as long as the mother breast feeds. The breast milk microbiome delivers hundreds of thousands of probiotic bacteria daily to the infant through mother's milk. Breast milk also contains **HMO (human milk oligosaccharide),** the ultimate baby prebiotic that promotes growth of the early beneficial gut bacteria, and lactose, which has some prebiotic effects and also promotes the growth of beneficial bacteria.

Past analysis comparing the intestinal microbiome of breastfed infants with formula-fed infants showed significant differences in bacteria, with a healthier microbiome profile and fewer harmful bacteria found in breastfed infants. These differences likely resulted from the from the large amounts of prebiotics as well as the lactose content in breast milk. (Many formulas use corn syrup solids instead.)

In light of this information, the more proactive formula companies are now adding prebiotics such as HMO and other **oligosaccharides,** switching back to lactose, and including other essential ingredients to try to mimic breast milk more closely and "close the gap" between formula and breast milk. Studies on how this impacts the infant microbiome and the future health of the child are ongoing.[27-31] For the mother who cannot breastfeed, the options for formula feeding continue to improve as new research is published. Formula that best supports the baby's microbiome with HMO and lactose should be considered for these parents.

However, breast milk will always remain the top choice for promoting the microbiome of the developing baby. Breastfeeding is highly encouraged by all major pediatric associations such as the **AAP** (American Academy of Pediatrics) as well as the **World Health Organization** (WHO). We will do a deeper dive into breast milk and formula in Chapters 8 and 9, so please refer to those chapters for more complete information and advice.

### The Standard American Diet (SAD)
The **Standard American Diet** is indeed SAD, high in sugar and processed foods, and low in vegetables and fruits. This diet is linked to most of the chronic diseases we see today affecting kids and adults, in large part because SAD damages the microbiome. The SAD is very low in fiber, especially prebiotic soluble fiber, the key fuel for probiotic bacteria in our intestines. Processing food removes most of the fiber and leaves the sugar, refined starches, and potentially harmful additives. This diet feeds harmful bacteria, starves beneficial bacteria, and causes **dysbiosis**. If we are not feeding our beneficial gut bacteria what they need (fruits and vegetables), they will not thrive. *If the good gut bacteria do not thrive, neither will your child.*[32-35] We will study diet in more depth in the chapters ahead.

### Antibiotics
Taking antibiotics, especially early in life, can be devastating to a child's healthy bacteria. Of course, antibiotics (which did not originate until World War II) have saved countless lives and changed the face of medicine. However, in the last 30 years antibiotics have become overprescribed and are sometimes less effective because of increased bacterial resistance. Antibiotics do not do *anything* to treat viral infections, which are the most common cause of ear infections and respiratory infections in children. All we get from treating these viral infections with an antibiotic is a damaged microbiome for our children.

Unfortunately, we are killing the good bacteria with the bad every time we take antibiotics, and this is only recently being recognized and researched. Links have been established between multiple rounds of childhood antibiotics and the development of **autoimmune diseases**, including inflammatory bowel disease and rheumatoid arthritis. The younger a child is exposed to antibiotics, the higher the risk.[36-39]

Antibiotic use also triggers most cases of the nasty intestinal infection *Clostridioides difficile*, known as *C. diff*, which was discussed earlier. However, good evidence shows that giving a probiotic during and after antibiotics significantly cuts the risk for *C. diff* infections in hospitalized patients by 50%. The suggestion by top adult gastroenterologists for probiotic use to become standard of care could save lives and hundreds of millions of healthcare dollars. The implications of this should be considered for pediatric as well as adult medicine.[40]

### Antibiotic and pesticide residues

Antibiotics are not only prescribed for illness but are also found in our food supply to wreak further havoc on our children's gut bacteria. Antibiotics are still used globally in livestock as well as in fish farming to accelerate weight gain, increase animal size, treat and prevent disease, increase feed conversion, and as a preservative. The misuse of antibiotics is leading to increased antibiotic residues and resistant bacteria in the environment and in our food. Antibiotic resistance is recognized as one of the most serious global threats to human health in the twenty-first century.[41]

If we feed the cattle, chicken, or fish antibiotics, the antibiotics do not magically disappear. They get into our food and into our environment and into our children. These antibiotics foster resistant "superbugs," strains of bacteria, viruses, parasites, and fungi that have become drug-resistant and are thought to disrupt the gut bacteria of our children when they consume foods with these antibiotic residues.[42]

In 2017, the FDA restricted antibiotic use in the U.S. for the purpose of fattening animals faster, but there is evidence that *70% of the antibiotics produced in the US are still used for food production rather than health care for humans.* This means that even if children have not taken these drugs, their beneficial bacteria may still be damaged by these antibiotics. When possible, choose meat, poultry and fish raised without antibiotics.

In addition to antibiotic residues, the role that pesticide residues play in the disruption of the child's microbiome is currently being investigated as a serious threat.[43,44] Increasing evidence shows that many pollutants found at unsafe levels in the food supply may be damaging our children's microbiome. Collectively, I refer to this group of chemicals as **microbiome** disrupting chemicals (MDCs) to mirror the dangers of **endocrine disrupting chemicals (EDCs)** also found increasingly in our environment. We will discuss more potential dangers of pesticides and chemicals in our food in later chapters.

### Food additives in highly processed foods

Other chemicals added to our food may damage the gut microbiome and can be considered MDCs.[35] These additives include anti-caking agents, artificial sweeteners, emulsifiers, colorants, artificial flavors, salts, preservatives, thickeners, and stabilizers—all ironically included in the Food and Drug Administration (FDA) "Generally Regarded as Safe" (GRAS) list. Any one or a combination of these substances may alter our gut bacteria in harmful ways and contribute to a **leaky gut**. This book discusses the dangers of endocrine disrupting chemicals (EDCs) in our diets, but we also need to be mindful of the many microbiome disrupting chemicals (MDCs) as well. Often, they can be the same items. Eating real food with a minimum of processing and chemical additives, and untainted by MDCs such as antibiotics, pesticides, and herbicides, can provide health benefits in a number of ways, not the least of which is a healthier gut microbiome.

### Antimicrobial soaps and cleansers

Soaps and cleansers with antimicrobial chemicals gained popularity over the past 20 years, but evidence shows that they are no more effective than regular soaps and cleansers at reducing bacteria and can disrupt our skin and gut microbiome. Luckily, the FDA banned several of the antimicrobial agents from household use in 2017. Choose soaps without antibiotics and antimicrobials for your house. To quote the FDA: "There isn't enough science to show that over-the-counter (OTC) antibacterial soaps are better at preventing illness than washing with plain soap and water. To date, the benefits of using antibacterial hand soap haven't been proven. In addition, the wide use of these products over a long time has raised the question of potential negative effects on your health."

# NUTRITION R$_X$

**1** A child's microbiome can be negatively impacted by an unhealthy maternal microbiome at delivery, C-section birth, formula feeding, perinatal antibiotics, and an early diet filled with processed food and little fiber.

**2** Choose vaginal birth when possible and safe, as this is the primary mode of seeding the infant microbiome with good bacteria. Discuss this decision with the obstetrician or midwife.

**3** If a child is going to be delivered by C-section, discuss with your OB, midwife, or pediatrician the possible methods to foster a healthy infant microbiome.

**4** Breastfeeding also delivers probiotic bacteria to the infant and can restore a healthy microbiome if the mother has a healthy microbiome herself.

**5** Discuss with the medical provider if you or your child really needs antibiotics for that ear infection, cold, or viral respiratory infection. Don't use them unless really needed.

**6** A whole food diet with lots of fiber and phytonutrient rich fruits and vegetables is crucial for maintaining a healthy microbiome.

**7** Choose meat, poultry, and fish raised without antibiotics.

**8** Choose soaps and cleansers without antibiotics or antimicrobial chemicals.

# CHAPTER FIVE

# BEING THE BEST STEWARDS OF OUR CHILDREN'S MICROBIOME

The child's **microbiome** could be viewed as a garden that needs to be planted (at birth) and tended over time with care. Just like our outer ecology, a healthy ecosystem is a diverse ecosystem in our children's inner gardens. "Monocropping" is not a sustainable farming technique and depletes the soil, leaving it barren. The same goes for your child's inner ecology—support a healthy, diverse microbiome by encouraging a diverse diet with a variety of fruits, vegetables, and high-fiber whole grains.

Before we discuss whether **probiotic** supplements may be helpful, we need to emphasize again the importance of being a "good steward" of our children's microbiome. Going back to the old adage of "an ounce of prevention is worth a pound of cure," it is far more beneficial to minimize lifestyle choices and environmental exposures that damage our children's microbiome while at the same time making dietary and health choices that have been shown to support growth of probiotic bacteria in the gut.

Stop for a second and think about how many kids in America are born by C-section, formula fed, or receive multiple rounds of antibiotics for recurrent ear infections, strep throat, or sinus issues, and also eat a poor diet with little fiber and few vegetables. The potential impact on their microbiome and the implications for their long-term health should not be underestimated.

## MICROBIOME BEATDOWN

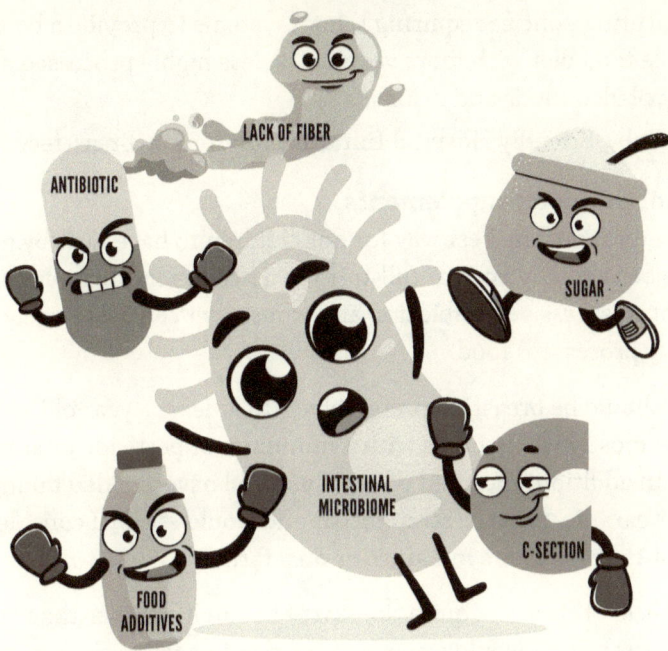

This common scenario leads to a major setup for **dysbiosis** for these children. A dangerously altered microbiome potentially opens the door to **autoimmune disease**, inflammatory disease, and quite possibly even impaired brain function and psychiatric disorders. Consider that the microbiome is now being viewed as another organ in our body, an organ which communicates directly with a child's developing brain. It is also one of the most important **epigenetic modifiers**. Alterations carry far-reaching effects that could negatively impact a child well into adulthood and affect almost every aspect of their physiology. *We need to be better stewards of our children's microbiome!*

Certain policy shifts and changes in medical practice would also help us collectively become better stewards of our children's microbiome. We should support policy and paradigm shifts such as:

+ Legislation to remove antibiotics from our food supply as much as possible.
+ Cutting back on the frivolous and unnecessary use of antibiotics, especially in pediatric medicine (for example, not using them for viral infections).

+ Minimizing harmful pesticide use, as recommended by the American Academy of Pediatrics (see Chapter 7).
+ Instituting policies requiring school systems to provide a better whole food diet with more vegetables, less highly processed and sugar-laden foods and drinks.
+ The Baby-Friendly Hospital Initiative to promote breastfeeding.

## The role of probiotic supplements

As reviewed earlier, the best way for our children to have healthy gut bacteria is to be vaginally born at full-term to a healthy mother who has not had recent or excessive antibiotics, and whose diet consists largely of real (minimally processed) food.

The child should be breastfed preferably until at least a year old and weaned to mostly whole foods with a minimum of pesticide or antibiotic residues. In addition, the child optimally would have avoided taking antibiotics for ear infections or strep throat and would spend a considerable amount of time outdoors in nature or on a farm.

Reality check—this is not quite the start I had in life (other than the outdoors part), and I would wager that many of us fall in the same boat. I am not bitter or upset about this, but my less-than-optimal microbiome history likely contributed to some health challenges along the road. However, as an adult, I am doing my best to be a good steward to my beneficial bacteria and try to raise my children in a better environment by keeping their microbiome and overall health in mind. Even in the best of circumstances, when we have done almost everything right, things can occur that potentially cause damage or disrupt our children's microbiome, such as infections and antibiotic use. So, what do we do if this happens? Can we repair the microbiome? Do we need to?

The use of probiotic supplements has become a controversial topic. Should you or your child take a probiotic? When is it appropriate? Opinions vary widely. On one hand, we have people who think probiotics should be placed in the drinking water. On the other, we have the "doubters and haters" who are very vocal in stating that probiotics are useless or even harmful. Who is right? Probably neither. Spoiler alert: there is not going to be a simple answer.

Reality in medicine is always more nuanced and individual, with truth somewhere between the extremes. Evidence does suggest benefit from probiotic supplementation in some cases, especially when the microbiome has been affected by antibiotics or other insults. However, more research is needed to hone the use of probiotics. For example, which probiotic species are useful for individuals in a given situation is not well known currently but is getting better thanks to researchers pushing the envelope. To say that probiotics are useless or have no effect is ignorant, closed-minded, and blatantly ignores the published evidence.

"**Precision Medicine**" is a newer concept often used in cancer treatment, Alzheimer's prevention, and other areas of medicine[1-3] but also applies to nutrition. Precision medicine looks at the patient as a unique individual and realizes that *a one size fits all approach to medicine is outdated*. Some of the authors and researchers on the cutting edge of this topic are pushing for a more individualized approach to probiotics, which I agree is where we need to head in science and medicine. One size does not fit all, especially in medicine and biology, and there are likely different probiotic species or combinations that may benefit different people depending on their medical condition and existing microbiome.

Clearly not everyone needs to be on a probiotic. However, as we will outline below, there is growing evidence that there are circumstances in which probiotic supplements appear to provide a health benefit. To do a full dive into this topic would be a book onto itself, so we will briefly review some of the more pertinent issues and related research.

### Are probiotics safe?

Could probiotics harm your child? The FDA approved the use of the probiotic bacteria *Bifidobacterium lactis* and *Streptococcus thermophilus* in infant formula as far back as 2002, but there is no official FDA regulation on probiotics currently. However, large studies and meta-analyses of pregnant women and infants, including premature newborns, have shown no reported adverse events with probiotic administration.[5-8] In the medical literature there are only scattered reports of possible "probiotic sepsis," where the probiotic bacteria get into the blood of very ill, mostly adult patients receiving probiotic supplements. However, the vast majority of probiotic studies in intensive care units for both adult and newborn infants showed no incidences of probiotic sepsis even in very sick patients. The studies are proving that for most people, including children, probiotic use is safe. Of course, caution and supervision are always warranted when giving any medication or supplement to a very young or ill child.

### Are probiotics useless?

Is it true that probiotics are "dead" and don't even get into the intestine of those children or adults who take them? Do probiotics pass right through the digestive tract without doing anything? Do we just poop them out?

Recent studies have shown that probiotic bacteria from a *good quality* supplement and probiotic foods can and do get into the intestines of the person ingesting them. Multiple past studies have shown increases in the *Lactobacillus* and *Bifidobacterium* counts in the research subjects taking a probiotic. Using the latest technology, the authors of a recent paper in one of the world's leading research journals proved that the probiotic bacteria used in their study were alive and viable and made it into the intestines of the study participants. This data debunks at least one of the common arguments that probiotics are dead or get killed by stomach acid and never get into our intestines and are therefore useless.[9] Additionally, a new study just published in 2020 provides evidence that fermented "probiotic" foods such as cheeses, yogurt, and fermented vegetables are a viable source of probiotic bacteria in the gut and may partially shape the microbiome.[10,11]

---

Scientific research is looking at both the *fecal (stool) microbiome* as well as the *mucosal (gut) microbiome*. Testing the poop for bacteria as most studies are doing—thereby reporting the **fecal microbiome**—may be useful but does not necessarily tell us which bacteria are living full time in that person's intestine, the **mucosal microbiome**. Some bacteria may be transient "guests" that are passing through and then end up in the toilet (or diaper as the case may be). What effect do these transient probiotic bacteria have on our health, versus the more "full-time" mucosal microbiome? Science is still working this out.

Additionally, the emerging field of **metabolomics** looks at the *functions* of the microbiome and of probiotic bacteria by analyzing certain chemicals in the blood, urine, and stool of the person taking these products. These studies give us not only the "who is in there?" data, which identifies bacterial species, but also gives us some of the "what are they doing in there?" data as well, to inform us of the functions of these bacteria.

---

A recent conclusion of one of these studies suggests that the intestinal mucosal microbiome may be somewhat "set" in certain adults and resist colonization by the "new guys" (a probiotic supplement or probiotic foods). However, the authors found that there were "resistant" and "permissive" individuals in their study that incorporated highly variable amounts of the supplemental probiotics into their microbiome. After taking the probiotic supplement, the bacteria in the intestines were different in *some but not all* individuals. This indicates that some people will respond to a probiotic while some will not. This fascinating data further lends credence to the personalized medicine approach.[9]

Also keep in mind that much evidence suggests that the *microbiome of an infant and child is far from "set"* and continues to be malleable for a good proportion of childhood. This important difference indicates that *infants and children may be more likely to respond (positively or negatively) to factors influencing their microbiome,* including probiotic foods and probiotic supplements. As in so many other ways, the pediatric axiom that "kids are not little adults" holds true.

### Should probiotics be given during or after antibiotics?

Let's consider what happens to the intestinal microbiome when someone is given antibiotics. As we discussed earlier, antibiotics have been around since the 1940s and have saved untold millions of lives from serious bacterial infections. They are probably the greatest invention of modern medicine. However, there is a dark side. The beneficial bacteria in the gut are wiped out along with the infection that is being treated with antibiotics, which may significantly damage the microbiome.

While some people may experience a spontaneous recovery of their healthy intestinal bacteria once antibiotics are discontinued, often there can be significant consequences. When antibiotics are stopped and unfriendly bacteria outgrow the good bacteria, an imbalance is created known as dysbiosis. The dysbiosis that can occur after antibiotic treatment may have wide ranging effects from relatively minor post-antibiotic diarrhea to longer term, more significant issues such as **irritable bowel syndrome**, **inflammatory bowel disease** (Crohn's and Colitis), autoimmune disease, and a potentially life-threatening intestinal infection known as *C. diff* (*Clostridioides difficile* infection). Clearly, these people did not have a spontaneous recovery of their healthy microbiome once antibiotics were stopped and may have benefitted from the use of probiotics.

The authors of the recent 2018 study published in *Cell* showed that probiotics taken after antibiotics can in fact take hold and effectively colonize the intestines of the person taking them.[9] They debunk the myth that probiotics don't do anything. However, findings by the same authors also showed that adults taking a probiotic may limit or delay their intestinal recovery to a full pre-antibiotic baseline microbiome. Conversely, these authors found that **fecal microbiome transplant (FMT)** offers a more complete, almost immediate post-antibiotic microbiome recovery.[12]

> Fecal microbiome transplant is a medically supervised procedure where the total microbiome from a healthy person's intestines is concentrated from the stool and then infused into another person's intestines. The primary use is as a cure for recurrent C. diff infections, but other applications are being examined.

This study raises some interesting questions:

+ Does the limited microbiome recovery seen in those taking a probiotic supplement after antibiotics somehow permanently limit the natural diversity seen in a healthy intestine? If so, why aren't we seeing negative health effects in people who have taken probiotics after antibiotics? In fact, we often see benefits as mentioned below.

+ A large number of people have some degree of dysbiosis at baseline even before taking antibiotics. In this case, do we *want* to keep their old microbiome by not giving probiotics?

+ How does a person's diet impact microbiome recovery after antibiotics? Can you shape the recovery by choosing more probiotic foods and prebiotic fiber-rich foods? It seems likely that you could.

+ Where do children fit into all this, given the more flexible nature of their developing microbiome? How much more vulnerable are children to the negative impact of antibiotic use?

So far, I have not seen good data that shows taking probiotics after antibiotics is harmful. In fact, large studies and **meta-analyses** are proving the effectiveness of probiotic supplementation for reducing antibiotic-associated diarrhea[13-15] and improving symptoms of irritable bowel syndrome,[16-19] which are common after antibiotic use or an infection.

Most importantly, recent studies and reviews show that the use of multispecies probiotics significantly decrease the rates of nasty antibiotic-associated *C. diff* infections that can be fatal in older adults. Given this information alone, I wouldn't be so quick to dismiss the use of a good probiotic while taking antibiotics.[20] Unfortunately, *C. diff* infections can be recurrent and cause long-term problems—an increasingly common issue due to antibiotic resistant organisms. Performing FMT rather than giving another round of antibiotics is known to be a cure for 80%–90% of recurrent *C. diff* infections.[21] Doing FMT may also offer a more complete microbiome restoration after the use of antibiotics according to the authors of the recent study mentioned earlier.[12] However, performing FMT in every person taking antibiotics is not really practical or appealing to the average joe. If you can't get most adults to eat a vegetable, selling them on the idea of getting someone else's poop infused into them is going to be difficult. It seems then that use of a multi-species probiotic may have a role in preventing unwanted side effects from antibiotic use, and ongoing research should help us to further improve this practice.

Many other circumstances in which probiotic supplements have shown benefit are found in peer-reviewed research studies. We do not have the space to review these in full detail but will highlight some relevant uses and cite the studies showing their effectiveness. This is not to say that probiotic use is warranted for every child. The use of probiotics for specific health conditions should be discussed with a child's primary medical provider.

## Other potential benefits from probiotic supplements

*Necrotizing enterocolitis*
As discussed earlier in the chapter, several large studies and meta-analyses have demonstrated a significant risk reduction in the development of **necrotizing enterocolitis** in premature infants in the NICU with no adverse events. The incidence of sepsis (a serious bacterial infection) was also reduced. It is worth noting that the studies that used multi-species probiotics found significant results, whereas those that used single species probiotics often found no effect. Based on this data demonstrating a 40% to 50% risk reduction with no adverse events, medical providers may consider the use of multi-species probiotics to protect these premature babies.[6,7,22-25]

*Constipation*
Also mentioned earlier in the chapter, mounting evidence suggests that probiotic use can improve chronic constipation related to dysbiosis in both children and adults. Studies have shown mixed results, but in general, those probiotics that contained *Bifidobacteria* or contained multiple species seemed to show more positive results.[26-29]

*Colic*
Four recent meta-analyses published in the past seven years all showed effectiveness of the probiotic *Lactobacillus reuteri* in treating infant colic. This treatment seemed to be more effective in breastfed infants than in formula-fed infants.[30-33]

*Allergy and eczema prevention*
Several recent meta-analyses have demonstrated a protective effect of probiotics on the development of allergies and eczema in children born to families with a strong history of allergic disease. It is interesting to note that the effect on allergy prevention was only significant if the pregnant mother and the child both received the probiotic supplements. Again, multi-species probiotic supplements seemed to show superior results compared with single species.[34-37]

*Anxiety and depression*
There is ongoing research into the role of the **brain-gut-microbiome axis** as it relates to mental health and cognitive disorders. While study results have been variable, as have the study design and the types of probiotics used, there is certainly enough evidence of a positive effect on mood to warrant further research and consideration of probiotics in treatment of mood disorders.[38-42] The effects of diet and probiotics on ADHD and autism will be discussed in a future chapter.

> If parents and healthcare providers decide that using a probiotic supplement for a child may be warranted, choose carefully. Choosing a probiotic can be daunting because so many products are available now. In general, studies using mixed probiotics with multiple strains of *Lactobacillus* and *Bifidobacterium*, plus a few other species, have shown the most promise in recent medical research. Look for a product that contains a mix of at least five strains of combined *Lactobacillus* and *Bifidobacteria* species. Refrigerated brands from a reputable company may help maintain potency and product integrity. Hopefully, future research will reveal which is the right combination of friendly bacteria for each individual.

Remember that if a child is eating a diet very low in prebiotic fiber and high in processed foods, then taking a probiotic supplement doesn't make a whole lot of sense. If we aren't feeding the beneficial bacteria, why bother taking them? Evidence shows that within 24 to 48 hours of a dietary shift, there is a considerable shift in the fecal microbiome. Eating a diet with lots of prebiotic fiber and phytonutrients from fruits and vegetables and fiber from whole grains can create a shift from an unhealthy to a healthy microbiome. **Always start with the diet first.**

Probiotic foods include high quality *low sugar* yogurt and kefir, as well as sauerkraut, kimchi, and naturally fermented "pickled" vegetables. These foods have all been eaten for thousands of years and provide a steady supply of probiotic bacteria to support our gut microbiome. Don't forget that a healthy microbiome must be *maintained* with lots of prebiotic fiber and **phytonutrients** too, so without those servings of vegetables, those good bacteria may starve!

# NUTRITION R$_X$

To foster a healthy microbiome in children, consider the following:

**1** Choose vaginal birth when it is safe and possible to do so to optimize the microbiome transfer to the child.

**2** Immediately after birth and during infancy have lots of skin-to-skin contact with your baby.

**3** Wait a minimum of 8 hours for the first bath after an infant is born to allow more time for the microbiome transfer from mother to infant occur. Delayed bathing also increases breastfeeding success. (The WHO and ICEA recommend not bathing the baby for the first 24 hours after birth. See www.icea.org and www.WHO.int)

**4** Choose to breast feed for the first year of life whenever possible, but consider a formula containing lactose and HMO if you cannot breastfeed.

**5** Mothers and children of all ages should spend time outside in nature. If possible, grow a small vegetable or herb garden for positive impact upon the microbiome. Healthy soil that has not been saturated with pesticides and artificial fertilizers has its own microbiome that will tie directly to the health of our own.

**6** Wean a child onto whole foods; avoid or minimize highly processed and high-sugar foods.

**7** Continue to feed children unprocessed whole foods: lots of vegetables (organic when possible), whole fruits, and whole grains, which are all full of prebiotic fiber and phytonutrients.

**8** Incorporate probiotic foods like whole-fat, low-sugar yogurt, kefir, sauerkraut, and fermented vegetables into a child's diet when it is age appropriate.

**9** Based on the medical literature, there are circumstances where probiotic supplements show potential benefit. These include premature delivery, antibiotic use, infant colic, chronic constipation, and possibly even allergy prevention and mood disorders.

**10** Probiotic supplementation is likely to do little if a child is fed a diet full of sugar and highly processed foods lacking fiber and phytonutrients.

# CHAPTER SIX

# NUTRITION ADVICE FOR THE EXPECTING MOTHER

Congratulations, you are expecting! Are you among the 85% of women who are not meeting current dietary recommendations during pregnancy?

We have all heard the expression "You are what you eat." Taken a step further, *the baby is what the pregnant mother eats and metabolizes,* for better or worse. The concept of "eat whatever you want... you're pregnant!" is outdated, erroneous, and dangerous. The mother's diet, starting on day one of pregnancy, is hugely important and has potential lifelong effects on that child. Rather than just worrying about providing calories for the child to grow and gain weight, we need to expand our focus.

In this chapter, we review what to eat during pregnancy to grow a healthy baby and avoid some of the risks in the modern diet. Given the current science on the impact of the mother's diet on the child's future health, we need to pay much more attention to maternal nutrition if birth outcomes and infant health are to improve.

In keeping with the **First Thousand Days** concept described in Chapter 2, feeding our children really starts at the moment of conception, with evidence suggesting that it may even begin in the months prior.[1-3] The developing baby is completely reliant on the dietary intake and nutrient stores of its mother and is exceptionally vulnerable to nutritional deficiencies and toxic exposures that may occur during this critical time.

> *"The clock for the first thousand days starts at conception."*

Pregnancy is a crucial window in the child's life for determining future health risks for a range of diseases, such as obesity, cardiovascular disease, **type 2 diabetes**, and **neurodevelopmental disorders**. Toxic exposures in the womb, poor maternal nutrition, unhealthy maternal microbiomes, and maternal trauma and stress, can negatively affect **gene expression** (**epigenetics**) and brain development during critical neurodevelopmental windows. Because this time period is so important, we need to take the necessary steps to give our children the best start possible. These include eating a healthy diet while pregnant, maintaining a healthy maternal **microbiome**, and doing our best to limit exposures to potentially toxic chemicals and toxic stress.

### MATERNAL FACTORS IMPACTING INFANT OUTCOMES AND EPIGENETICS

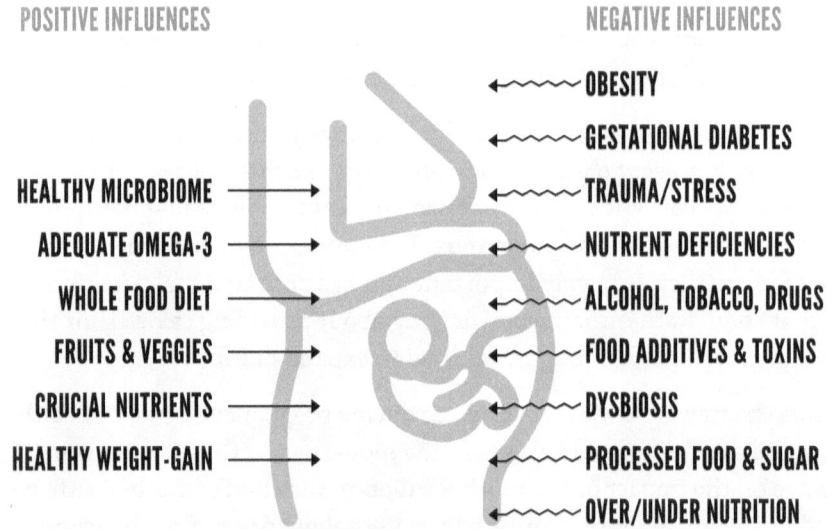

| POSITIVE INFLUENCES | NEGATIVE INFLUENCES |
|---|---|
| | OBESITY |
| | GESTATIONAL DIABETES |
| HEALTHY MICROBIOME | TRAUMA/STRESS |
| ADEQUATE OMEGA-3 | NUTRIENT DEFICIENCIES |
| WHOLE FOOD DIET | ALCOHOL, TOBACCO, DRUGS |
| FRUITS & VEGGIES | FOOD ADDITIVES & TOXINS |
| CRUCIAL NUTRIENTS | DYSBIOSIS |
| HEALTHY WEIGHT-GAIN | PROCESSED FOOD & SUGAR |
| | OVER/UNDER NUTRITION |

## THE CURRENT STATE OF MATERNAL NUTRITION

Despite better access to prenatal and medical care, all is not well for many mothers in the US and in other industrialized countries. According to research, only a small proportion of pregnant mothers (less than 16% in one study) are meeting the overall recommended dietary guidelines for pregnant women, and less than half of pregnant women were eating the recommended amounts of fruits and vegetables.[4,5]

High-calorie malnutrition is rampant in Western culture and is characterized by a diet with too many calories but not enough key nutrients. This modern diet leaves the unborn child at risk for the negative consequences associated with a lack of vital nutrients needed for growth and brain development, some of which may be irreversible. Processed food and high amounts of sugar also contribute to excessive weight gain and **gestational diabetes** during pregnancy, both of which increase lifelong health risks for the unborn child.

In the United States, about 1% to 2% of pregnant women have *type 2 diabetes* at the time of pregnancy, an increase of 37% in recent years. In addition, 6% to 9% of pregnant women develop *gestational diabetes* during pregnancy, and the numbers are increasing. In the ten years between 2000 and 2010, the percentage of pregnant women with gestational diabetes increased 56%!

Why are the rates of diabetes in pregnancy increasing? For starters, many pregnant women consume far too much sugar and highly processed "convenience foods." Also of concern are the increased levels of **endocrine disrupting chemicals (EDCs)** to which pregnant mothers are exposed. As described in the following chapter, EDCs such as BPA and phthalates are widespread and may alter the hormones and glucose **metabolism** of mothers and children, potentially predisposing them to the development of diabetes.[6,7] We will take a closer look at these chemicals in the next chapter. Unborn children and their mothers are exposed to thousands of chemicals that have *never been tested for safety in humans,* many of which have potential effects on the endocrine system (hormones) and brains of the pregnant mother, infant, and child.

Currently 50% of women gain excessive weight during pregnancy, and 25% of pregnant women are obese. This is not fat shaming and has nothing to do with body image or aesthetics. There are both short and long-term health risks to the baby of an overweight or obese mother or one with diabetes, including

+ Childhood obesity
+ Early type 2 diabetes
+ Developmental delays
+ Learning disabilities
+ Large for gestational age (LGA) babies

+ Increased rates of C-section
+ Maternal complications during childbirth
+ Iron deficiency in both mother and infant

What can we do to mitigate these risks?

In addition, environmental factors that affect epigenetic programming during pregnancy, such as toxic exposures, nutritional deficiencies in the womb, and altered maternal microbiomes are suspected to contribute to rising rates of several disorders including

## Pediatric autoimmune diseases

+ Type 1 diabetes
+ Thyroid disease
+ Crohn's disease
+ Celiac disease

## Neurocognitive disorders

+ Developmental delays
+ ADHD
+ Autism

When I was growing up, only a few kids in my entire school took ADHD medications; Special Education (SPED) classrooms were relatively small. Now, incredible numbers of children are taking stimulant ADHD medication, and the SPED programs are overloaded and understaffed. More children are taking antidepressant medications and rates of depression in children continue to rise with one in five teens experiencing depression before they are 18, and 10% of teens diagnosed with major depressive disorder.[17,18] The "new normal" is anything but.

Some physicians and scientists argue that the reported rise in these disorders results from "detection bias," an ability to better screen and diagnose these disorders. While this may account for some proportion of the rise in reported rates, there is no "detection bias" with autoimmune disorders like **type 1 diabetes** or Crohn's, just like there is no detection bias with type 2 diabetes and obesity. Either you have it or you don't, and more and more kids are developing these disorders by the day.

Many physicians and scientists, including myself, are convinced that we have a real increase in these disorders and need to ask *why*. Something is happening to our children early in their lives, starting in the womb, that is potentially leading to impairments in their brain, immune system, and metabolic functioning. The increase in these disorders should be a call to arms immediately to begin reversing these trends. This starts with improving nutrition during pregnancy.

# IT ALL STARTS WITH DIET

Feeding our children starts at, or prior to, conception. Proper maternal nutrition is crucial to giving each child the best start possible. During those first thousand days, diet can impact three important developmental targets. **Food choices for both mother and child are**

1. **Feeding the brain (neurodevelopment)**
2. **Feeding the gut (microbiome)**
3. **Feeding the genes (epigenetics)**

Let's explore each of these target areas and how making the right food choices supports proper development and a happier, healthier child.

# FEEDING THE GROWING BABY BRAIN

As we have discussed, the most rapid brain growth and neurodevelopment in a child's life occurs in the first thousand days. Most of the **neurons** (brain cells) and the highest number of **synapses** (connections between neurons) are formed in a process called **synaptogenesis** during this period. We start out as a single cell that divides and differentiates into all the tissues and organs of the body, including the brain and nervous system. The brain continues to grow and develop after birth and *doubles in weight* by 6 months of life. This phase of rapid brain growth occurs until the age of 2 to 3 years, although the process of synaptogenesis continues throughout life. During this time there are *critical developmental windows* that if missed or damaged by nutrient deficiencies or toxic exposures can lead to neurological or developmental deficits in our children.

Given the rapidity of growth and the complexity of the brain and nervous system, the child's brain is extremely vulnerable to nutritional deficiencies and toxic insults during these times. Both serious and more subtle impacts on brain development and future academic outcomes can occur during those first thousand days; mom's diet can play a big role in making sure her child's brain is equipped with what it needs to perform at its best.

However, a deficiency of key nutrients or exposure to **toxic chemicals** during this time can lead to cognitive and behavioral issues that may be difficult or impossible to overcome down the road.[1,2,8-16] Key nutrients for brain development such as iron, zinc, essential fatty acids (**EPA/ DHA**), and choline are commonly deficient even in the diets of mothers in modern industrialized countries like the US.[1,2,13,19,20] In addition, research shows that exposure to neurotoxic and endocrine disrupting chemicals such as BPA, phthalates, pesticides, and heavy metals such as lead and arsenic may harm brain development during this critical window.[8–12,14–16]

## KEY BRAIN NUTRIENTS FOR THE DEVELOPING BABY

A recent policy statement by the American Academy of Pediatrics asserts that "Although all nutrients are necessary for brain growth (in babies), key nutrients that support neurodevelopment include protein, zinc, iron, choline, folate, iodine, vitamins A, D, B6, and B12, and long-chain poly-unsaturated fatty acids (**EPA/DHA/ARA**)."[1] As proper maternal nutrition supports and protects the developing brain of the baby, we will focus on these brain nutrients, along with calcium and magnesium. The following section is divided into crucial micronutrients (minerals and vitamins) and crucial macronutrients (protein, fat, and carbohydrate).

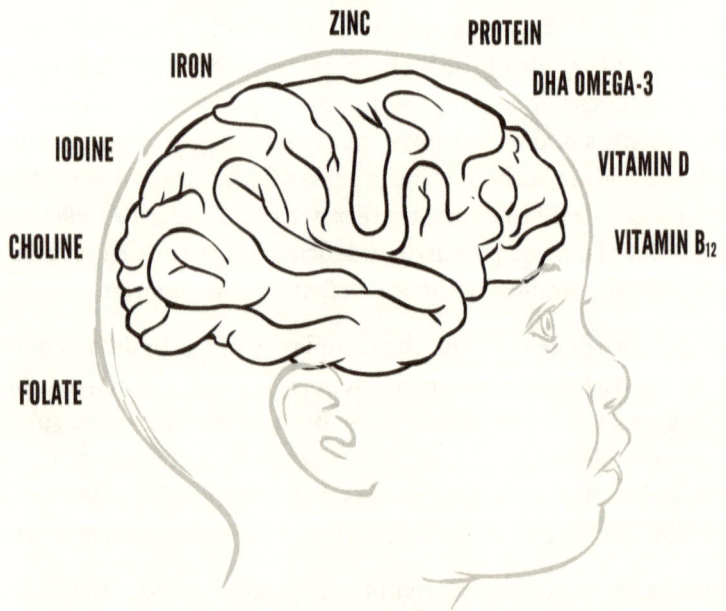

IMPORTANT PREGNANCY NUTRIENTS FOR THE BABY'S BRAIN

ZINC

PROTEIN

IRON

DHA OMEGA-3

IODINE

VITAMIN D

CHOLINE

VITAMIN B12

FOLATE

# CRUCIAL MICRONUTRIENTS: MINERALS

## Iron

Worldwide more than one in four pregnant women suffer from anemia during pregnancy, with rates approaching 50% in developing countries. Anemia during pregnancy is defined as a blood **hemoglobin** level less than 11 g/dL (110 g/L) and is primarily caused by low iron levels in the body. At least 40% to 50% of all pregnancies suffer from *iron deficiency*, which may or may not result in anemia. A low iron intake or low iron stores during pregnancy can have profound effects on the development of the unborn child as well as putting the mother at increased risk of complications.[23,25-27] Prenatal iron deficiency doubles the risk of prematurity and triples the risk of having an underweight baby.

Despite knowing for decades about the developmental importance of iron, 25% of US children are still deficient in this vital mineral, often starting in the womb. The biggest predictor of infant iron deficiency is maternal iron deficiency. This deficiency has the potential to cause lifelong learning and developmental disabilities in the child. We have discovered that infants born to mothers who are obese or have diabetes, mothers who smoke, mothers with iron deficiency, as well as infants born prematurely, are at higher risk for iron deficiency. Iron deficiency in the US is increasing, in part because obesity and gestational diabetes interfere with the mother's iron metabolism, leaving iron less available for the developing baby. The standard policy of delayed umbilical cord clamping during childbirth can help improve an infant's iron stores but is not always adequate or possible during high-risk births or C-sections.

Besides the vital role in forming blood (hemoglobin), iron is essential for the formation and development of brain cells and their insulation (myelination). Iron deficiency during critical periods of brain development can have harmful and irreversible effects, resulting in decreased IQ and increased learning and behavioral disabilities.

Iron deficiency also causes epigenetic modifications that span generations, making it more likely that the iron deficient child will bear children who are also iron deficient. Even mothers who are not anemic may have inadequate iron levels and low iron stores that put their developing babies at risk. Maintaining adequate iron levels during pregnancy is a top priority for having better child outcomes.

*Testing for deficiency*

The Institute of Medicine recommends that mothers in the US should be screened for anemia with a **complete blood count (CBC)** including a hemoglobin in each trimester, but other guidelines suggest screening CBC at the initial visit and between 24 and 28 weeks of gestation. Generally, if a mother is not obviously anemic (that is, her hemoglobin levels are greater than 11 and considered in the normal range on standard blood tests), her iron levels will not be routinely checked, *missing up to half of the cases of prenatal iron deficiency* that could benefit from more aggressive supplementation or dietary alteration.

---

## HOT TOPIC

Iron deficiency during pregnancy, while increasingly recognized as a major issue, currently lacks international consensus. Iron levels are not routinely checked during pregnancy. Research shows that among pregnant women in the first trimester who were screened and found not to have anemia, *42% had evidence of low iron levels in their bodies* putting their child at risk.[21,22]

According to guidelines from the British Society for Hematology, iron deficiency during pregnancy can be defined as a **serum ferritin less than 30 ug/L regardless of hemoglobin level**. This cutoff level is more sensitive at picking up mothers who have depleted their iron stores and may not be delivering optimal amounts of iron to the baby. However, ferritin levels are not routinely checked in pregnant mothers unless they are obviously anemic. In some countries such as the US, even when ferritin levels are checked the guidelines are less stringent and use 10 to 15 ug/L as the cutoff for iron deficiency. Past research suggests that when mom's ferritin is below 15, the baby is already getting iron deficient.

Top iron researchers are suggesting that perhaps all pregnant women be screened for iron deficiency AND anemia to optimize infant neurodevelopment. I would tend to agree, given the lifelong ramifications.[191-202]

I am among a growing group of doctors who feel that *all* pregnant mothers should be screened for iron deficiency regardless of their hemoglobin status because of the potential impact on the baby's brain. At the very least, mothers who are anemic and those at increased risk for iron deficiency should be screened. This list includes women with

+ Twins or multiple pregnancy
+ Short time between pregnancies (less than 1 year)
+ Obesity
+ Gestational diabetes
+ Use of nicotine products
+ Vegetarian/vegan diet or low meat intake
+ History of anemia
+ History of being born to an anemic mother
+ History of GI disease: celiac, Crohn's, colitis, reflux requiring acid blocking medication

Early in the pregnancy, as well as the second trimester, it may be advisable for the obstetrician, midwife, or PCP (primary care provider) to check the mother's hemoglobin as well as other iron markers such as **serum ferritin**, and possibly **transferrin saturation**. If these tests indicate that iron levels are low, supplementation should be started immediately, and iron levels rechecked periodically to make sure levels are normalizing. Iron screening, supplementation, and retesting should all be done under the guidance of the obstetrician, midwife, or PCP to optimize iron stores and avoid iron overload. Adding a ferritin level to the hemoglobin tested during pregnancy would detect a great many cases of maternal iron deficiency that could be corrected, thereby protecting the brain of the unborn child.

*Food sources*
The best food sources of iron are meat, liver, and shellfish (which contain **heme iron**); in plant sources, iron is less concentrated and less available to the baby. We will discuss this further in the section on baby's first foods, but vegetarian and fortified sources of iron (**non-heme iron**) are not as well absorbed and often contain plant compounds that can block absorption of iron and zinc, so the vegetarian and vegan mother or the mother who rarely eats meat is *highly encouraged* to get her **hemoglobin** *and* iron levels monitored to avoid potential damaging effects of iron deficiency on the unborn child.[25–27]

**Omnivorous** mothers are at somewhat lower risk for low iron but are not exempt by any means. Pregnant mothers need to make sure they are getting enough iron to support the developing baby, which can be difficult without supplementation in the best of circumstances. Examine the iron rich foods list below for dietary iron sources.

### TABLE 6.1 IRON RICH FOOD SOURCES

| Heme Sources (per 2.5 oz serving) | Iron (mg) |
| --- | --- |
| Ground beef | 2.0 |
| Beef (steak/various cuts) | 2.0–2.4 |
| Liver (chicken) | 9.2 |
| Liver (beef) | 4.8 |
| Chicken thigh | 1.0 |
| Chicken breast | 0.8 |
| Turkey dark meat | 1.1 |
| Turkey white meat | 0.8 |
| Oysters/mussels | 5-6 |
| Salmon | 0.6 |
| Trout | 1.4 |
| Sardines | 2.0 |

| Non-heme Sources | |
| --- | --- |
| Fortified breakfast cereal* (1 cup) | 7-10 |
| Black beans* (½ cup) | 2.5 |
| Refried beans* (¾ cup) | 2.7 |
| Lentils* (¾ cup) | 4.9 |
| Spinach ½ cup (cooked)* | 3.4 |
| Quinoa (½ cup) | 1.4 |
| Enriched rice (½ cup) | 1.0 |
| Egg (1)* | 1.0 |
| Raisins* (¼ cup) | 1.0 |

Data from National Institutes of Health (www.NIH.gov), USDA Nutrient Database (https://fdc.nal.usda.gov/), Health Link British Columbia, (www.healthlinkBC.ca), Linus Pauling Institute (https://lpi.oregonstate.edu/mic/minerals/iron)[203-206]

*Non-Heme iron sources are significantly less well absorbed. Absorption may be enhanced with vitamin C or by including sources of heme iron.

### Supplementation

To prevent the negative outcomes that are associated with prenatal iron deficiency, oral iron supplements are recommended for the iron deficient mother to normalize her iron levels, and intravenous iron for women in the second and third trimester if they are not responding to oral iron supplements.[23,24] Intravenous iron is proven to be safe and effective if new guidelines are followed. It is recommended that all pregnant women take a daily prenatal vitamin with iron to make sure that at a minimum they achieve the **RDA of 27 mg per day**, but the iron content of prenatal vitamins is highly variable. The **Center for Disease Control and Prevention (CDC)** currently recommends 30 mg iron be taken daily by US mothers, starting in early pregnancy. The WHO recommends an iron supplement of 30 to 60 mg of elemental iron daily for pregnant women internationally living in areas with less access to heme-iron rich foods. Too much iron is potentially harmful to mother and baby, so high-dose iron should not be taken indiscriminately.

Checking a ferritin level would help determine which mothers need extra iron and which ones have adequate iron stores for the baby. Ferrous sulfate, gluconate or fumarate are all approved forms of iron during pregnancy. Newer guidelines suggest that taking iron just once a day or every other day may improve absorption and decrease stomach upset. Take iron on an empty stomach if tolerated and avoid taking iron with dairy products or calcium supplements that block absorption. Iron supplementation should be done under the guidance of a qualified health professional.

*Bottom line on iron*
Iron deficiency and anemia are very common in pregnancy and can have long-term impacts on the baby's brain development. Many mothers who are not yet anemic may still have low iron levels that can potentially harm the baby. Make a conscious effort to incorporate iron-rich foods into a pregnancy diet. Based on the evidence and expert opinion of the top iron researchers, many if not most mothers should be screened for low iron levels with a serum ferritin in addition to screening for anemia to identify women who need more iron in their diet or additional supplementation.

## Zinc
Zinc plays a key role in immune system function and is required for the protein and DNA formation necessary for proper growth and development of the baby. This crucial mineral is also required for the healthy functioning of more than 300 enzymes in our bodies.[28]

The **World Health Organization** (WHO) states that 80% of pregnant women worldwide are likely not getting adequate zinc from lack of animal-based proteins in their diet,[29] and that well over 500,000 maternal and child deaths annually are due to zinc deficiency.[30]

Based on these grim statistics, and the fact that zinc supplementation improves the growth of children in nutritionally high-risk areas, United Nations Children's Fund (UNICEF) supports supplementing zinc for pregnant mothers in all developing countries.

Zinc deficiency in pregnancy is associated with[13,30–34]

+ increased risk of preterm birth
+ fetal loss (miscarriage)
+ growth impairments, including
+ small for gestational age (SGA)
+ low birth weight (LBW)
+ neurodevelopmental disorders
+ altered microbiome
+ increased inflammation
+ impaired immune function in the child

Effects of maternal zinc intake on the infant's immune system and risk of infections are subjects of investigation. It is known that zinc deficiency negatively affects the ability of the immune system to function, leaving children more prone to infections. Animal models have shown that zinc deficiency is likely an **epigenetic modifier**, persistently impairing immune function *for three generations* in offspring of a zinc deficient mother.[36]

A few smaller studies looking at the effect of zinc supplementation in pregnant moms from developing countries showed a decreased incidence of diarrheal illness in their babies. Zinc supplementation in older infants and children in developing countries show a clear immune benefit and reduced risk of infections like pneumonia and gastrointestinal infections. More research in this area needs to be done, especially on milder forms of zinc deficiency or insufficiency seen in more developed countries like the US. Nutritional support of the infant's immune system is crucial to fighting off potentially dangerous infections in the first months of life. Additionally, prevention of infection likely plays an important developmental role, as significant infections during the first year of life can be associated with developmental delays.

*Recommended daily amount*

Getting adequate zinc in the diet should be a primary goal for a pregnant mother. **The RDA for pregnant women is 11 mg daily.** The WHO estimates average worldwide intake at around 10 mg, but US estimates average 12 mg daily. However, the recommended or estimated intakes do not take into account the percentage of dietary zinc that is actually absorbed or how much is blocked by **anti-nutrient** compounds in food called **phytates.** Grains, beans, and seeds contain a substance known as *phytate*, which is a naturally occurring chemical that partially blocks absorption of the zinc (and hence is labeled an anti-nutrient). A high intake of grains, beans, and seeds without the presence of adequate seafood or meat in the diet increases risk of inadequate zinc levels, and potentially increases zinc requirements especially during pregnancy.

*Detecting deficiency*

Unfortunately, testing mothers for zinc deficiency is not as straight-forward as testing iron levels. Currently, blood tests for zinc levels are unreliable in determining whether the mother is truly low in zinc unless deficiency is more severe. There is no accurate testing method for milder zinc deficiency that I endorse currently. Risk of deficiency is based on reported dietary intake and underlying medical conditions that may increase zinc requirements, such as Crohn's or colitis, celiac disease, and patients with reflux disease taking proton pump inhibitors (PPIs).[37,38]

## TABLE 6.2 ZINC FOOD SOURCES

| Food (per 3 oz serving unless otherwise specified) | Zinc (mg) |
|---|---|
| Oysters (1 oz) | 25 |
| Beef (steak/roast) | 7.0-8.7 |
| Ground beef | 5.3 |
| Liver (beef) | 4.5 |
| Chicken thigh | 1.8-2.4 |
| Chicken breast | 0.75 |
| Turkey dark meat | 3.0 |
| Turkey white meat | 1.5 |
| Salmon/trout | 0.6 |
| Sardines | 1.0 |
| Fortified cereal – All Bran (1 cup) | 7.6 |
| Pumpkin seeds (1oz) | 2.2 |
| Sunflower seeds (1 oz) | 1.5 |

| Food (per 3 oz serving unless otherwise specified) | Zinc (mg) |
|---|---|
| Cashews (1 oz) | 1.6 |
| Almonds (1 oz) | 0.9 |
| Peanut butter (2 tbsp) | 0.8 |
| Black beans/kidney beans (½ cup) | 0.9 |
| Baked beans (½ cup) | 0.7 |
| Chickpeas (½ cup) | 1.2 |
| Spinach (cooked) | 0.6 |
| Greek yogurt (1 container) | 1.2-1.7 |
| Cheese (1 oz) | 1.0 |
| Egg (1) | 0.6 |

Data from National Institutes of Health (www.NIH.gov), USDA Nutrient Database (https://fdc.nal.usda.gov/), Health Link British Columbia, (www.healthlinkBC.ca), Linus Pauling Institute (https://lpi.oregonstate.edu/mic/minerals/iron)[203-206]

Most non-fortified grain products are only a moderate source of zinc but have a high phytate level. Nuts, seeds, and beans, while good sources of zinc, also contain phytates that will bind up some of the zinc and reduce absorption (less **bioavailable**). Moms who eat a lot of beans and grains and no meat or seafood are therefore likely at risk for suboptimal zinc intake for their baby.[39,40] Zinc absorption from highly processed foods may also be impaired by certain chemicals commonly found in these foods.[41] Soaking, rinsing, and sprouting seeds, nuts and grains can reduce the phytate content to some degree and allow better absorption of zinc, as can adding some animal protein to the meal. Unfortunately, in contrast to iron, vitamin C does not enhance the absorption of zinc.[41] I don't think we should take it for granted that pregnant women in developed countries are necessarily getting adequate zinc for the developing baby. The best bet to ensure adequate zinc for the baby is to incorporate zinc rich foods in the pregnancy diet such as red meat, shellfish, seeds, and nuts *and* take a good quality prenatal vitamin.

*Supplementation*
Interestingly, even though we know the negative effects of *dietary* zinc deficiency during pregnancy, the data on benefits of zinc *supplementation* during pregnancy are mixed. This may indicate that getting zinc from food sources is better than getting it from a supplement, but that supplements for mothers at risk for low zinc can have benefits. In the zinc studies done exclusively on zinc deficient mothers, a positive effect of taking a zinc supplement on babies birthweight was shown.[35]

Low to moderate dose supplementation (10–15 mg) in a prenatal vitamin is safe. The safe upper limit of total zinc intake (food plus supplements) for pregnant women is estimated at a maximum of 40 mg per day.[34] (Vegetarian and vegan mothers need to take special precautions to ensure adequate zinc intake and may want to err on the side of a higher amount of zinc in their prenatal vitamin.)

Also note that zinc oxide is not as well absorbed as other forms of zinc and is not the optimal supplemental form.[42] Zinc forms such as citrate, aspartate, gluconate, or other **chelated** forms are better absorbed. It is also worth noting that taking a prenatal vitamin containing zinc at the same time as an iron supplement may not be a good idea, as absorption of the zinc may be blocked by a high dose iron supplement.[34] It is best to take the prenatal vitamin and the iron supplement at different times to improve zinc absorption.

*Bottom line on zinc*
Zinc is very important for the baby's growth and immune system and many mothers are not getting enough in their diet. Make an effort to incorporate zinc rich foods into the pregnancy diet. Plant sources of zinc are partially blocked by natural compounds in the plants making them less absorbable. A good prenatal supplement should have a safe amount of zinc (10–15mg), but be aware that zinc oxide is not as well absorbed as other forms.

## Iodine
Iodine is a key component of thyroid hormones and essential for the baby's neurological development. Iodine requirements are significantly increased during pregnancy and breastfeeding, up to 50% higher than baseline. It is now thought that even mild iodine deficiency during pregnancy may result in IQ loss for the baby. Starting in the 1920s by the Swiss to prevent cretinism (severe retardation caused by iodine deficiency), table salt often has iodine added to it, labeled as iodized salt. However much of the salt added to processed foods is not iodized and there is renewed worry about milder forms of iodine deficiency in pregnant moms in the United States. Other than seaweed, plant foods are poor sources of iodine.

*Recommended daily amount*
The WHO recommends an intake of **250 micrograms (mcg) per day of iodine** and the **RDA is set at 220 mcg per day for pregnant women**. The

Endocrine Society recommends a prenatal supplement containing 150 to 200 mcg daily to prevent thyroid issues and promote optimal brain development. It may also be advisable to use iodized salt during pregnancy and lactation, but don't be excessive about salt usage at these times. A little goes a long way, and too much iodine (intakes over 500–1000 mcg/day) could have negative effects.

*Food sources*
Iodine rich foods include:

+ seaweed (highly variable in the content from 16 up to 3000 mcg/1 gram serving)
+ seafood such as oysters (30 mcg/oz) and cod (100–150 mcg/3 oz serving)
+ yogurt (116 mcg/cup)
+ milk (38–159 mcg/8 oz)
+ eggs (25 mcg per egg)
+ iodized salt (77 mcg per 1 gram salt)

*Supplementation*
Most good quality prenatal vitamins will have an adequate but not excessive amount of iodine in them, and I recommend all pregnant women take a good quality prenatal vitamin with the recommended level of iodine immediately before becoming pregnant, during pregnancy, and while breastfeeding.

*Bottom line on iodine*
Iodine is needed in increased amounts during pregnancy and is important for thyroid function and brain development. Make sure you are getting some good dietary sources but take a prenatal that has a safe but adequate amount (around 150 mcg) of iodine to prevent deficiency.

## Calcium
Calcium, as we all know, is important for bones. Building a baby skeleton takes a significant amount of calcium over the course of a pregnancy.

However, there are multiple other roles of calcium in maternal and fetal health. Low calcium intakes by pregnant mothers are associated with increased risk of **preeclampsia, pregnancy induced hypertension,** and **preterm delivery**.[43] Low intake is typically defined as less than 500 mg of calcium daily and is relatively common among pregnant women worldwide. The metabolism of calcium in a pregnant mother is very complex, and precise intake recommendations have been debated.

*Detecting deficiency*
There are no good laboratory methods for checking a mother's calcium status, which also makes it difficult to tell who may need more calcium. A mother's body adapts during pregnancy, increasing her intestinal absorption of calcium and releasing more calcium from her bones for the benefit of the baby. Surprisingly, despite the increased bone turnover during pregnancy, having multiple children does not appear to increase a woman's risk for osteoporosis as long as the mother is physically active and has good overall nutrition (including adequate intake of vitamins D and K, magnesium and calcium).

*Recommended daily amount*
Calcium requirements for pregnant mothers over 18 years of age are listed at 1,000 mg per day by the US and most European countries, while the WHO lists 1200 mg daily as their international recommendation.[44] Teen mothers need 1300 mg per day, which almost surely requires a calcium supplement to achieve.

## TABLE 6.3 CALCIUM FOOD SOURCES

| Calcium Source (serving size) | mg |
|---|---|
| Yogurt (8oz) | 415 |
| Cheddar cheese (1.5 oz) | 300 |
| Milk (8oz) | 300 |
| Fortified almond/soy milk (8oz) | 300 |
| Tofu (½ cup) | 430 |
| Canned salmon (3oz) | 180 |
| Sardines (3oz) | 325 |
| Fortified orange juice (1 cup) | 350 |
| Turnip greens (½ cup) | 100 |
| Collard greens (½ cup) | 180 |
| Bok choy (½ cup) | 80 |
| Kale (½ cup) | 90 |
| Broccoli (½ cup) | 30 |
| Orange (1) | 55 |

Data from National Institutes of Health (www.NIH.gov), USDA Nutrient Database (https://fdc.nal.usda.gov/), Health Link British Columbia, (www.healthlinkBC.ca), Linus Pauling Institute (https://lpi.oregonstate.edu/mic/minerals/iron)[203-206]

*Supplementation*

For mothers achieving around 1000 mg of calcium from their daily diet, likely no calcium supplementation is needed. In women with low dietary calcium intake, especially those at higher risk for developing hypertension, calcium supplements are recommended during the latter half of pregnancy to try and prevent the development of preeclampsia and high blood pressure. The WHO recommends 1500 to 2000 mg of calcium daily in divided doses, while a recent Cochrane review listed potential benefits of supplementation of 1,000 mg (or higher) in women with low calcium intake, and even potential benefits from lower dose supplementation (500–600 mg).[45,46] Some researchers feel all pregnant women should be advised to take 1,000 mg calcium supplementation daily as a cost-effective preventive measure[47] but this is not universally accepted, as there are women with adequate dietary calcium who may not see a benefit. The amount of calcium found in most prenatal vitamins is typically small and will not contribute much to total daily requirements. *Ultimately the decision about whether to take a calcium supplement should be a conversation with the OB, midwife, or primary care provider based on the mother's current diet and risk factors.*

*A word of caution: Calcium in higher doses and high intake of cow's milk have the potential to impair iron absorption in a pregnant woman.[48-51] Be aware of the timing of calcium supplements and milk ingestion, especially if a mother is anemic or iron deficient requiring iron supplementation. I also have concerns that high dose calcium could impair magnesium status and cause an imbalance unless care is taken to ensure adequate magnesium intake (see section on magnesium). Taking steps to improve calcium intake could put a pregnant woman at higher risk for iron deficiency if not done correctly. As we have shown, iron deficiency is very common during pregnancy and can have negative lifelong effects on the child. Try to avoid taking a calcium supplement or drinking cow's milk at the same time as a prenatal vitamin or iron supplement in an effort to maximize the iron absorbed. Calcium citrate can be taken between meals as opposed to calcium carbonate, so it may be a better choice to optimize both calcium and iron status during pregnancy. Women on acid blocking medication for GERD should also opt for calcium citrate, as the carbonate form of calcium needs stomach acid to absorb it. Avoid the high doses (over 1,500 mg) unless specifically advised by a provider.

*Bottom line on calcium*

Calcium is important for building the baby skeleton, but also for preventing high blood pressure and premature birth. Incorporate calcium rich foods into the pregnancy diet but consider supplements if intake falls short of 1,000 mg daily. High calcium intake can block iron, so take these supplements at different times.

## Magnesium

Magnesium is another vital mineral during pregnancy that does not get enough attention. It is involved in well over 600 reactions in the body, including a number of processes that are absolutely crucial during pregnancy:[52-54]

+ Supports cardiovascular health
+ Prevents high blood pressure
+ Prevents preeclampsia
+ Supports proper placenta functioning
+ Helps prevent premature uterine contractions that can lead to preterm birth
+ Plays a role in bone formation and health
+ Is involved in energy production in our cells
+ Maintains insulin sensitivity to prevent type 2 diabetes and gestational diabetes[54-57]

In addition, magnesium has neuroprotective effects, and the WHO strongly recommends the use of magnesium sulfate in mothers imminently delivering a premature baby to protect the brains of premature infants. Magnesium may also act as an epigenetic modifier and getting adequate magnesium while pregnant may help prevent future development of cardiovascular disease and type 2 diabetes in children.[56,58]

*Recommended daily amount*

**The RDA for magnesium during pregnancy is 350 to 400 mg per day.** Unfortunately, most women of childbearing years are not getting adequate magnesium in their diet because of our overreliance on processed foods. This likely has negative consequences, including increased risk for poor fetal growth, gestational diabetes, preterm birth, and preeclampsia. *Consuming magnesium-rich whole foods such as leafy greens, whole grains, and nuts should therefore be a high priority for mothers.*

*Detecting deficiency*

Knowing which mothers are truly low in magnesium could help target those most likely to benefit from supplementation, but testing is uncommon. Blood tests looking at *serum magnesium* levels are notoriously inaccurate for detecting magnesium deficiency, but *red blood cell magnesium* levels are likely a better screening method for deficiency although mostly used in research studies.

### TABLE 6. 4 MAGNESIUM FOOD SOURCES

| Food Source (serving size) | mg |
|---|---|
| Cashews (1 oz) | 83 |
| Brown rice (1 cup) | 86 |
| Quinoa (1 cup) | 118 |
| Oats/oatmeal (1 cup) | 57 |
| Almonds (1oz) | 80 |
| Peanuts (1oz) | 48 |
| Pumpkin seeds (1oz) | 156 |
| Spinach/chard/greens (½ cup) | 78 |
| Black beans (½ cup) | 60 |
| Pinto/refried beans (½ cup) | 43 |
| Lentils (½ cup) | 36 |
| Cod/salmon (3 oz) | 25–30 |
| Mackerel (3 oz) | 82 |
| Baked potato w/ skin (1 med) | 48 |
| Peanut butter (2 tbsp) | 50 |
| Raisins (1 cup) | 46 |
| Yogurt (1 cup) | 43 |
| Banana (1) | 32 |
| Avocado (1) | 58 |
| Lima beans (½ cup) | 63 |

Data from National Institutes of Health (www.NIH.gov), USDA Nutrient Database (https://fdc.nal.usda.gov/), Health Link British Columbia, (www.healthlinkBC.ca), Linus Pauling Institute (https://lpi.oregonstate.edu/mic/minerals/iron)[203-206]

*Supplementation*

While magnesium supplementation is currently recommended only for mothers with severe preeclampsia to prevent seizures (**eclampsia**), more research is needed on lower-dose magnesium supplementation for preventing high blood pressure, preterm birth, and gestational diabetes. However, there is much promise; magnesium supplements have been shown in recent research to improve glucose control and insulin sensitivity in pre-diabetic patients and pregnant mothers with gestational diabetes, as well as lowering blood pressure in pregnant mothers in the third trimester while also potentially helping prevent leg cramps.[55-57,59-66]

Given these health benefits from magnesium, some researchers feel that a low dose supplement of 100 to 200 mg daily could be warranted for pregnant women with questionable dietary intake of magnesium. Magnesium oxide and sulfate are not well absorbed orally; opt for the citrate, lactate, chloride, and **chelated** forms like glycinate.

*Bottom line on magnesium*
Magnesium is important for a litany of functions in the human body and deficiency is very common. Adequate intake may help prevent high blood pressure and gestational diabetes. Make an effort to incorporate plenty of magnesium rich foods into the pregnancy diet. If dietary intake is questionable, a supplement of 100 to 200 mg of magnesium citrate or chelated form could be considered.


# CRUCIAL MICRONUTRIENTS: VITAMINS

## Choline
Choline is a B vitamin that is crucial for brain and nervous system development. It is a key component of the outer packaging of our cells (cell membranes) as well as brain signaling molecules like **acetylcholine**, known as **neurotransmitters**. Choline is involved in the growth and development of the brain and spine and may be as equally important for preventing **spina bifida**, a birth defect of the spine, as folic acid. In one study, women in the lowest percentiles for choline intake had four times the risk of having a child with spina bifida as women who had a high choline intake.[67]

Choline, folate, $B_6$, and $B_{12}$ are all part of an important group of interrelated nutrients known as **methyl donors**, which are involved with certain detoxification processes as well as the process of epigenetic modification and regulation of gene expression. Deficiency of any of these nutrients during pregnancy or lactation could make the infant more susceptible to toxic exposures, and ultimately affect expression of certain genes in the crucial first thousand days. However, with any of the methyl donor nutrients, more is not always better, as there are concerns of *over-methylation;*

high doses may suppress important genes. There is likely a sweet spot for intake of nutrients like choline, B12, and folate that may differ based on individual genetics and environment. However, research shows that most people, especially pregnant mothers, may not be getting enough choline in their diet.

*Recommended daily amount*

The demand for choline is high during pregnancy and lactation, and maternal stores can easily be depleted if dietary intake is not sufficient. There may be a synergistic effect between choline and the vital **omega-3** fatty acid **DHA**, improving absorption and accumulation in the baby brain. Like omega-3 DHA, the placenta is known to pump choline and concentrate it in the amniotic fluid and blood supply to the baby, which demonstrates its importance to the growth and development of that infant. Adequate dietary intake levels for choline were set by the Institute of Medicine as **450 mg per day for pregnant women**, and 550 mg per day for lactating women, with a recommended upper limit of 3.5 grams per day (3500 mg).[68,69]

Several studies in pregnant women have shown low dietary intake of choline in at least one out of four women (at levels 25% to 50% below the recommended intake). According to Dr. Marie Caudill, an expert in choline metabolism from Cornell University, *less than 10% of pregnant mothers in the US are meeting the recommended intake for choline and could be putting their child at increased risk for adverse outcomes.* The average intake of choline for a pregnant woman in the US is reported as 220 to 300 mg daily, which could be putting a significant number of infants at risk for neurological and developmental disorders as well as birth defects such as cleft lip, spina bifida, and heart defects.

Recent evidence shows that increasing maternal intake of choline above 500 mg per day and closer to 1000 mg may have lasting cognitive benefits to the baby that are still detectable up to age 7 with improved childhood attention and memory.[75-77] Not all studies have shown a benefit with increased choline, but the majority of studies seem to show a positive effect.

*Food sources*

Choline from foods is found in the highest amounts in liver, meat, seafood, and eggs and is typically low in vegetarian/vegan diets. It is also high in human breast milk but less so in some formulas. Amounts in breast milk can vary based on the intake of the mother, so choline intake for breastfeeding mothers is also crucial.[20, 69-74]

### TABLE 6.5 CHOLINE CONTENT OF FOODS
### (PER 3 OZ PORTION UNLESS OTHERWISE SPECIFIED)

| Food | Total Choline (mg) |
|------|---------------------|
| Liver (beef) | 350–430 |
| Egg (1) | 150–225 |
| Steak | 104–117 |
| Ground beef | 72 |
| Salmon | 90 |
| Cod | 71 |
| Pork | 78 |
| Chicken breast | 62–72 |
| Baked potato (1 large with skin) | 20–57 |
| Almonds (1 oz) | 15 |
| Quinoa (1 cup) | 43 |
| Yogurt (1 cup) | 38 |
| Broccoli (½ cup) | 31 |
| Brussels sprouts (½ cup) | 32 |
| Cauliflower (½ cup) | 24 |
| Peas (½ cup) | 24 |
| Baked beans (½ cup) | 31 |
| Black beans (½ cup) | 28 |
| Tofu (3oz) | 30–90 |
| Milk (1 cup) | 40 |
| Peanut butter (2 tbsp) | 20 |

Data from National Institutes of Health (www.NIH.gov), USDA Nutrient Database (https://fdc.nal.usda.gov/), Health Link British Columbia, (www.healthlinkBC.ca), Linus Pauling Institute (https://lpi.oregonstate.edu/mic/minerals/iron)[203-206]

*Supplementation*

Don't rely on most prenatal vitamins to deliver adequate choline. It is hard to get adequate choline in a prenatal vitamin as it can make that prenatal vitamin roughly the size of a golf ball. Based on the recent research, if a mother is not regularly eating the foods with the highest choline content, (especially for vegetarian moms), I would recommend considering a supplement to make sure they are getting the 500 to 1000 mg of total dietary choline per day for that growing baby brain.

> *"There is evidence to support choline supplementation in all pregnant mothers in the range of 300 to 600 mg daily to support placental health and proper brain development of the infant."*
>
> – Dr. Marie Caudill, Division of Nutritional Sciences, Cornell University

I recommend pregnant mothers discuss with their healthcare provider adding a supplement like choline bitartrate or choline chloride as these forms in the recommended dosages are safe, inexpensive, and readily absorbed and available to the body.

In a 2018 study out of Cornell University, Dr. Caudill and her co-investigators gave pregnant women in the third trimester a choline supplement to get their choline intake to 930 mg per day and followed the cognitive development of the children. They found faster brain processing speed in the high choline group as compared to the average choline groups, but also found that even getting 480 mg per day showed benefit above the average intake of 300 mg per day. A seven-year follow up study looked at these same infants as schoolchildren and found a lasting benefit on memory and brain functioning in the high choline group.[77]

*Bottom line on choline*
Choline is underrecognized as an extremely important nutrient for infant brain development and well as detoxification. Many if not most mothers are low in choline. Make every effort to incorporate choline rich foods into the pregnancy diet. FYI: 1 egg (yolk) contains 150 to 200 mg of choline, so three eggs a day will pretty much get you most of the way to meeting the basic requirements! Leading researchers are suggesting that all pregnant mothers consider a choline supplement at a safe level to prevent deficiency and to optimize infant brain development.

## Liver in the pregnancy diet

Although not high on many people's "comfort food list," liver can be a nutritional powerhouse food that contains many important nutrients like all the B vitamins, iron, zinc, folate, choline, Vitamin A and D. Ounce per ounce, it is the most concentrated of any foods for many vital pregnancy nutrients. When a lion or large predator takes down an animal, what do you think is the first thing that animal eats? The liver. There are several cautions with eating liver during pregnancy however, as some animal liver is super-concentrated in vitamin A at doses that could be toxic to the developing baby if over-consumed.

If you are part of the Paleo/Ancestral health movement, then liver is likely something you have delved into. If you hunt, or have access to sustainably raised animals, you could consider having liver as part of your diet but do so with a bit of caution if you are pregnant. Watch portion sizes to make sure they are not excessive and check the vitamin A content. A little bit of liver goes a long way nutritionally. Also consider that commercially raised animals could have an increased toxic burden in their livers. Conventionally raised animals exposed to high amounts of antibiotics, pesticides, and hormones likely have far too many **toxicants** in their liver and could put the baby at risk.

## Folate

Folate is a B vitamin found in plant foods and liver that was originally discovered for its roles in promoting growth and preventing *macrocytic anemia* during pregnancy. In **microcytic (iron deficiency) anemia,** there are not enough red blood cells being made. It is characterized by cells that are smaller than normal. In contrast, macrocytic anemia results from $B_{12}$ or folate deficiency and also impairs red blood cell production. Cells in this case are larger than normal. The damaging effects of both anemias can be similar on the growing baby. However, the link between dietary folate deficiency and the birth defect of the spinal cord known as spina bifida was discovered in the 1960s and led to the fortification of processed grains with folic acid (the synthetic form of folate) in an attempt to decrease the occurrence of this disorder.

Folate is needed for the manufacture of the baby's genetic material (DNA) as well as being important for brain and nerve development. Folate, along with its business partners vitamin $B_6$, $B_{12}$, and choline, are classified as "methyl donors," supplying the body with important compounds called methyl groups that are vital for growth at the level of DNA as well as detoxification of certain metabolic **toxins.** Low levels of these key methyl donor nutrients can lead to a buildup in the body of a toxic metabolite called **homocysteine**. Increased levels of homocysteine in pregnant mothers have been implicated in complications like preeclampsia and preterm birth as well as birth defects like spina bifida.[212] As epigenetic modifiers, low intake of folate, $B_6$, $B_{12}$, and choline can potentially alter the baby's gene expression in unfavorable ways.[83]

Folate is vital at every life stage, from early development in the womb through birth and all the way through adulthood, and low folate intake in adults is linked to cancer and cardiovascular disease as well as depression.

*Recommended daily amount*

The current **RDA for folate during pregnancy is 600 mcg/day.** In the early 1990s the CDC began recommending folic acid (the synthetic form of folate) supplementation for pregnant mothers in prenatal vitamins at the level of 400 mcg but recommended higher doses (4,000 mcg daily) if there was a prior birth with spina bifida. ACOG (American College of Gynecology) currently recommends 400 mcg per day of supplemental folic acid for pregnant women. The US Preventive Services Task Force recommends that any woman even *thinking* about getting pregnant should be taking 400 to 800 mcg of folic acid daily as a supplement. Supplemental folic acid in early pregnancy has been effective in reducing the incidence of spina bifida in babies. Studies have shown reduced risk for having a child with autism with folate supplementation of at least 400 mcg *before* pregnancy and with higher intake of folate (600 mcg) during the first month of pregnancy.[84] However, more is not always better, and recent concerns have been raised over excessive folic acid supplementation during pregnancy. The US Institute of Medicine recommends no more than 1,000 mcg (1 mg) daily unless specifically advised by a healthcare provider.

*Food sources*

First and foremost, pregnant mothers will benefit from incorporating ample leafy green vegetables and other folate-rich foods into their diet to ensure good baseline folate intake. Dietary folate is naturally found in leafy greens (think foliage), beans/lentils, avocado, and liver, and was commonly low in the diet of pregnant women prior to the era of food fortification and nutritional supplementation with the synthetic form of folate known as folic acid. It is strongly recommended that pregnant women consume a diet rich in naturally occurring folate from high folate foods, as the fortified foods are more of a backup plan for those mothers not consuming enough of these natural folate foods.

## TABLE 6.6 FOLATE FOOD SOURCES

| Source | Qty | Folate (mcg) |
|---|---|---|
| Lentils | ½ cup | 179 |
| Chickpeas | ½ cup | 141 |
| Spinach, cooked | ½ cup | 130 |
| Brussels sprouts | ½ cup | 78 |
| Broccoli | ½ cup | 52 |
| Green peas | ½ cup | 47 |

| Source | Qty | Folate (mcg) |
|---|---|---|
| Beef liver | 3 oz | 215 |
| Enriched spaghetti | 1 cup | 167 |
| Enriched rice | 1 cup | 153 |
| Fortified cereals | 1 cup | 100 |
| Avocado | 1 whole | 122 |
| Orange | 1 whole | 29 |

Data from National Institutes of Health (www.NIH.gov), USDA Nutrient Database (https://fdc.nal.usda.gov/), Health Link British Columbia, (www.healthlinkBC.ca), Linus Pauling Institute (https://lpi.oregonstate.edu/mic/minerals/iron)[203-206]

Folate is the food form of this vitamin. Folic acid is the synthesized version of folate, made in the lab and is the form usually found in prenatal vitamins and fortified foods, but this may not be the optimal form of this nutrient for some people. The active form of folate in the body is not folic acid, it is actually *L-methylfolate* also referred to as *5-methylTHF*. The body needs to convert supplemental folic acid or dietary folate to 5-methylTHF for it to be able to perform its roles in reducing homocysteine, manufacturing neurotransmitters, and repairing and epigenetically modifying DNA. The enzyme that makes the active form of folate is called **MTHFR (methylenetetrahydrofolate reductase)**, and it has recently been discovered that many people carry forms (variants or mutations) of this gene that makes the MTHFR enzyme not as efficient or effective, potentially putting them at risk for a host of disorders related to the decreased ability to use dietary folate, or synthetic folic acid. The two most studied of these MTHFR genes that affect folate metabolism, often reported on popular genetic/ancestry screening tests are called C677T and A1298C.

In fact, it is thought that *up to 60%* of the population have one of these genes and are not *fully* effective at converting folate to its active form. A surprising number of people may have two copies of these genes leaving their ability to use folic acid *significantly impaired*, and putting them at increased risk for conditions like heart disease, cancer, poor pregnancy outcomes, depression, ADHD, autism, and blood clots.[78] According to the research and data published by the National Institute of Health (NIH), 10-15% of Caucasians, up to 20% of Italians, and *25% of Hispanics* have the severe form of the MTHFR mutation referred to as being C677T *homozygous* (two copies of the mutation). These genes are relatively uncommon in Africans and African Americans (1%–2%), but somewhat higher in Asians (8%–20%).[85-88]

This means there are many mothers with these genes whose bodies are not able to efficiently use the folic acid commonly found in standard prenatal vitamins or fortified into foods. These mothers may require a higher amount of dietary or supplemental folate to keep their levels adequate for a healthy growing baby. Millions of mothers and millions of babies are therefore potentially at risk of the consequences of low folate and high homocysteine levels in the body including preeclampsia, premature birth, spina bifida and heart defects. Mothers carrying the 677T (homozygous) form of MTHFR have double the risk of having a child with spina bifida, which may increase to seven-fold if the unborn child is also homozygous.[209,210]

## HOT TOPIC

One way to bypass the dysfunctional MTHFR enzyme is to supplement with a moderate dose of L-methylfolate (the biologically active form of folate) instead of folic acid. L-methylfolate has shown to be at least as effective at boosting mother and baby's levels of folate and in reducing levels of homocysteine in the general population and may more effective in those carrying the MTHFR mutations. The other advantage with L-methylfolate is that it does not result in increased levels of unmetabolized folic acid in the body, as do folic acid supplements above 400 mcg per day.[207,208] While still under investigation, there are health concerns with high levels of *unmetabolized synthetic folic acid* from *high-dose* folic acid supplementation in the bodies of pregnant mothers and their offspring, including masking of $B_{12}$ deficiency, impairments of the immune system, increased risk of fetal loss, and negative effects on children's metabolism in later life.[78,89,208,213,214] L-methylfolate or naturally occurring folate do not carry any of these same concerns.

Several higher quality prenatal vitamins are now incorporating L-methylfolate for this very reason to more effectively boost levels of biologically active folate in the mother and unborn child. To be clear, supplemental folic acid at 400 mcg is still the standard and is absolutely useful for the prevention of birth defects in mothers with and without MTHFR mutations.

The CDC currently does not support the use of L-methylfolate during pregnancy as it has not specifically been tested for the prevention of spina bifida. While this is true, the fact remains that it is the biologically active form of folate used in the human body, whereas folic acid is not. It is worth mentioning that the FDA approved use of L-methylfolate in several oral contraceptives, which now also contain L-methylfolate to reduce the incidence of birth defects including spina bifida. There is a confusing disconnect here, as evidently the FDA feels the evidence is strong enough to approve the use of L-methylfolate for prevention of birth defects. This is a hot topic and worthy of further investigation.

*Supplementation*
Folate supplementation during pregnancy helps prevent spina bifida and heart defects in the baby, and may help prevent preterm birth, perhaps even autism.[78-82] All pregnant and breastfeeding moms should continue to take a good quality prenatal vitamin with some form of folate (L-methylfolate or folic acid) in the standard dosing of 400 mcg, as well as a safe adequate dose of $B_{12}$ and dietary or supplemental choline to maximize effectiveness in the body. I fully support current guidelines that suggest that *any woman of childbearing years, even teenagers* take a multivitamin containing 400 mcg folate/folic acid or a 400-mcg folic acid tablet daily (as well as eating lots of vegetables) prior to pregnancy to improve outcomes for our future children. I feel that at-risk mothers (see hot topic discussion) should discuss taking a prenatal with the L-methylfolate form of folate at a safe dose (400–800 mcg), for a little extra insurance that mom and baby are getting the most benefit from this essential nutrient. Hispanic mothers, mothers carrying the C677T/A1298C mutations, or those who have a family history of spina bifida, cleft lip or palate, or early onset heart disease or stroke, could potentially benefit from L-methylfolate, but this remains controversial. Prescription prenatal vitamins may contain high dose folic acid (1000 mcg or more) but I would not recommend high dose folic acid *unless specifically advised* by the obstetrician, midwife or PCP.

*Bottom line on folate*
Adequate folate is needed during pregnancy to prevent anemia and birth defects like spina bifida. Eat plenty of vegetables and incorporate some legumes or liver while pregnant to ensure good dietary intake. Adequate choline and $B_{12}$ intake is crucial to maximize benefit from folate. Many mothers carry a genetic variant of the MTHFR gene that makes it harder for their body to use folate or the synthetic form folic acid, increasing the risk for birth defects and pregnancy complications. These mothers especially need to focus on dietary sources of folate, $B_{12}$, and choline and may consider a prenatal containing the active form of folate called L-methylfolate.

## Vitamin A
True deficiency of vitamin A still occurs in the developing world but is rare in the developed world because the body gets Vitamin A in two ways. One way is through preformed Vitamin A (retinol/retinoic acid) found in animal foods (meats, fish, liver) and also found in vitamin supplements

and cod liver oil. The body also makes vitamin A from beta-carotene, which is actually two molecules of vitamin A stuck together. B-carotene and its cousins the carotenoids are **antioxidant** compounds found in a variety of brightly colored fruits and vegetables, the most common of which are the orange vegetables like carrots, squash, and sweet potato, but also the green leafy vegetables. Pre-formed vitamin A (retinol/retinoic acid) is one of the fat-soluble vitamins, meaning it is absorbed with dietary fat, and is stored in our fat cells.

> FYI: Cooking vegetables with some healthy fat like olive oil dramatically increases the absorption of carotenoids and makes them more available to the body.

Vitamin A is crucial for vision, skin maintenance, respiratory and gastrointestinal tract health (mucosal integrity), and the immune system. Deficiencies of vitamin A increase susceptibility to infections in the infant and child. Vitamin A is also known to be a potent signaling molecule in our cells and plays a role in brain development. It helps the body regulate DNA expression, including those genes involved with the growing brain. Research in this area is somewhat lacking, but there is no doubt of the importance of vitamin A in proper growth and development.

*Recommended daily amount*
The **RDA for Vitamin A intake for pregnant women is 750 mcg/day or 2,500 IU**. A good prenatal vitamin will supply a moderate, safe amount of beta-carotene, and certainly no more than 1,000 to 2000 IU of pre-formed vitamin A to ensure adequate but not excessive amounts for the baby.[90] More is not better! *Vitamin A can be toxic to the developing baby in higher doses* (above 10,000 international units (IU) per day), so this is another nutrient where *adequate but not excessive* intake is key. In the developed world, there is no evidence to support isolated vitamin A supplementation. The WHO advises against giving preformed vitamin A during pregnancy because of the potential damage to the baby with excessive doses.

*Food sources*
Mothers are encouraged to eat lots of colorful vegetables containing beta-carotene so their bodies can make plenty of vitamin A for their babies. Recall the caution for mothers eating liver during pregnancy, as some animals will have very high vitamin A content in the liver which could have toxic potential to the baby. If using liver during pregnancy to boost nutrient intake, my advice is to look up the vitamin A content on

the USDA nutrient database website to ensure levels are not exceeding 10,000 IU per day.

*Bottom line on vitamin A*

Emphasizing a pregnancy diet with lots of vegetables will ensure that a mother gets plenty of beta-carotene which is then converted to vitamin A in the body. Excessive vitamin A (over 10,000 IU) daily during pregnancy could damage the baby, so more is not better. Prenatal vitamins should not have more than 1,000 to 2000 IU of preformed vitamin A for this reason.

## Vitamin D

Vitamin D status in pregnancy is becoming an increasingly hot topic. Unlike other vitamins where deficiencies can be more subtle or *subclinical*, frank (overt) vitamin D deficiency is relatively common in the general population and *a large proportion of expectant mothers are found deficient or insufficient in vitamin D—up to 70% of mothers in the US!*

Vitamin D is a fat-soluble vitamin that is unique in that it is made from cholesterol by the human body when exposed to adequate sunlight. Historically, this has been the main source of vitamin D in our bodies, as opposed to dietary sources. Those of us living in northern climates who don't see the sun for four to six months out of the year are prone to deficiency, and I see a large number of young children with low levels of vitamin D, so it is likely their mothers are low as well. People of color with darker skin pigment are further prone to deficiency, as they do not make as much Vitamin D when exposed to sunlight.

Food sources are limited but include salmon and herring, cod liver oil, and to a lesser degree pork, eggs, butter, and cheese. Therefore, many mothers, but especially vegetarian or vegan mothers in northern climates who are not getting dietary sources or adequate sun exposure, are at increased risk for deficiency. Since the 1930s, Vitamin D has been sup-plemented in milk. At that time, the main concern was bone formation because Vitamin D deficiency in infants and young children was known to cause rickets, a condition of weakened bones leading to a bowing of the legs. Since then, additional research has shown that vitamin D has major importance for every cell in our bodies.

Recent research is looking at Vitamin D's role in infant neurodevelopment as well as immune function and inflammation. Like vitamin A, vita-min D is a cellular signaling molecule and a powerful epigenetic modifier, turning genes on and off, and has influence on immune system function and regulation.[91,92]

Poor maternal vitamin D status has been shown in some studies to be related to low birth weight, preeclampsia, gestational diabetes, increased risk of C-section birth, increased risk of autism and psychiatric disorders in the child, as well as delays in cognitive and language development. Low vitamin D status in the baby is also associated with childhood asthma, respiratory syncytial virus (RSV) and other respiratory infections in the infant. Maternal supplementation with vitamin D potentially reduces the risk of preeclampsia, gestational diabetes, preterm birth, and having a low-birth-weight infant, but more research is needed.[93-98]

*Recommended daily amount*
The Institute of Medicine set the RDA at 600 IU vitamin D daily for pregnant women. However, as discussed below, the actual requirements for vitamin D are going to vary depending on a mother's genetics, ethnicity, and sunlight exposure.

*Detecting deficiency and supplementation*
Currently, despite reports of high rates of deficiency, screening tests for vitamin D deficiency during pregnancy are somewhat controversial. On one hand, major OB/GYN groups such as the American College of Obstetricians and Gynecologists (ACOG) and UK based Royal College of Obstetricians and Gynecologists (RCOG) do not recommend general screening of pregnant women for vitamin D deficiency (through testing blood levels of 25-OH Vitamin D), but rather endorse universal vitamin D supplementation at the level (400 IU) that is found in most prenatal vitamins. In the UK, women deemed at high risk for deficiency (obese, dark skinned, or low sunlight exposure) are recommended by the RCOG to take 1000 IU daily as opposed to having levels checked.

## HOT TOPIC

In the US, ACOG does not make a strong recommendation to screen for Vitamin D deficiency, but rather lists it as a consideration.[99] However, when scrutinized, their official statement would suggest that perhaps *all pregnant women living in northern climates, with darker skin, or with limited sun exposure (women who work indoors) should be screened for deficiency*. Vegetarian and vegan women should also be screened. This practice does not seem to be the case currently, and a great many at-risk pregnant women are not being tested. Whether or not this leaves a large number of mothers with vitamin D deficiency or insufficiency is unknown. If a woman's blood level of vitamin D is 20 ng/mL (50 nmol/liter) or less, ACOG recommends vitamin D supplementation in a dosage of 1,000 to 2,000 IU daily.

On the opposite side, the Endocrine Society's expert committee on vitamin D recommends *universal screening* during pregnancy and that **blood levels of vitamin D in a pregnant woman be above 30 ng/ml.** They recognize pregnant women are at high risk for vitamin D deficiency and 600 IU of vitamin D per day for a pregnant woman may not be enough because of the large variability between women for the amount of vitamin D required to get blood levels into the normal range.[98] Some scientists believe vitamin D levels should be above 40 ng/ml, as it was felt to be historically, in people with adequate sun exposure before we stopped working and spending lots of time outdoors.

## TABLE 6.7 VITAMIN D STATUS

| Vitamin D Levels | 25-OH Vitamin D Blood Level (ng/ml) |
| --- | ---: |
| Deficiency | Less than 20 |
| Insufficiency | 21-30 |
| Normal | >30 |
| Optimal | 40-70 |
| Potentially toxic | >100 |

There is a lot of fear about sun exposure and skin cancer, but the reality is that most pregnant mothers should probably be taking sun breaks with a considerable portion of their skin exposed for brief periods (30 min in off-peak times of day) without sunscreen to maximize their body production of Vitamin D. The WHO advises that sunlight is the most important source of vitamin D for a pregnant mother, but the amount of time in the sun needed is variable depending on skin color and latitude.

Is the 400 IU of vitamin D in the standard prenatal vitamin enough? Top researchers in this field have doubts about the adequacy of standard Vitamin D dosing during pregnancy.[98] Without routine testing there is no metric to tell us if Vitamin D levels in most pregnant women are optimal. My inclination is that perhaps all pregnant women should be screened, but even if we followed more conservative ACOG recommendations, we should be screening *at least half the population*: those living in the northern hemisphere, as well as all *non-white mothers*. When we also factor in the women who work and spend most of their time indoors, we include pretty much the entire population. Widespread screening is not happening currently.

If a pregnant mother feels she could be at risk for deficiency for any of these reasons, she should consider asking her OB or midwife to have levels screened with a blood level of 25-OH Vitamin D. If levels are significantly less than 30 ng/ml, it should be discussed with the provider whether to start additional supplementation with vitamin $D_3$ (I prefer vitamin $D_3$/cholecalciferol over vitamin $D_2$/ergocalciferol, as $D_3$ is better utilized by the body). The dose can be adjusted to get blood levels above 30 ng/ml, but not higher than 70 ng/ml. Vitamin D supplementation is viewed by both major obstetric groups (ACOG/RCOG) as safe in the recommended doses (generally up to 2000 IU daily), and that high doses can be safe in deficient mothers if monitored.

*Bottom line on vitamin D*
The majority of mothers are likely low in vitamin D, potentially impacting the baby's brain and immune system. Adequate but not excessive sunlight exposure is the best way to get vitamin D. At risk mothers should be screened for vitamin D deficiency and supplementation started and monitored by their healthcare provider if they are deficient. All pregnant women are recommended to take 400 to 600 IU vitamin D in their prenatal vitamin.

## Vitamin $B_{12}$
Vitamin $B_{12}$ is a nutrient found in several forms: cyanocobalamin (the synthetic form) or the naturally occurring co-enzyme forms adenosylcobalamin and methylcobalamin. $B_{12}$ is an important member of the group of methylation vitamins ($B_6$, $B_{12}$, choline, and folate). $B_{12}$ is important for the growing baby and is needed for nerve growth and myelination (brain insulation), for DNA and red blood cell formation, and for certain detoxification reactions.

Low maternal vitamin $B_{12}$ levels are associated with preterm birth, spina bifida, and developmental issues.[100-102] The effect of milder deficiency on infants has not been well studied, but several trials of supplementation in mildly deficient pregnant mothers improved developmental outcomes in their children.[103]

*Recommended daily amount*
The Recommended Daily Allowance (RDA) for pregnant women is **2.6 mcg/day**. It has been previously reported that $B_{12}$ intake among those who consume animal products varies from 3 to 32 mcg/day, which typically meets requirements depending on how much of the vitamin is absorbed.

*Detecting deficiency*
B$_{12}$ levels in the blood can be tested, as can a marker of B$_{12}$ status called a *methylmalonic acid (MMA)*. When B$_{12}$ levels are low, MMA levels increase, so this can be an additional screening for deficiency. There is a third marker felt to be more accurate in older populations in detecting low B$_{12}$ called holotranscobalamin (HoloTC), but it is not as widely available at present and may not hold advantages over standard B$_{12}$ and MMA testing for younger females.[109-110] Changes in B$_{12}$ metabolism during pregnancy affect absorption and transport, and concentrations in the blood are known to drop, so it is important to *use reference values for pregnant women during each trimester if you are getting tested.*

Strict vegetarians intake an average of 0 to 0.25 mcg of B$_{12}$ per day; it is easy to see that this is a high risk group for deficiency.[105] Marginal B$_{12}$ depletion is more common than previously thought even in younger (largely omnivorous) populations, with one large survey reporting 14% to 16% of people of childbearing age having lower than optimal levels.[105] A recent Canadian study showed that a third of all pregnant women studied had marginal B$_{12}$ levels in the first trimester and almost 40% of pregnant women were deficient in B$_{12}$ by the third trimester, potentially putting the baby at risk.[102] Further research in this area is needed.

Mothers taking long-term acid blocking medications for GERD increase their chances of B$_{12}$ malabsorption and B$_{12}$ deficiency.[106]

*Food sources*
B$_{12}$ is mainly found in foods of animal origin, (meat, fish, eggs and dairy products), and therefore is commonly low or deficient in pregnant populations who culturally avoid or don't have access to these foods.[100] With the exception of the seaweed purple nori and possibly shitake mushrooms, plant and algae products claiming to have B$_{12}$ activity actually have little to no biologically active B$_{12}$ and are not adequate sources.[104] While some B$_{12}$ can be manufactured by certain (**probiotic**) bacteria in the intestines, most of this is in the large intestine and is not able to be absorbed or utilized by humans. B$_{12}$ as cyanocobalamin is supplemented in some foods to augment people's intake of B$_{12}$ but is largely found in more processed grain products.

*Supplementation*
Given the critical brain development that occurs in the first thousand days and the importance of myelination (brain insulation) to proper nerve and

brain function, efforts should be made to ensure adequate $B_{12}$ intake while pregnant and breastfeeding both from food and prenatal supplements.

Regardless of dietary preferences, I recommend all pregnant mothers take a good prenatal vitamin that includes $B_{12}$. Prenatal vitamins have a variable amount of $B_{12}$ in them, generally ranging from 8 mcg up to 25 mcg, but blood levels potentially plateau at intake levels above 10 mcg per day.[105] Both common forms of $B_{12}$, cyanocobalamin and methylcobalamin, do the same thing in the body and prevent or correct deficiency and one form is not clinically superior to the other. However, there is some evidence that the methyl form may be slightly better absorbed and retained in the body.[107,108] As with any vitamin during pregnancy, excessive doses can potentially be harmful. Higher doses should only be considered for those mothers deficient in $B_{12}$ and under the supervision of an OB or primary care provider (monitoring levels closely).

*Bottom line on $B_{12}$*
$B_{12}$ is important for infant brain development and is only found in adequate amounts from animal foods like meat and eggs. Vegetarian sources are typically not adequate during pregnancy. Most prenatal vitamins should have an adequate amount of $B_{12}$.

## CRUCIAL MACRONUTRIENTS

### Protein
Adequate protein and calories are fundamental to the growth and brain development of the unborn child. Protein in the diet is digested into building blocks of amino acids, and these amino acids are then used to grow the uterus, placenta, and baby during pregnancy. Inadequate protein intake during pregnancy is associated with low birthweight babies and poor cognitive and developmental outcomes. It is uncommon for someone in the Western world to suffer from inadequate *calorie* intake during pregnancy, with the exception of those mothers with "hyperemesis gravada"—an extreme form of morning sickness. However, insufficient protein intake during pregnancy may be more common than we previously thought.

Mothers with increased risk of inadequate protein intake for the baby include strict vegetarians or vegans, those diagnosed with hyperemesis, or mothers who are on a very carbohydrate-heavy diet without a steady intake of high-quality protein sources. All pregnant mothers must get adequate, high-quality protein to ensure they provide the full spectrum of amino acids required by growing babies.

*Recommended daily amount*
Current RDA recommendations are for pregnant mothers to get 60 to 70 grams of protein per day.[111] My analysis is that these recommendations are low based on average pregnancy weights in the US and a number of studies. Protein requirements for pregnant mothers had previously been set at 1.1 grams of protein per kilogram of body weight daily, which is about 80 grams per day for the average 75 kg pregnant woman. A recent study using a more accurate assessment of maternal protein status revised this requirement to 1.2 to 1.5 grams/kg/day, which means a 75kg/165 lb. pregnant woman would need **90 to 110 grams of quality protein daily**.[112.113]

*Detecting deficiency*
It has been estimated that the average American woman is getting about 75 grams of protein per day, according to data from the National Health and Nutrition Examination Survey (NHANES), which implies that many women fall short of these updated recommendations.

To take this a step further, current recommendations and intake estimates do not take into account the *quality* and *digestibility* of the protein consumed. The overall quality of a protein source and how well it can be digested have potential effects on how well the growing baby can use protein from the mother's diet. Scientists have recently developed scoring methods for protein quality, which tell how well the body can use the protein from certain foods. Studies to measure the true *digestibility and bioavailability* of foods showed that less than 60% of protein from beans and legumes are absorbed by the gut.[114] By comparison, meat, fish, and eggs are known to have a higher quality and digestibility score of greater than 90%.

Studies looking at poor growth in infants and children demonstrated that protein *quality* is associated with risk of stunted growth, and that the incorporation of animal foods decreased the risk of growth failure.[115] Studies in which supplemental protein was supplied (as food) to at-risk mothers eating questionable amounts of dietary protein showed significant reductions of the number of babies with restricted growth.[112]

Non-vegetarian mothers who eat a balanced diet with an *adequate but not excessive* amount of high-quality protein foods should not have an issue getting to an adequate level of intake. However, we should not take for granted that most pregnant mothers are meeting these protein requirements, especially when protein *quality* is considered. Too much protein is bad, too little protein is bad. Balance is the key, as always.

### TABLE 6.8 PROTEIN FOOD SOURCES

| Protein | Quantity approximates |
|---|---|
| 3 oz of fish, meat, or poultry | 25 grams |
| One egg | 6–7 grams |
| 2 tbsp peanut butter | 6–7 grams |
| 1 oz almonds | 6 grams |
| 1 cup of milk or 1 oz of cheese | 7–8 grams |
| 1 serving of Greek yogurt | 17 grams |
| ½ cup of beans or tofu | 10 grams |
| 1 cup cooked quinoa | 8 grams |

## HOT TOPIC

A word of caution for those using soy products for a large proportion of their protein intake. Soy protein, unlike most other plant proteins is considered "complete," which means it contains all essential amino acids. However, there are certain compounds in soy that might not be good for the mom or the baby in higher amounts. Soy contains substances called isoflavones that have estrogen-like effects on the body and may have some health benefits in lower amounts, but high intake of soy raises concerns of potential hormonal disruption in the pregnant mother. The effects that higher amounts of these phytoestrogens have during pregnancy on the developing fetus are not well studied, but there are some concerns worthy of note.[116-119]

In addition, soy contains a fairly high amount of **anti-nutrients**. The two anti-nutrients of concern are phytates that block the digestion and absorption of zinc and iron, and trypsin inhibitors that decrease the digestion of the protein itself. High intake of soy protein that contains substances that blocks its own digestion and absorption of iron could be potentially problematic for the pregnant mother.

Lastly, soy may contain the highest plant levels of the herbicide glyphosate, which has been found in the urine of 90% of pregnant women in one recent study. In this study levels correlated with shorter pregnancy lengths.[120] Small to moderate amounts of organic soy may be acceptable during pregnancy, but a high soy diet should be avoided for the reasons already mentioned.

*Bottom line on protein intake*

Updating protein intake recommendations from a range of 60 to 70 grams to closer to 100 grams daily could mean that some pregnant women's diets may be marginal for protein. Inadequate protein intake can have negative effects on the growth and neurodevelopment of the unborn child. If the mother is vegetarian or vegan, or doesn't eat much meat, fish, or poultry, I would advise working with a dietician trained in pregnancy requirements to make sure the mother is getting adequate quality protein to support the growth and development of the baby. However, excessive protein intake is likely not good for the baby either and may mean that other macronutrients (healthy fats and carbohydrates) are lacking in the mother's diet. Like most nutrients, balance is key, and more protein is not always better.

## DIETARY FATS AND ESSENTIAL FATTY ACIDS: A PRIMER

Dietary fats (also referred to as lipids) and their role in health is a fascinating topic, and one I spent a great deal of time researching. My master's thesis was a project looking at brain accumulation of **omega-3** fatty acids and the effect on learning. This research convinced me of the importance of essential fatty acids (EFAs) in human health. Fast forward twenty years, and unfortunately omega-3 fatty acid insufficiency is still rampant in our children and may be contributing to the neurodevelopmental issues we are seeing today.

First off, let's clarify some confusion and misconceptions about fats. Thanks in part to some highly questionable research in the 1960s and 1970s, fat and cholesterol have been maligned and falsely accused as the cause of much human disease.[121] With the exception of **trans fat** (partially hydrogenated oils) and damaged (**oxidized**) polyunsaturated fats, this is not true. (Trans fats were the worst health experiment of the twentieth century as we will discuss below.) Otherwise, fats, including cholesterol, eaten in the right amounts are not bad for us. They are essential for a child's growth and brain development both in the womb and beyond. Pregnancy and childhood are not the best time for a low-fat diet, and the use of such a diet at any stage in life should only be medically prescribed for specific reasons.

Fats come in many sizes and configurations, all of which have different important roles to play in a growing child. Fats can be classified under one of several headings: sterols (cholesterol), phospholipids, **saturated fats,** and unsaturated fats. None of these fats, other than trans fats, are "bad" and several are absolutely critical for proper brain development in the baby.

---

### HOT TOPIC

The negative effects toxic trans fat may have on the developing baby brain are not well studied but can't be good. Given the suspected link between trans fat and adult neurodegenerative disease like Alzheimer's, there could be potential associations between trans fats in the mother's diet and neurodevelopmental disorders in children as well. Trans fats in the mother's diet cross the placenta and are incorporated into the baby's brain and other tissues. Trans fats are known to interfere with the crucial long-chain omega-3 fats EPA/DHA found in fish oil, which are vital to the developing baby brain (see below). Eating foods high in trans fat in the first thousand days could potentially damage the developing brain and should be avoided. Maternal intake of trans fats also increases the risk for premature delivery and preeclampsia, a dangerous condition of very high blood pressure during pregnancy.[122,123]

Given these dangers, every step should be taken to avoid these trans fats during pregnancy. They are now technically outlawed from the US and Canadian food supply, but there are often loopholes and ways around the enforcement of these types of laws. The **World Health Organization** (WHO) is trying to create a worldwide ban on trans fats in food by 2023. Despite being outlawed in the US, I would still make sure you read food labels, and if the food has trans fat or partially hydrogenated oil, put it down before it has a chance to harm you or the baby.

---

In addition to **trans fat**, mothers should try to avoid other potentially damaging fats and oils during pregnancy. Eating high amounts of deep-fried foods (French fries, onion rings, deep fried chicken or chicken strips, doughnuts, fried tortilla strips) could pose a potential risk to the unborn child when pregnant. Although slightly different than hydrogenated oils, deep fried foods often contain potentially dangerous damaged oils from the high heat and prolonged exposure to air from the frying oil. These damaged oils are referred to as "**oxidized**" and pose many of the same health risks as hydrogenated oils, such as increased risk of heart disease, cancer and diabetes as well as other inflammatory conditions.[124-126] They are also potentially damaging to the developing baby brain for the same reasons that trans fats are, and have been shown to increase the risk of gestational diabetes in the mother.[127,128] Deep fried foods are potentially bad news for the baby brain and for the mother, so really try to minimize intake of these foods while pregnant. Eating them once in a while is no big deal, but they should not be a regular part of a pregnancy diet.

## Cholesterol

Although continuing to be vilified by the media, cholesterol is vitally important for human health and the growth and development of your child. Dietary cholesterol is *not* bad for you. It *does not* cause heart disease or any other health malady, and the Dietary Guidelines Advisory Committee (DGAC) dropped limitations on dietary cholesterol and total dietary fat in 2015 because of the lack of evidence of harm.[129] In fact, cholesterol is made by every cell in our bodies and is necessary for life. It is the basis for many of the hormones made by the body, as well as the main component of cell membranes (the coating on the outside of cells) and the protective insulation around nerve cells called **myelin**. Do you think a growing baby brain might need some cholesterol? Mother nature seems to think so as she puts it in breast milk in considerable amounts. It is advisable to *eat eggs* when pregnant and breastfeeding (unless allergic) largely for protein, the B vitamin choline, and important fats called phospholipids. Don't be afraid of dietary cholesterol!

## Saturated Fats

**Saturated fats,** as opposed to unsaturated fats, are structurally different, changing their properties in the body. They tend to be found more in animal food products (meat) but also in coconut and palm oil and even in an appreciable amount in olive oil—arguably the healthiest oil on the planet! Saturated fats, like cholesterol, have been maligned and associated with heart disease and increased risk of other health conditions. This is a controversial topic, but I trust the work of Dr. Ronald Krauss, among others, who have been researching fats since before many of us were born. His work and the work of others indicate that saturated fat (in moderate amounts and in the context of a healthy overall diet) may not cause heart disease or "clog your arteries" as previously claimed.[130] In fact, *most of the saturated fat in our bloodstream is made in our liver from carbohydrates*.

Saturated fats can be burned for energy but have numerous more complex roles in the human body including strengthening our cell membranes and taking part in the communication between our cells. The growing baby brain uses saturated fat as well as cholesterol and polyunsaturated fats; all have important roles. Breast milk contains a fairly high proportion of both cholesterol and saturated fat, so clearly there is an ongoing role for these fats in infant development.[131] Saturated fats should not be strictly avoided in the maternal diet, nor should they be excessive. The nice thing about saturated fats is they are more stable when cooking and do not oxidize like vegetable oils. Have a steak, cook with coconut oil or butter. As long as saturated fat intake is not excessive, it isn't going to hurt the baby, but it needs to be in balance with the other healthy items in the diet. We will go into the hot topic of saturated fat a bit more in later chapters.

### Polyunsaturated fats

**Polyunsaturated fats (PUFAs)** are among the most important nutrients for the developing baby brain.

Unsaturated fats are those containing one or more double bonds (see PUFA diagram). There are monounsaturated fats containing only one double bond (think olive/avocado oil), or polyunsaturated fats containing multiple double bonds. These seemingly small differences have a huge impact on how these fats behave in the body. Monounsaturated fats are great and have some health benefits (olive oil) and are among the best oils to cook with, but we are going to focus on the polyunsaturated fats here, as they are more vital to the developing infant brain.

PUFAs fall into two families: omega-6 and omega-3. **Omega-6** and **Omega-3** fats are the Yang and Yin of fatty acids, and a balance of the two is needed (as everything in life) to maintain health. Omega-6 is found in plant oils like corn, sunflower, safflower, vegetable oils and in its longer form (**ARA**) in meat, poultry, and eggs, and are very prevalent in the Western diet. Omega-3s are scarcer in the modern diet and found in flax, chia, and hemp seeds, walnuts, and other nuts, as well as in smaller amounts in canola and soybean oil. The longer form omega-3s (**EPA/DHA**) are found mostly in fish, but also in lower amounts in game meat, beef, and eggs.

The only fats that are considered truly essential are omega-6 **linoleic acid (LA)** and omega-3 **alpha linolenic acid (ALA)**. LA and ALA are true *essential fatty acids (EFAs)* because the body cannot manufacture these like it can with other fats. We need to get these EFAs from our diet, or we can become EFA deficient. Classic essential fatty acid deficiency is rare, especially of the omega-6 fats like LA because LA is *everywhere* in the highly processed American diet. Overt and relative omega-3 deficiency is more common, as the foods that contain omega-3 are not consumed as commonly in the Western diet. One of the many issues with the modern diet is that we have tons of omega-6 fats from vegetable oils and processed foods in our food supply, but very little omega-3 fats, pushing us way out of balance.

## POLYUNSATURATED FATS IN THE HUMAN BODY (PUFAs)

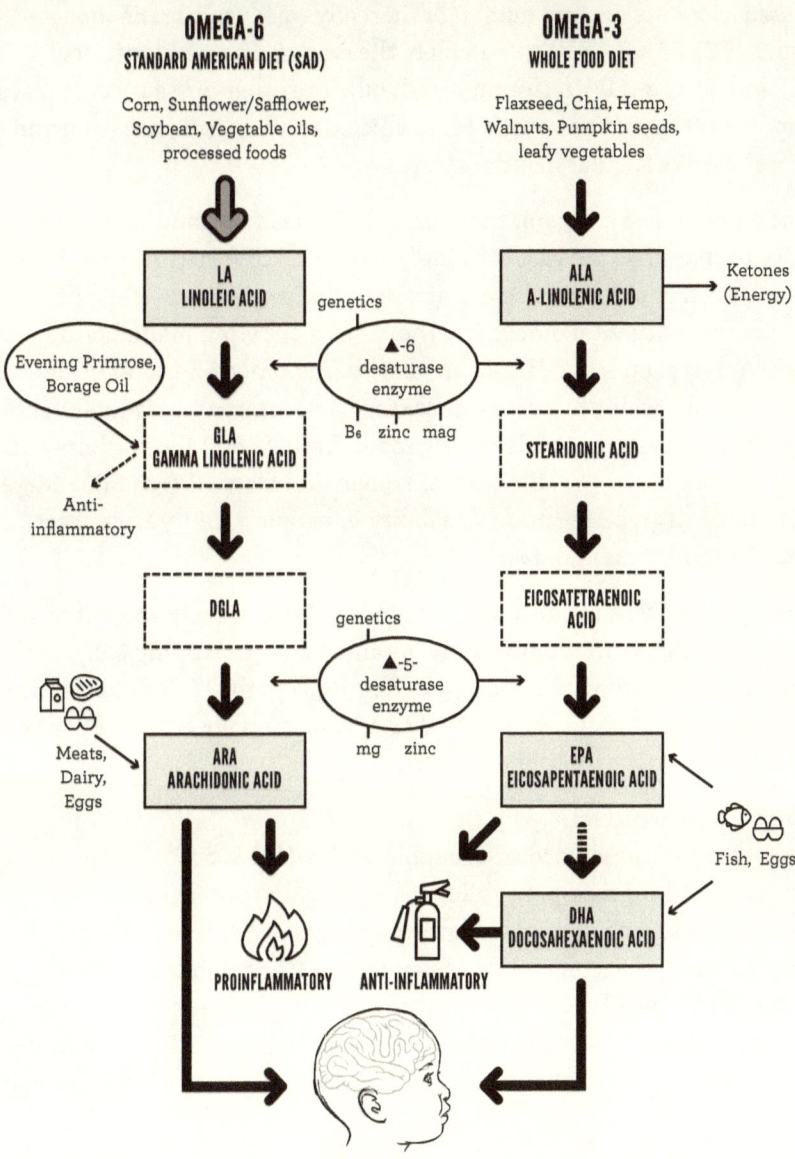

**BABY'S BRAIN & EYES**

ARA, DHA – delivered via umbilical cord, breastmilk/formula, and first foods

Short chain PUFAs in the diet can be converted to ARA, EPA, DHA in the body. This process is inefficient and the modern diet is very high in Omega-6, shifting the balance toward inflammation. Whole food diets containing fish shift the balance to block imflammation, and support the baby's brain and eye development. The ability of the desaturase enzymes to convert ALA to EPA is affected by the type of fat in the diet, nutrient deficiencies (zinc, magnesium, B₆) and to some degree genetics.

The essential PUFAs *LA and ALA are not the biologically active forms of fatty acids used in our bodies.* The human brain really wants to use the longer versions of PUFAs (LCPUFA)—namely the omega-6 **arachidonic acid (ARA)** and omega-3 DHA (found in fish oil). The other omega-3 that plays an important role in the body is EPA, which decreases inflammation and promotes cardiovascular health.

As illustrated in the diagram, the human body has the somewhat limited capacity to manufacture the *biologically active* LCPUFAs (ARA, EPA, DHA). However, even in the best of circumstances this process is inefficient, especially for those vital omega-3s. The human body can manufacture some EPA, but even less DHA, from plant-based omega-3 found in soybean oil, canola, walnuts, chia, and flaxseed. In fact, multiple studies show no significant amounts of DHA being made from ALA in most adults and a range of only 1% to 8% efficiency of conversion from ALA to EPA. There is likely some degree of genetic variability in people's ability to convert ALA to the longer chain omega-3.

The amounts of DHA produced in the modern human body are paltry and not sufficient for optimum brain development in a developing baby.[139-144] Recent scientific evidence could make the case why the biologically active omega-3 fat DHA should be classified as a "conditionally essential" fatty acid for the pregnant mother and infant.

### The importance of DHA
The omega-3 fat called docosahexaenoic acid (DHA) is arguably the most important for the developing child. DHA is highly concentrated in nerve cell membranes, especially at the growing edges of brain cells that are seeking to make new connections (synapses). Who might have a high need for DHA? The obvious answer is the growing infant and their rapidly expanding brain, which is making 40,000 new synaptic connections *per second* during the first two years of life. Their brains are like a sponge for DHA.

DHA is essential for the brain and eye development of the unborn and young child. Insufficient DHA during pregnancy or childhood could leave that child's brain and eyes structurally unsound and more prone to visual or cognitive impairment, neurodevelopmental disorders, and behavioral or mood issues. Omega-3 LCPUFA are so important to the baby that biological systems have evolved to maximize the amount of this fatty acid that the fetus receives from the mother. DHA is preferentially transferred from mother to child across the placenta and into the baby's brain. If the body must substitute another type of fat in the baby's brain because there is not enough DHA, this could have potential long-term consequences.

While there is little doubt that omega-3 fats play an important role in the developing brain, studies looking at omega-3 intake, brain development, and academic outcomes have been variable. Multiple studies have linked higher seafood and omega-3 intake during pregnancy as well as DHA content of breast milk to improved developmental measures and academic performance of the child.[140,141,147-150] One recent study showed a lower risk of children developing ADHD if the mother had better omega-3 intake during pregnancy.[154] However, other studies on DHA supplementation of pregnant mothers have not consistently shown a significant measurable cognitive benefit in children, making the importance of supplemental DHA for pregnant mothers not uniformly accepted; the debate is ongoing.[151-153] The data on DHA and infant brain development was strong enough to prompt most infant formula companies to start putting DHA and ARA in their formulas, so the importance of DHA in the brain is not fringe by any means and is well recognized. Maternal diets that are not adequate in DHA may lead to less than optimal neurodevelopmental, behavioral, or psychological outcomes for the child.

Having researched this for the past twenty years, I fully believe in the importance of DHA for the baby brain and made sure my pregnant wife was getting salmon or trout several times a week and taking a cod liver oil supplement on the days without fish in her diet.

What else do the omega-3 EPA and DHA do in the pregnant body?

+ Maintain healthy cell membranes (keeps them flexible and not brittle)
+ Support growth and development of infant brain cells
+ Facilitate communication between cells of the body
+ Control inflammation in the body and brain (omega-3 are anti-inflammatory)
+ Decrease inflammation of the placenta to maintain good blood flow to the baby
+ May help prevent premature uterine contractions and decrease risk of premature birth.[138]
+ May help prevent preeclampsia

+ Assist in regulation of gene expression (epigenetic modification), turning off genes for inflammation and turning on genes for brain growth.[145-147]

*How to get your omega-3s*

Currently there are no RDA levels set for EPA and DHA omega-3. *The Dietary Guidelines for Americans* from 2015 to 2020 recommended **12 oz of seafood weekly** to improve a pregnant mother's intake of EPA/DHA which would approximate 375 mg omega-3 daily. Currently mothers in the US are getting 3 oz or less per week of fish, falling far short of the recommendations.

The **World Health Organization** recommends at least **500 mg combined EPA/DHA daily** for pregnant mothers, containing at least 200 mg DHA, but average omega-3 intake in pregnant mothers in the US, Canada and Australia is 78 to 90 mg at best.[155-157] Recent studies of maternal intake as well as their tissue and blood levels of EPA/DHA have confirmed that **the majority of mothers are not getting enough long chain omega-3.**[140,141145,156,158]

EPA and DHA are found in cold water fish, but also to some degree in pasture-raised or omega-3 enhanced eggs, with smaller amounts found in red meat and game meat. They are not found in plant sources, although DHA can be manufactured by algae for a vegan source of DHA. There is a high variability in the amount of omega-3 in fish, and the best and safest sources are listed in Table 6.9. I would recommend every non-vegan pregnant mother eat safe sources of high omega-3 fish several times weekly or take a fish oil supplement (EPA/DHA) for the benefit of the unborn child. Tragically, this is getting more complicated, as our seas are becoming increasingly polluted. Fish from cold waters are by far the best source of DHA, but because mercury levels in our oceans are rising (largely from atmospheric mercury contamination from coal burning), many of these fish should not be consumed by pregnant women for risk of harming the baby's brain.

A few servings of safe high omega-3 fish each week will go a long way to provide a healthy dose of DHA that goes straight to the brain of a developing baby. Bake or grill some salmon or trout. Have some pickled herring on a whole grain cracker as a snack. You can use a can of sardines or salmon just like you would use tuna and make a sardine or salmon salad sandwich that tastes similar with significantly more omega-3 and less mercury than any tuna sandwich. Even if you are not a huge fan of fish, try to "doctor it up" in a way that is palatable for you (see recipe section on the book website) and know that getting your omega-3 is one of the most important things you can do for your baby for the rest of their life!

*Vegetarian Omega-3*
Vegetarian and vegan mothers are typically the lowest in DHA, potentially putting their babies at the highest risk for deficiency if efforts are not made to supplement this crucial fat. In a recent study, DHA levels were found to be seven to eight times lower in vegetarian and vegan moms, as compared to moms consuming fish and other sources.[149] Unfortunately, trying to increase intake of flaxseed oil and chia seeds is not likely to increase DHA levels enough for optimal infant development.

Strict vegetarians and vegans can opt for an algae source DHA of 200 to 500 mg to improve their levels and should also consider taking cold-pressed flaxseed oil (refrigerated to prevent rancidity), approximately 1 to 2 tbsp per day. To maximize the conversion of ALA from flaxseed to EPA, it is advisable for a pregnant mother to limit her intake of the high omega-6 vegetable and seed oils like corn oil, sunflower and safflower oil, soybean oil, and vegetable oil which can block the omega-3 if excessive. In addition, common deficiencies in nutrients such as zinc and magnesium make it more difficult for the body to make EPA, so these nutrients need to be in adequate supply in the diet.

*Other fats matter*
The other fats that a pregnant mother consumes can affect her body and that of her baby. Excessive omega-6 fats, as well as trans fat and damaged (oxidized) vegetable oils all push the body toward more inflammation and displace the vital omega-3s.

Optimum ratios of omega-6 to omega-3 in the diet are debated but felt by experts to be in the range of 2:1 to 4:1. Current dietary patterns in the US skew this ratio to more like 10:1 to 20:1 in favor of the omega-6 fats.[132-136] This imbalance can have serious health implications for the pregnant mom, the unborn child, and the infant. Omega-6 fats tend to promote inflammation (pro-inflammatory) in the body, and omega-3 suppresses inflammation (anti-inflammatory). Having a state of *relative* omega-3 deficiency creates a predisposition toward excessive inflammation, which can affect the uterus, placenta, and the growing baby. In the average diet, the small amounts of omega-3 fats are not able to do what they are designed to do because they are being crowded out by the proinflammatory fats listed earlier. The higher amounts of unhealthy fat a pregnant woman has in her diet, the more omega-3 she will need to overcome this deficit to deliver healthy fat to that precious baby brain.[137] It is advisable to limit the proinflammatory fats in the diet, especially while pregnant.

### TABLE 6.9 FISH WITH HIGH AND LOW MERCURY LEVELS

| Fish to Avoid or Minimize (high mercury) | Safer Fish (low mercury) |
| --- | --- |
| Tilefish | Shellfish (shrimp/clams/oysters/scallops) |
| Swordfish | Sardines* |
| Shark | Tilapia |
| Tuna (most species) | Anchovies* |
| Orange roughy | Pollock |
| Grouper | Haddock |
| Mackerel (except North Atlantic) | Butterfish |
| Bluefish | Salmon and trout* |
| Sea bass | Herring* |
| Halibut | Mackerel (North Atlantic)* |
| | Whitefish* |
| | Flounder |
| Cod* and light tuna have more moderate mercury levels | Sole |

*denotes high Omega-3 fish

### TABLE 6.10 OMEGA-3 LEVELS OF FOOD SOURCES

| Qty/Source | Omega 3 (EPA/DHA) |
| --- | --- |
| 3 oz fresh, canned or frozen salmon | 1100–1900 mg EPA+DHA |
| 3 oz trout or steelhead | 840 mg EPA + DHA |
| 3 oz sardines | 1000 mg EPA+DHA |
| 3 oz herring or whitefish | 1300–1700 mg EPA+DHA |
| 1 omega-3 egg* | Variable: 60-100 mg DHA per egg (read labels) |
| 1.5 tbsp flaxseed oil | 10,000 mg ALA yields 100–600 mg EPA/ 0-100 mg DHA |
| 1 tsp cod liver oil | 1100 mg omega-3: 400mg EPA/500 mg DHA |

*some omega-3 eggs contain mostly ALA, and little DHA. Look for the DHA content on the label.

*Omega-3 Supplements*
If someone really can't tolerate fish, I recommend a high-quality fish oil/cod-liver oil, rich in EPA and DHA to augment Omega-3 intake. I often use

the lemon-flavored liquid fish oil by Carlson's or Nordic Naturals mixed in a smoothie, yogurt, or "magic applesauce." In my opinion, a high-quality fish oil is one of the most important supplements. One teaspoon of cod liver oil contains 1,000 mg of EPA/DHA omega-3 and can be used to improve the omega-3 intake of pregnant mothers. It is important not to overdo it, so I recommend staying in the 500 to 1000 mg EPA/DHA range daily unless otherwise advised by the mother's healthcare provider.

A word of caution on omega-3 supplements: very high intake of omega-3 could potentially act like a blood thinner, which would not be advisable during pregnancy. Limit daily intake to the amount you would find in a nice piece of salmon (up to 1000 mg or so). Another caveat is there are also reportedly high number of rancid fish oil and flaxseed oil supplements on the market, which can be harmful to mother and child. I advise sticking to a trusted high-quality brand and if the supplement has a sharp/rancid or very fishy odor it needs to be returned and replaced with a better-quality supplement. Refrigeration before purchase for flax oil and after purchase for both flax and fish oil is essential. Nordic Naturals, Barlean's, and Carlson are trusted brands of oils.

*Bottom line on omega-3*
DHA is vital for the growing baby brain. DHA should be supplied in the diet directly either through fish, eggs, or from a supplement. Because our bodies can only produce limited amounts, **pregnant mothers should supply their growing babies with pre-formed EPA and DHA and not rely exclusively on plant-based omega-3 fats like canola or flaxseed oil.** A minimum of 200 mg DHA daily is recommended for the baby brain but don't discount the importance of EPA in supporting a healthy placenta and uterus during pregnancy.

## Carbohydrates
**Carbohydrates** can be described as simple (dietary sugars such as fructose, glucose, sucrose) and complex (vegetables as well as starches such as breads, pastas, and grains made from oats, wheat, rice, quinoa). Complex carbohydrates can further be described as **low glycemic index** (they are digested more slowly into sugar) or **high glycemic index** (starches that turn into sugar very quickly in the digestive tract). Fiber is referred to as a non-digestible carbohydrate but has important health benefits as outlined below. There is also **resistant starch**, which is a carbohydrate usually found in grains that is not digested by humans but is a prebiotic that can feed the microbiome.

Each of these classes of carbohydrates can have important effects on the pregnant mother and the unborn child. A diet too high in sugar and highly processed (high glycemic index) carbohydrates and low in fiber is damaging to the maternal microbiome and can promote excessive weight gain and gestational diabetes, which program the unborn child for future disease. Emphasizing a diet rich in vegetables, whole grains, and whole fruit and low in highly processed foods will ensure that the mother gets adequate fiber and low glycemic index carbohydrates that are associated with better pregnancy outcomes.[159]

*Feeding the Gut: Supporting a Healthy Maternal Microbiome*
The mother's microbiome during the period of pregnancy and delivery is of vital importance to both the mother and the infant. Several of the most important roles of the maternal microbiome are outlined below. Refer to the previous chapter for more information on all the benefits of a healthy microbiome for the baby. How does a mother best support her microbiome and become a good steward of these probiotic bacteria?

First and foremost, the mother needs to feed her microbiome with plenty of fiber-rich fruits and vegetables as well as choosing whole grains during the pregnancy, and limit sugar and processed foods that can damage her microbiome (see the previous chapters). "Eating the rainbow" of a variety of colorful fruits and vegetables also supports microbiome diversity because of the presence of important **phytonutrients** found in these foods. Remember that a diverse microbiome is a healthy microbiome. A pregnant mother should also consider eating plenty of probiotic foods such as high quality, low sugar yogurt, kefir, or fermented vegetables like sauerkraut. Consider a multi-species probiotic supplement if there were antibiotics involved during the pregnancy.

*A word on Fiber and Prebiotics*

The term fiber refers to carbohydrates in our food that are not digestible by humans but provide several health benefits, one being helping with eliminating waste and having regular bowel movements. Many mothers experience the discomfort of constipation during pregnancy. High estrogen and/or progesterone levels contribute to slowed motility of the colon, and the pregnant mom has a large growing object in her uterus pressing on things like her bladder and colon. Fun! Adequate dietary fiber can help prevent or decrease the constipation associated with pregnancy.

More importantly, ensuring proper fiber intake will not only help to prevent constipation and hemorrhoids, but soluble fiber is also the main food **(prebiotic)** for the probiotic bacteria living in the intestines that create the maternal microbiome. As discussed previously, during the optimal birthing process, the mother passes a healthy microbiome to the infant. This healthy infant microbiome is vitally important for their health and development. Low fiber intake by mom means less food for the good bacteria, potentially impacting her ability to pass along healthy bacteria to her child. A high fiber diet during pregnancy may also help to decrease the incidence or severity of gestational diabetes and preeclampsia, potentially by mechanisms involving the microbiome and its metabolism of soluble fiber.[173-175]

Pregnant women should get 25 to 30 g per day, but unfortunately adults in the US typically get less than 15 g of fiber daily. Please refer to the page on high fiber foods to help make dietary choices that increase your daily fiber intake. There are many fiber supplements on the market that may provide health benefits as well, but whole food sources are always best. For supplemental fiber, I often recommend psyllium-based products as they have a high proportion of soluble fiber and can be mixed in a smoothie, yogurt, applesauce, or taken as capsules, but inulin and pectin-based products also act as prebiotics and may help with constipation. Ramp up on fiber slowly over the course of weeks to avoid bloating and be sure to drink plenty of water.

The mother's gut and vaginal microbiome are interrelated and play a number of roles that are extremely important for her health and the health of the infant. Several of the most important reasons to protect and support a healthy intestinal and vaginal microbiome are listed below. Research shows:

+ Vaginal infections are a common cause of preterm birth. High *Lactobacillus* (probiotic bacteria) counts in the vagina are protective against vaginal infections that lead to preterm birth. These probiotic bacteria lower the vaginal pH and increase antibacterial factors that fight off bad bacteria to help prevent these infections.[160]

+ An altered maternal microbiome, vaginal infections, and inflammation are implicated in 30% of preterm births.

+ Bacterial vaginosis, a form of vaginal dysbiosis, is associated with a 40% increase in preterm birth. Low levels of *Lactobacillus* probiotic bacteria have been found in women with bacterial vaginosis and are associated with increased risk. There was an 81% reduction in bacterial vaginosis with probiotic supplementation in one recent study.[161]

+ A healthy microbiome and probiotic supplementation may help reduce risk of preeclampsia, a condition of dangerously elevated blood pressure in the mother, which can lead to premature birth.[162]

+ Probiotic bacteria may help prevent preterm birth by reducing vaginal inflammation. By lowering the body's production of hormone-like inflammatory chemicals called **cytokines**, probiotics help to decrease inflammation in the vagina and further decrease chances of preterm birth.

+ It also appears that probiotic bacteria in the mother positively affect the breast milk by lowering inflammatory cytokines and increasing anti-inflammatory cytokines, which may have positive effects on the infant.[160,163,164]

+ A healthy maternal microbiome helps prevent Group B strep (GBS), a potentially harmful bacteria to the baby. A few smaller studies show that probiotic use by pregnant mothers in some cases may help eradicate GBS colonization and eliminate the need for maternal antibiotics around the time of the birth. Recall that antibiotics near the time of delivery wipe out mom's and baby's microbiome and can lead to dysbiosis.[165,166]

+ Maternal probiotic bacteria from the mother's microbiome can be passed through breast milk, which becomes another vehicle to continue probiotic inoculation in the infant gut. Maternal diets with probiotic rich foods or probiotic supplementation increase the amount of *Lactobacillus* bacteria in breast milk and increase the amount of healthy *Bifidobacteria* in the baby. These "hand me down" probiotics from mom increase an important immune system protein called Immunoglobin A (IgA) found in the baby's gastrointestinal tract that is a first-line defense against invaders.[167-169]

+ Some evidence suggests probiotic use by pregnant moms helps reduce the baby's risk of developing allergies and atopic disease (asthma and eczema) in highly allergic families. The results were stronger for prevention of eczema but seemed to only be effective for reducing allergy if the probiotics were given to mom during pregnancy and also baby after birth.[170]

+ Probiotics may help improve or prevent gestational diabetes.[171]

+ Most importantly, the pregnant mother will pass along either a healthy or unhealthy microbiome to the baby during the birth process! The infant is initially "inoculated" with the mother's microbiome during the passage through the birth canal. If the mom is colonized with healthy bacteria, this will be passed along to the infant. This is why it is tremendously important for pregnant women to ensure that they have a healthy microbiome to pass along to their child.[172]

## FEEDING THE GENES: SUGAR, EPIGENETICS, AND THE UNBORN CHILD

Unfortunately, there still seems to be a common sentiment that pregnancy gives you free license to eat whatever you want because the baby needs the calories. While a growing baby does need calories, as with most nutrition, there is also a sweet spot of sufficient but not excessive calorie intake. Calorie restriction and starvation during pregnancy has been found to have negative long-term effects on babies that last through adulthood, and studies on children born during famine and starvation periods led to some remarkable insights starting with the "Barker Hypothesis."[176] A low calorie/low protein diet while pregnant can lead to a child with developmental delays and low birth weight, yet paradoxically put that child at future risk for obesity and diabetes later in life due to epigenetic programming. Similarly, excessive calories, especially excessive sugar and excessive weight gain during pregnancy, can program that child for future heart disease, diabetes, and obesity, also through the process of epigenetic programming discussed earlier. And for the record, "a calorie is not a calorie," in contrast to what some food companies have been pushing. Different types of fats and carbohydrates are metabolized very differently and have different metabolic and epigenetic effects. Vegetables and soda are both carbohydrates; some food industry marketers will try to tell you they do the same thing in the human body, but this myth has been debunked by many experts in medicine and science.

See Dr. Robert Lustig's "A calorie is not a calorie" infographic: https://robertlustig.com/calorie_en/

Fructose is a sugar historically found in natural fruit, but is now available in high amounts year-round in the modern diet, mostly from sucrose (table sugar) and high fructose corn syrup. The main foods contributing to added sugar in our diet are highly processed foods and sweetened drinks (added sugar is found in 75% of all the processed food products available in the US). Fructose is metabolized very differently than other sugars (see Chapter 17 on metabolic health) and there are growing links between high fructose intake and risk of obesity, diabetes, and heart disease. Evidence is growing that high sugar intake during pregnancy adversely affects both the mother and the unborn child.

In animal models, a high fructose diet in the pregnant mother results in higher blood pressure and **insulin resistance (prediabetes)** in the offspring, and increased fat storage and obesity in females.[177] There is an increased risk of fatty liver, present in epidemic levels in children, especially in the offspring of mothers on a high fructose diet. In humans, a high maternal carbohydrate intake during pregnancy, especially from sugar sweetened drinks (including fruit juice), is associated with an increased infant and child **body mass index (BMI)**, which is a marker for obesity, and higher fat storage lasting far into childhood. These associations suggest that the mother's sugar intake may program that child for future obesity.[178-181]

It has also been shown that high sugar intake during pregnancy leads to excessive weight gain in the mother, increasing her risk for gestational diabetes, which further increases the risk of her children developing obesity and type 2 diabetes. Animal models show alterations of the *maternal microbiome* with a reduction in healthy probiotic bacteria in the mother fed high amounts of fructose during pregnancy. Offspring of mothers who consumed high amounts of fructose and who were also fed fructose rich diets experienced increased incidence of **"leaky gut,"** as well as weight gain and insulin resistance (prediabetes). These results likely stemmed from an altered microbiome.[182]

Studies examining the epigenetic effects of high sugar or fructose intake by pregnant mothers show alterations in gene expression in multiple organs of their offspring, including brain, heart, and kidney, as well as alterations in genes regulating sugar and fat metabolism. A high fructose diet during pregnancy increases risk factors for high blood pressure in the offspring from effects on the kidney.[183-186]

A high intake of refined grains by the mother (baked goods made with bleached flour, including most breads, pastas, cookies, cakes, and crackers), may act to program the child for obesity as well. Highly refined or *high glycemic index* carbohydrates essentially turn into sugar very quickly in the digestive system, causing metabolic stress on the mother and child and can lead to epigenetic changes that may increase the risk for obesity and diabetes. Researchers found the negative effects of the mother's high glycemic diet could be reduced in children who were active and ate a healthy diet low in sugar and refined flour products. In contrast, the negative effects of this maternal diet were amplified in children who were sedentary and also ate a high glycemic diet.[187]

It is important to mention that these negative dietary effects can amplify across the generations, and that epigenetic alterations that are occurring in the child of a mother with an unhealthy diet can in turn be handed down to their children and grandchildren, creating a legacy of obesity, type 2 diabetes, and metabolic dysfunction. But the cycle can be broken by adoption of a diet low in sugar and refined carbohydrates and an active lifestyle in our children. People in medical research and healthcare policy are starting to realize the implications of this concept. We need to make every effort to break this cycle now, before it is too late.

*The bottom line on sugar and carbs*
The take home message is clear: pregnant mothers should avoid eating or drinking a high amount of sugar, and specifically should avoid the sugar sweetened drinks and soda that constitute the bulk of the excessive fructose in the diet. Eating nutrient dense whole fruit is fine and rec-ommended, but juice should be minimized since it has all the sugar and none of the intact fiber found in whole fruit. Choose 100% whole grain and high fiber options when it comes to selecting healthy carbohydrates in your diet. Supporting a healthy microbiome through dietary choices during pregnancy is important to the health of the mother and child and decreases the risk of epigenetic programming for disease in future generations.

# VEGETARIAN AND VEGAN MOMS

Vegetarian and vegan mothers are advised to take special care to provide adequate nutrition to the unborn child and avoid deficiencies during the pregnancy. This can take extensive planning and assistance to get it right. Work with a qualified dietician and don't just "wing it." Pay special attention to ensuring that iron, zinc, B12, choline, DHA and protein levels are adequate, and not just on paper; remember that to benefit the baby these nutrients need to be digested and absorbed. Take into account that digestion and absorption of several important nutrients from plant-based sources are not as efficient as those from animal sources. Some special considerations are listed below.

## Iron

Special care needs to be taken to maximize the absorption of the non-heme iron in a vegetarian or vegan diet.

+ Extensively rinse and soak beans and nuts
+ Cook in cast iron
+ Eat iron-rich green leafy vegetables
+ Ingest vitamin C in either citrus fruit, lemon or lime juice, or an ascorbic acid supplement, with meals. This will help boost iron absorption that is partially blocked by the phytates in foods, but not as much as previously hoped.[188-190]

Megadosing with high amounts of vitamin C during pregnancy in an effort to increase iron absorption is not recommended. It is therefore essential for vegetarian and vegan mothers to choose a prenatal supplement with higher iron support, as some prenatals will contain up to 28 mg of iron. Despite this, getting iron levels tested and monitored by a qualified healthcare provider is required to know if extra supplementation is needed.

## Zinc

Soaked and rinsed beans and lentils, nuts, and seeds are the best bet for getting zinc in a vegan/vegetarian diet, but amounts may not be enough given that requirements are 50% to 70% higher in a vegetarian diet because of the anti-nutrients that block absorption. Pescatarians will not have as much of an issue with zinc, as shellfish and seafood are good sources. Having 10 to 15 mg of zinc gluconate, glycinate, aspartate, or other chelated form in a prenatal vitamin is likely to be important. Zinc oxide is not as well absorbed so consider another form of zinc.

## Choline

For those vegetarian mothers not willing to eat eggs, other foods such as baked potato, quinoa, brussels sprouts, and broccoli are decent sources of choline and should be incorporated regularly. However, getting to 500 mg daily will likely require a choline supplement. Choline chloride or bitartrate are both good supplemental forms.

### B12

Even if Nori seaweed and shitake mushrooms are incorporated regularly in the pregnant vegan diet, B12 levels and/or MMA levels should still be tested in the mother, and a good prenatal vitamin with B12 is a must to prevent deficiency.

### Vitamin D

Sunshine exposure is still the best bet to boost vitamin D levels, but a supplement of 400 to 800 IU of vitamin D3 daily is warranted for all mothers, including vegetarian and vegan mothers. It may be more important to get blood levels tested for 25-OH Vitamin D for these women.

### Protein

Getting the 80 to 100 grams of quality protein needed during pregnancy may require supplementation for the vegetarian or vegan mother. Vegetarians can consider frequent intake of eggs and dairy products to boost protein intake, some may consider fish as well if they are pescatarian. For vegans, don't rely on soy for all your protein needs; consider a pea/rice-based protein or alternate supplement instead. Continue to eat complementary protein foods in your daily diet—beans and rice or quinoa—but keep in mind the lower digestibility factor of the protein in these foods.

### Essential Fatty Acids

For those opposed to high omega-3 eggs or eating fish or taking a fish oil supplement, consider a daily vegetarian or vegan source for DHA of 200 to 500 mg daily. Cut way down on the omega-6 oils in the diet to make way for more omega-3. Don't use significant quantities of corn, soybean, sunflower, safflower, or vegetable oil for cooking. Use olive, avocado, or coconut instead. Ground flaxseed and flaxseed oil can boost levels of EPA somewhat, and can be incorporated, but these will not boost DHA levels to an appropriate level for a growing baby brain. Consider a refrigerated high-quality flaxseed oil supplement 1 to 2 tablespoons per day along with a vegan source of DHA to get both EPA and DHA for the baby

For a sample menu of what to eat when you are expecting, check on the book website.

## RECOMMENDED READING

1. Thousand Days non-profit organization: www.Thousanddays.org.

2. Center for Disease Control and Prevention- Maternal and Infant Health Information: https://www.cdc.gov/reproductivehealth/maternalinfanthealth

3. For more information on vitamin D in pregnancy: www.endocrine.org

4. For more information on choline during pregnancy: https://www.human.cornell.edu/dns/research/profiles/groups/choline-cognition

5. For more information on mercury in seafood: https://www.nrdc.org/stories/smart-seafood-buying-guide https://www.fda.gov/food/metals-and-your-food/ mercury-levels-commercial-fish-and-shellfish-1990-2012

# NUTRITION $R_X$

Many topics were covered in this chapter. It may seem overwhelming, but don't give up! Even a series of small changes can accumulate to give the baby a better start in life and decrease the risks that result from poor nutrition.

**1** Take a good quality prenatal vitamin even when thinking about getting pregnant! Most should contain folate, $B_{12}$, zinc, iodine, and iron in recommended amounts and 600–800 IU of Vitamin $D_3$.

**2** Consider taking a prenatal vitamin that has the L-methylfolate form of folate rather than folic acid for increased protection if you fall into one of the high-risk groups described in this chapter.

**3** Take steps to ensure adequate iron and zinc intake during pregnancy as these minerals are crucial to the developing child.

**4** Many pregnant women are at risk of iron deficiency during pregnancy with lifelong effects on the child's brain. Consider getting screened for iron deficiency with a serum ferritin level even if you are not anemic. Optimal maternal ferritin level is greater than 30 ug/L.

**5**  Consider having your vitamin D levels checked with 25-OH Vitamin D if you are a woman of color, live in a northern climate, or work inside. If levels are low (below 30 ng/ml, but especially below 20 ng/ml) then work with a healthcare provider for aggressive supplementation to get levels above 30 ng/ml.

**6**  Eat EPA/DHA rich foods like sardines, salmon, trout, herring, or anchovies at least 2 to 3 times per week. Avoid high mercury fish.

**7**  If eating fish isn't an option, consider an omega-3 supplement with EPA/DHA in it for the baby's brain. Minimum intake should be 200 mg DHA daily, preferably 500 to 1000 mg of combined EPA/DHA daily.

**8**  Eat plenty of choline-rich foods: 3 eggs a day is great; red meat and liver are also good sources. If the intake of choline rich foods is questionable, consider a choline chloride or bitartrate supplement of about 500 mg daily to support the baby's brain growth.

**9**  Protein requirements during pregnancy may be closer to 90 to 100 mg per day for the average pregnant mother based on recent studies. Be conscious about getting adequate amounts of high-quality protein in the diet to support proper growth and development of the baby.

**10**  Soda, juice, candy, sweets, and sweetened drinks should be avoided as much as possible. Focus on whole grain and vegetable carbohydrates during pregnancy to decrease risk of gestational diabetes and decrease fetal programming for future obesity and type 2 diabetes.

**11**  Cook for yourself as much as possible—it is the best way to know exactly what mother and baby are consuming!

**12**  Minimize exposure to environmental toxins and pollutants when pregnant. We devote the entire next chapter to raising awareness of the ways a pregnant mother can decrease toxic exposures.

# CHAPTER SEVEN

# MINIMIZING EXPOSURE TO TOXINS AND POLLUTANTS

We as modern humans are swimming in a soup of potentially toxic elements every day. Pregnant mothers and young children are unwittingly exposed to a host of concerning chemicals through our air, water, food, and cosmetics. Modern chemistry and technology have benefited mankind in many ways. However, products of modern science can be a double-edged sword, and we need to consider the risks as well as the benefits, especially to a vulnerable developing child.

There is a new field of science that examines the **"exposome"**—the sum total of all environmental influences affecting our health, and the combined potential impact of our chemical exposures throughout our lifespan.[1-3] Historically, most studies have looked at these health factors and environmental exposures in isolation but not in relationship to each other (and how they interact in the human body). How these chemicals affect and potentially damage an unborn or young developing child has only recently come under increased scrutiny.

Currently in Europe, a large project is underway to better assess these exposures in early life. Dubbed "HELIX" (Human Early Life Exposome), this project is collecting data on tens of thousands of mothers and children to better understand the health impact of environmental exposures.[4,5] In this chapter, we focus primarily on the effects of toxic exposures on infant and child brain development, but it is important to note that science is also examining the role of the exposome in the epidemics of obesity and **type 2 diabetes**, cancer risk, and multiple other health outcomes in children and adults.

More than 80,000 chemicals are currently used in US industries and agriculture; very few are tested for safety in humans. Among the ones that have been tested in animal studies, more than one thousand have been shown to be toxic to the brain. Among these neurotoxins, two hundred are known to affect humans, which is surely a vast under-representation.[6] None of these chemicals have been tested for safety in unborn children or pregnant mothers. In general, our government adopts a policy of "innocent until proven guilty." This might be appropriate for an individual involved in a legal struggle, but not for evaluating a potentially harmful chemical.

For example, through a legal loophole, many food additives are automatically granted Generally Recognized As Safe (GRAS) status by the FDA with no testing, and rely on food manufacturers to make their own safety determinations with no FDA involvement. Another list called EAFUS (Everything Added to Food in the US) includes 3976 substances directly added to food, most of which have names that people can't even pronounce. In addition, the FDA approved over 3000 substances for use in food packaging, including potential endocrine disruptors and neurotoxins, without any research into their cumulative effect in humans, much less the developing baby during the critical windows discussed earlier in the book.

We are apparently expected to believe that all these chemicals are safe for the youngest, most vulnerable members of our society with absolutely no testing. This is not a scientific approach. For decades, the growing concerns and lack of data about the health impacts of these chemicals among physicians and scientists have largely been ignored. As a physician, pediatrician, and father to two young children, I find this kind of cavalier attitude toward the health of our children reprehensible. Toxic exposures and the downstream health effects is a subject that brings out the disinformation artists, the skeptics, the doubters, and the haters. There are industry forces that try to label such concerns as alternative quackery; however, a growing movement of critical thinkers are seeing through this illusion and lack of transparency.

The simple fact is that unborn babies and young children are being exposed to a large number of untested chemicals with potentially significant consequences. Several studies in the early 2000s showed more than two hundred potentially toxic chemicals in the umbilical cord of unborn children, several of which had been outlawed for decades. More recent research is verifying these findings and showing that the unborn child may in fact be exposed to higher levels of these chemicals than their mothers because they are concentrated in the fetal bloodstream.[7–10] Toxic compounds are routinely found in maternal breast milk and urine.

How do we minimize these exposures and potentially damaging effects?

For now, it is up to us to educate and protect ourselves and our children from potentially harmful chemicals. Thankfully, there is increased research on several potentially harmful items, which are discussed below. The curtain is being pulled back so now we can see what the great Oz has been up to all these years. A great resource on how to protect oneself and loved ones is the Environmental Working Group (found at www.EWG. org), a nonprofit group dedicated to consumer protection from harmful effects of chemicals, food additives, and pollutants. Their website is a treasure trove of information that can be used every day to protect the family. Among the most important information they put out is the "Dirty Dozen" list of the fruits and vegetables with the highest pesticide residues. Avoiding these Dirty Dozen conventionally grown foods and choosing organic alternatives can go a long way to reduce pesticide exposure for the entire family. They also provide information on safer cleaning products, cosmetics, and other ways to reduce exposure to potentially toxic agents.

### Oxidative Stress

**Oxidative stress** is an imbalance between the production of damaging chemicals known as free radicals in the body and the ability to neutralize them with **antioxidants.** Excessive free radicals damage our cells and their **mitochondria**; our brains may be especially susceptible.

The harmful effect of oxidative stress is one of the common denominators of all **toxins**. Increased oxidative stress can contribute to any number of diseases, including neurologic and neurodegenerative disease (autism, Alzheimer's), heart disease, cancer, and **autoimmune disease.**

Foods rich in antioxidants and phytonutrients protect the body from oxidative stress; highly processed foods contribute to oxidative stress.

## THE MULTIPLE HIT HYPOTHESIS

**System Overload!**
Kids at greater toxic risk than adults:
- Toxic dose per weight is much higher
- Less able to detoxify some chemicals
- Immature brain and rapid growth
- Critical development windows

SAD diet low in vital brain
and detoxification nutrients:
- Iron, zinc, magnesium,
  DHA, folate, choline, $B_{12}$,
  phytonutrients

IMMATURE/
DAMAGED BBB

INADEQUATE NUTRITION
FOR BRAIN DEVELOPMENT

INADEQUATE
PROTECTIVE NUTRIENTS

INCREASED OXIDATIVE STRESS

LEAD
MERCURY
ARSENIC

DETOXIFICATION
PATHWAYS

BPA
PHTHALATES
PFOS

PESTICIDE
RESIDUES

(DYSBIOSIS)
LEAKY GUT &
ENDOTOXINS

# DETOXIFICATION

Currently, much more emphasis is placed on avoiding exposure to dietary and environmental **toxicants** in alternative medicine than in Western medicine. In the eyes of the average physician, the term "detoxification" is stigmatized because of the focus on "detoxing" and "doing a cleanse" to reduce the body burden of toxins (naturally occurring) and toxicants (man-made) in integrative and alternative medicine circles. The health impact of toxic exposures often gets downplayed and attempts at discussion often result in eye-rolling and head shaking from many dubious, conventionally trained medical doctors.

Failing to recognize how multiple toxic substances may be interacting and catalyzing negative health effects, medical practice is lagging behind a growing base of evidence that a very real toxic threat exists to our children and our species, especially among our youngest and most vulnerable.

Over fifty years ago, Rachel Carson wrote her landmark book *Silent Spring* as a wakeup call that we still have not heard, a warning that has often been deliberately silenced. This worry about our physical environment is not "alternative pseudoscience" as vocal skeptic groups declare. The National Institute of Environmental Health Sciences division of the NIH, the Harvard and Yale Schools of Public Health, Duke University Integrated Toxicology and Environmental Health Program, NYU Department of Environmental Medicine, Imperial College London, King's College London, are not quacks. These and multiple other highly respected institutions, physicians, and researchers provide reliable evidence pointing to the serious hazards threatening our children's health.

The mounting evidence provided by scientists with impeccable research integrity is too extensive to ignore any longer, even for skeptics. I would also remind the skeptics that toxins, toxicants, and detoxification are fundamental physiological concepts we as doctors all learned in the first year of medical school. Environmental toxins have the capacity to harm the human body and detoxification is a basic biological process, essential to our health and survival. Let's review it here quickly to get the basics down in the context of children's health and why the infant and young child are at such high risk from toxic exposures.

## Detoxification Strategies

The human body tries to protect itself from potentially toxic compounds in several ways. In the mature GI tract, **probiotic** bacteria are a front-line player in the initial detoxification process, helping to bind or degrade certain compounds such as pesticides and heavy metals to make them less toxic and more easily excreted from the body.[12–14] The integrity of the gut barrier (those tight junctions we talked about earlier in Chapter 3) also helps to keep unwanted compounds out of the body.

However, the leading detoxification center of the body is the liver. Despite even the most vigilant efforts, any number of toxic compounds will enter our body and our bloodstream from our air, water, cosmetics, food, and medications. The liver is the vital organ that filters these toxic compounds as they are recognized in the blood and then metabolizes them in a two-phase detoxification process for elimination from the body.

*Phase 1 detoxification* uses special enzymes called cytochrome p450 (CYP) that start the detox process. CYP are known as a "superfamily" of over fifty enzymes that metabolize thousands of chemicals: toxins produced in the body and toxicants we are exposed to in our environment. These enzymes, present in most tissues of the body but highly concentrated in the liver, also play important roles in hormone synthesis and breakdown.

However, the initial Phase 1 process is incomplete and can temporarily make a substance more toxic until Phase 2 detoxification takes place.

*Phase 2 detoxification* involves one of several neutralizing compounds (sulfur compounds, methyl groups, glucuronic acid, glutathione, amino acids) being attached to the toxin by other enzymes in the liver, which limits damage to the body and allows the substance to be flushed out. Neutralized toxins can be excreted from the liver in the bile and pooped out, or they can be filtered from the blood and flushed out by the kidneys. Given the constant flow of toxicants, the liver takes a beating, but as long as it is not pushed too far, it has an amazing ability to regenerate itself and keep working.

Keep in mind that these detoxification enzymes cannot function without the help of vital nutrients acting as "coenzymes" and "co-factors" that help the enzymes work. Iron, zinc, magnesium, vitamin A, C, E, selenium, $B_6$, $B_{12}$, choline and folate are all essential to these detoxification processes. Many of the foods associated with improved health and longevity (i.e., fruits and vegetables) enhance the body's detoxification system, potentially enhancing both phase 1 and phase 2 detoxification.[15] Deficiencies in any of these crucial nutrients reduce the body's ability to eliminate toxic compounds and open the door to increased oxidative stress and damage. Also, some people may be more susceptible to certain toxins or have adverse reactions to certain medications because genetically (or epigenetically) they don't make one or several of the CYP detoxification enzymes, or a specific phase 2 detoxification process may be partially defective.

"Houston, we have a problem." When combining the toxic burden created by our increasingly compromised environment with a susceptible host (such as a baby) without the proper defense mechanisms and a nutrient deficient diet, we open the door for problems.

When the unborn or newborn child is hit with multiple toxic exposures, the dangers of this scenario worsen. Here are several reasons why the infant's brain is even more susceptible to these deficiencies and toxins than adults:

1. **They are small**. This means the *dose per weight* of the toxic insult is *much* higher in children than adults. Substances that might not affect an adult because they are present in less concentrated

amounts may be significantly more problematic to an infant or unborn child.

2. They have an **immature detoxification system** (Phase 1 and 2).[16,17] Our bodies have evolved amazing systems to neutralize and get rid of a large number of toxic compounds. Unfortunately, these detoxification systems take several years to mature. From basic pharmacology we know that an infant cannot clear medications as effectively as an adult can; their "machinery" isn't fully functional yet. For this reason, pediatric dosing for medications is often quite different than adult dosing.

   The same principle applies to other toxic insults to which the fetus or baby is vulnerable. Babies are not equipped to get rid of all the toxic elements they are being exposed to in the modern world, and so these chemicals have the capacity to do more damage in their developing bodies and brains. And contrary to previous thinking, the placenta does NOT filter out most toxins, so the unborn child is impacted by the same exposures as the mother.

3. They have an **immature blood brain barrier**. The blood brain barrier refers to the single layer of cells in the blood vessels of the brain that provide a screen between circulating blood and the brain cells. Optimally, it only allows key nutrients (glucose, vitamins, **ketones**) to pass into the brain and tries to keep out unwanted metabolites and toxicants. While present at birth, there are components of this barrier system that potentially do not mature until the child is at least 2 years old, and some evidence suggests even 20 years old.[18] This means the infant brain is potentially exposed to more toxins than an adult who has a fully developed blood brain barrier and detoxification system. A leaky or dysfunctional blood brain barrier in later life, which facilitates additional exposure of toxins to the brain, is now being implicated in autism and several adult neurological disorders, including Alzheimer's. Interestingly, a leaky brain may also be linked to a **leaky gut** and an altered **microbiome**.[19-23]

4. They are going through **critical neurodevelopmental windows** in the first thousand days that leave their infant brain especially vulnerable to toxic "hits" that occur during these developmental phases.[24] If a **neuron** (nerve cell) is damaged when it is new and growing and trying to make connections, it can die or

"short circuit." When this is done to millions of neurons, a developmental or neurological disorder may develop.

5. Infants cannot make their own healthy dietary choices. The unborn child and infant are reliant on the mother's dietary choices to supply their nutrient needs. **Common deficiencies of certain key nutrients** in the maternal/infant diet (zinc, iron, magnesium, folate, choline) further impairs their detoxification systems, leaving them more vulnerable to toxic insults. Highly processed food eaten by the mother may contain high levels of multiple harmful compounds that are delivered directly to that baby.

Taking into account the whole picture, we have a potential recipe for neurological disaster during the most vulnerable period of a child's life: multiple toxins, nutritional deficiencies, and an immature blood brain barrier and detoxification system—all impacting the baby brain. I agree with a growing number of physicians and researchers who believe these are the root causes in the rising incidence of neurodevelopmental and other brain disorders.

## How do parents protect their developing children?

1. Make sure that the mother is getting adequate nutrition, especially key nutrients that support the brain and detoxification during the pregnancy by taking an effective prenatal vitamin and following the dietary guidelines outlined in the previous chapter.

2. Avoid foods and beverages with potentially high toxicant levels and avoid using cosmetic or cleaning agents that contain neurotoxic or **endocrine disrupting chemicals**. Choose organic when possible to replace the Dirty Dozen fruits and vegetables to reduce the baby's exposure to pesticides. There are several apps available that help screen for cosmetics and foods that are considered "clean."

3. Support a healthy microbiome during the pregnancy, so these beneficial microorganisms can be passed on to the baby since their microbiome is a first line of defense.

4. The pregnant mother and child should eat a variety of fruits and vegetables as the antioxidants and **phytonutrients** contained in these foods have beneficial effects on detoxification pathways and are **epigenetic modifiers** (substances that modify gene behavior)

that can "turn down" inflammation and potentially activate genes involved with detoxification.[15,25]

5. Pay attention to the containers and packaging for foods and drinks. They often contain a significant amount of endocrine disrupting chemicals (EDCs) and other toxicants. Eating fewer processed foods will also lower these exposures.

---

## The 2020 "Dirty Dozen" highest pesticide foods by EWG

- Strawberries
- Spinach
- Kale
- Nectarines
- Apples
- Grapes
- Peaches
- Cherries
- Pears
- Tomatoes
- Celery
- Potatoes

## The 2020 "Clean Fifteen" lowest pesticide foods by EWG

- Avocados
- Sweet corn
- Pineapple
- Onions
- Papaya
- Sweet peas (frozen)
- Eggplants
- Asparagus
- Cauliflower
- Cantaloupes
- Broccoli
- Mushrooms
- Cabbage
- Honeydew melon
- Kiwi

---

## HOT TOPIC

### Are Organic Foods Better for You?

One of the most hotly debated topics of recent years has been whether organically grown foods are better, or if claims are all hype. Research coming out of the nation's top institutions suggests that commonly used pesticides pose a clear and present danger to a developing child. Not only are organically grown fruits and vegetables markedly lower in pesticide residues, but they are higher in antioxidants and phytonutrients, some of the most beneficial food components for our health.[26,27]

Some of the more dangerous pesticides are known as organophosphates (OP) but others have toxic potential as well. OPs have been mostly banned by the FDA for residential use because of their potential dangers but unfortunately are not banned in industrial agriculture.

Unless produced organically or locally from small farms, it may be difficult to determine whether fruits and vegetables have a significant amount of pesticides not only on but also in them. Washing food does not necessarily remove the pesticides.

These pesticides kill insects because their chemical compounds disrupt brain cells and nervous systems. In fact, OPs are also the key ingredients in nerve gas used in chemical warfare. The nervous systems of animals and humans share similar chemistry to insects. Scientific evidence shows that the growing infant may also be affected by these toxic chemicals, even with low levels of exposure. These toxic substances can affect the growing infant's brain cells and **neurotransmitters,** impacting neurological, mental and behavioral development.[28-30] Research and policy statements by the American Academy of Pediatrics and numerous public health groups support these concerns and are calling for widespread reform of OP pesticide use.[28,31]

OP pesticides can cross the placenta, directly exposing the unborn child. Remember that given their small size, immature detoxification routes, and critical developmental windows, the unborn child is more susceptible to toxic exposures. Early research focused on concerns related to pregnant mothers who were exposed while working and living in areas where industrial agriculture was predominant, notably with the heavy application of agrochemicals.

Numerous studies have linked OP pesticide exposures at levels commonly found on fruits and vegetables to birth defects, impairment in **neurodevelopment**, and loss of IQ points in the child. Exposure to these pesticides, as measured by detectable urine levels in children, has been associated with doubling the risk of having ADHD.[32-34] This does not prove causation, but is a concerning link worthy of further investigation. In fact, *all but one of 27 studies from 2002 to 2012 looking at OP pesticides and neurodevelopment in children showed a significant negative effect on children's brains, both in learning and behavior.*[30,35-38]

Recent research also suggests that OP pesticides harm the gut microbiome, promote "leaky gut," and are being linked to increased inflammation and development of obesity through several mechanisms.[41] Exposure to pesticides has been linked to leukemia and brain tumors in multiple studies.[35] On a reassuring note, five days on an organic diet eliminated detectable levels in children's urine.[27] There is also increasing evidence that even low levels of pesticide exposure in adult females may increase the risk of miscarriage, infertility, and difficulty conceiving a child.[42] In addition to food consumption, pesticides and herbicides can be absorbed through the air or skin. Having the lawn sprayed for weeds or the house sprayed for ants while pregnant is something to avoid.

To reduce exposure to organophosphate and other potentially dangerous pesticides

+ Choose organic when possible, especially for the "Dirty Dozen" fruits and vegetables. Don't worry as much about choosing organic for the "Clean Fifteen" fruits and vegetables.
+ Don't spray the lawn or garden with pesticides or herbicides when pregnant or when young children are active in the yard.
+ Maintain a healthy microbiome to help detoxify some of these compounds.

## Minimizing exposure to endocrine disrupting chemicals

In addition to the direct negative effects on the nervous system, OPs and other pesticides may also be endocrine-disrupting chemicals (EDCs). EDCs are a group of chemicals that have the capacity to mimic hormones and trigger or block hormone receptor sites, altering the body's natural balance of hormones. This can include disruption of thyroid hormones, estrogen and testosterone, and other crucial systems involved in the child's growth and brain development during the critical first thousand days.[39,40]

Food packaging may also contain endocrine disruptors that leach into food, into the body of a pregnant mother, and into the growing baby. Other routes of exposure can be plastic bottles, non-stick pans, cosmetics, sunscreens, flame retardants on clothing or furniture, and unfortunately, drinking water.

There are many important reasons why toxic exposures and EDCs are a serious concern for pregnant mothers and children in the first thousand days. EDCs have the potential to cause harm even at very low levels, making their damage even more insidious.

> Contrary to the "dose makes the poison" theory of toxicology, recent research refers to a non-monotonic dose response curve (NMDRC) which has been used to show that even low level human exposure to certain toxins can result in a physiological response (rising rates of disease) that appears to contradict a flawed assumption—that only high-dose hazards can be harmful to humans.[43-45]

Endocrine Disrupting Chemicals have the potential to[46,47]

+ Cross the placenta into the developing baby
+ Cause harm even at low doses
+ Disrupt critical developmental windows, which may cause irreversible damage
+ Trigger epigenetic programming for future disease
+ Place undue toxic burden on unborn and young children that do not have the ability to filter and eliminate these chemicals

Describing EDCs and their dangerous impact on children in the detail they deserve is beyond the scope of this book. To learn more about environmental impacts on our children in depth, see the referenced studies, journal articles, and books by leaders in this field at the end of this chapter. Here, I will focus on a few EDCs that deserve special attention: BPA (and its close relatives, BPS and BPF), Phthalates, and PFAS.

*Bisphenol A, Bisphenol S, and Bisphenol F*
Bisphenol A (BPA) is a chemical found in many plastics, microwave cookware, baby bottles, food can liners, plastic food packaging, and the paper receipts that get handed out with every store purchase. BPA is *everywhere*. BPA and its relatives BPS and BPF are insidious, entering the body from many sources, and research is showing that there is almost universal exposure in every human in this country and on the planet. This chemical is known for disrupting the endocrine system, potentially disturbing hormonal balance in both mother and child. BPA from mom's exposure crosses the placenta and is also delivered to the baby in breast milk.

There are numerous important reasons why we should be concerned about how these chemicals affect the child. BPA and its cousins BPS and BPF can affect sex hormones (like estrogen and testosterone) as well as thyroid hormone **metabolism**. A healthy balance of hormones is needed during the baby's development to help guide proper brain development and significantly impacts later learning and behavior. We do not want to disturb the hormonal balance in unborn or growing children, as disruption of the endocrine system during early development can have lifelong effects.

BPA and BPS are now suspected to be epigenetic modifiers, altering DNA expression in the unborn child.[48] Exposure during pregnancy is potentially linked to abnormalities in childhood behavior and brain function.[49–52] It is still unclear if there are particularly critical periods of prenatal exposure, and there may be differences in effects between boys and girls. A growing body of research indicates there is an association between BPA and autism spectrum disorder. A recent **meta-analysis** links early life BPA exposure to development of ADHD.[52] BPA and BPS can alter insulin production and release from the pancreas, raising concern that it contributes to type 2 diabetes and obesity.[53,54] There are also possible links between BPA exposure and certain cancers, many of which are hormone related, such as breast cancer, ovarian cancer, uterine or endometrial cancer, and prostate cancer.[55-57]

While BPA products are rapidly eliminated in the urine, it does not mean they don't interfere with hormones. Mothers and children are bombarded with these chemicals daily, exposing the baby to a constant dose of hormone-altering chemicals.

To minimize exposure

+ Avoid drinking out of plastic bottles. Use glass, ceramic, or stainless-steel containers.
+ Decrease intake of canned foods and look for BPA/BPS-free packaging.
+ Opt for electronic store receipts to avoid handling the printed receipts coated in BPA.

*Phthalates*
Phthalates are chemicals found in *plastics, cosmetics, perfumes, shampoos, body lotions, and sunscreens.* A mother can absorb these EDCs through the skin as well as through the digestive tract. Like BPA, phthalates are a known endocrine disruptor, are rapidly excreted in urine, and almost every person in the Western world has been exposed. Similar to BPA, phthalates are thought to interfere with thyroid metabolism, estrogen and testosterone, and alter adrenal hormones. There is also research looking into the role phthalates may play in **insulin resistance** and obesity.

The European Union (EU) classifies phthalates as a "reproductive toxicant" because of their ability to alter estrogen and testosterone metabolism. There are concerns and some studies showing potential association with phthalate exposure and infertility, as well as maternal exposure and birth defects like undescended testicles and hypospadias (in which the opening of the urethra is on the underside of the penis instead of at the tip) in boys.[58]

Prenatal exposure to phthalates is possibly linked to neurodevelopmental and behavioral issues in children in some studies, including risk of ADHD, autism, and reduced IQ although results have been inconsistent.[49,51,59–61] Male babies could be more adversely affected than females to phthalate exposure.

To minimize the baby's exposure to phthalates,

+ Purchase phthalate-free cosmetic products, shampoos, lotions, and sunscreen.
+ Don't microwave foods in plastic or pour hot liquids into plastic containers.
+ Reduce the amount of processed, prepackaged food in the diet; certain packaging materials can leach phthalates and other EDCs into the food.

### PFAS and PBDEs

This alphabet soup refers to a group of particularly nasty compounds including Perfluoroalkyl Substances (PFAS) and PolyBrominated Diphenyl Ethers (PBDE). These are chemicals found in nonstick coatings on cookware, flame retardants, and stain resistant coatings on clothing and furniture. These are potentially dangerous compounds because they do not rapidly excrete from the body or the environment and can last for *decades* in the soil, water, and the human body, which is why they are referred to as POPs (persistent organic pollutants). Exposure to these chemicals has increased markedly in the past twenty to thirty years and people in the US have the highest exposure in the world, at levels ten times greater than people living in Europe and Asia. American infants and toddlers have higher exposures than adults in the US as these chemicals are in mom's breast milk and also because of the amount of household dust that babies and toddlers are exposed to while crawling around on the floor.[62,63]

Household furnishings and clothing coated with flame retardant are thought to provide 80% of exposure. PFAS and PBDE from these items get into house dust on the floor, transferring from the baby's hands into their mouths. These extremely toxic chemicals are now known to contaminate drinking water in the US. EPA testing from 2013 to 2015 found significant amounts of PFAS in public water supplies in 33 US states (with increased contamination near industrial sites and military bases). More information about this alarming reality can be found in the recommended reading section.

These chemicals present a danger to our babies because they are known neurotoxins and endocrine disruptors. Exposure at vulnerable periods could affect the growth of infants, their brain development, immune function, and potentially predispose them to obesity by acting as an epigenetic modifier that turns on genes related to weight gain. They are known to disrupt thyroid metabolism which is essential for proper brain development in the growing baby. Three US studies and a meta-analysis have shown decreasing brain function as levels of these chemicals increased in the body.[64,65] There is also fairly conclusive evidence of negative effects on immune system function.[66-68]

> *National Toxicology Program director Linda Birnbaum testified before congress in 2019: "PFAS are extremely persistent in our environment, they are transported globally with widespread human exposure, and we are learning more each day about PFAS toxicity. PFAS ... affect multiple tissues in both males and females, of multiple species, at all developmental life stages, it's not just cancer. It's not just effects on the immune system, it's not just effects, for example, on the kidney or the liver, it's also effects on development and reproduction, and pretty much almost every system that you can think of."*

Based on the increasing evidence showing the potential damaging effects of these chemicals on our children, we should minimize exposure.

+ Drink filtered water as much as possible.
+ Eliminate the nonstick pots and pans, especially if they are scratched. Use stainless steel or cast-iron cookware instead.
+ Avoid clothing and furniture that contain flame retardant and stain-resistant EDCs.
+ Wash your baby's hands well before feeding. Damp mop floors frequently to catch more of the dust containing POPs.
+ Decrease your intake of fast food and take-out food as the packaging at many establishments contain PFAS.[69]

## Heavy Metals

Lead, arsenic, and mercury are elements known as heavy metals. Unlike iron and zinc, there is no use for these metals in the human body. They are all known to be significantly toxic to the brain of the child. The US Department of Health and Human Services ATSDR (Agency for Toxic Substances and Disease Registry, found at (https://www.atsdr.cdc.gov/) has made these metals a top priority of concern based on the frequency with which they occur in our environment and their potential for toxicity and human exposure.

### Lead

Lead has been notorious for decades as a common cause of brain damage and loss of IQ in children. Because of concerns about the impact of lead on our children, leaded gas was outlawed in the 1970s and leaded paint was outlawed in 1978. However, harm from elevated levels of lead on child development, including the loss of intelligence, is ongoing and has really only been recognized by the government in the last decade.[6] There are still a large number of children in the US being exposed to and harmed from lead, mostly by paint residues from older housing and tainted water. Lead levels of children can be found through routine testing by pediatricians who are concerned about exposure.

An estimated 18 million people are served by water systems that violate lead rules, and there are 6 million lead pipes in operation serving over 10 million people in the US. A Reuters study found 3000 areas in the US worse than Flint, Michigan, known for its public health water crisis of national infamy, which began in 2014 and is still unresolved. In the period from 1999 to 2010, an unbelievable 1.2 million children were estimated to be lead poisoned, and an estimated 500,000 kids under the age of 5 have elevated lead levels in the US.[70]

It is now thought that *significant loss of IQ points occurs at blood lead levels far below the previous acceptable cutoff of 10ug/dl*. In fact, the **CDC** admits that there is no safe lead level for children. The new CDC level for poisoning is now a blood level greater than 5 ug/dl. Many researchers are concerned about low-level exposure and what is referred to as *subclinical toxicity*—leading to behavioral and learning impairment without the other clinical symptoms of lead poisoning at blood levels as low as 2 ug/dl and below. Low-level lead exposure down to a blood level of 1.3 ug/dl is associated with ADHD, and low-level exposure is linked to increased delinquency and aggressive behavior in children.[6,70,71] *Top scientists are* *clearly stating there is no safe level of lead exposure*, especially to the baby in the mother's womb and the young child.

> Lead and other heavy metals are now also known to be transgenerational epigenetic modifiers, meaning that they can alter the genetic expression for generations to come. It is an unwanted gift that keeps on giving.

Take steps to reduce lead exposure in the home. If residing in older housing, watch for peeling and chipping paint that could end up in the dust and in the baby's mouth. Be very cautious if conducting any renovations on an older house, especially when pregnant or raising young children. I had a pair of lead-poisoned twins come into my office whose parents were renovating a 1930s house, stirring up enough old paint and dust to dangerously spike their kids' lead levels.

They moved the family out to continue the rest of the work, and their levels returned to a safe level. Home dust lead-testing kits are available if there is concern for contaminated dust in the house. (Go to www.nchh.org for more information on how to test house dust for lead). I would strongly suggest drinking filtered water for any pregnant mother or young child, or for any human for that matter.

*Arsenic*
Arsenic may be the "new lead." Exposure is rampant. This toxic metal contaminates 13% to 19% of US wells, with 40 to 50 million Americans currently relying on well water. This means millions of Americans may be getting slowly poisoned from their water. The **Natural Resources Defense Council (NRDC)** one of the nation's most powerful non-profit environmental watchdog organizations, calculated a much higher estimate of this danger, indicating that 30 to 50 million Americans were getting slowly poisoned by arsenic in tap water. The **World Health Organization** states that 200 million people worldwide are exposed to potentially harmful levels of arsenic.[72]

Arsenic is a naturally occurring metal in the soil, and elevated levels in drinking water are often caused by high soil concentrations rather than contamination. Known arsenic "hotspots" across the US have high soil levels of arsenic that can leach into well water making it too dangerous to drink. Mining, smelting, and industry are other known causes of arsenic contamination in the soil and water.

Because of its toxicity, the EPA lowered acceptable water levels of arsenic from 50 ug/L to the WHO recommended limit of 10 ug/L. However, Canada dropped the acceptable level to 5 ug/L. It is worth noting that the WHO adopted the current drinking water arsenic limit of 10 ug/L based on practical considerations of worldwide water quality, but recognize that optimal levels are likely much lower based on the associated long-term health risks.[72]

If arsenic is "naturally occurring," is it really something we should be concerned about? Various industry representatives might argue "no," completely disregarding the danger to our children. Arsenic is a serious concern. Arsenic damages the brain and causes cancer and immune-system impairment leading to increased risk of infections. It is also a "gateway toxin" and damages the protective blood-brain barrier (especially in the unborn child) and depletes glutathione, the main detoxification enzyme in our bodies, leaving us more susceptible to other toxic exposures.

Arsenic is now thought to be a powerful epigenetic modifier, turning on some genes linked with increased inflammation, poor birth outcomes, preterm birth, impaired lung function, neurodevelopmental impairment, increased susceptibility to infections, and future development of heart disease and cancer.[72,73] In adults, arsenic exposure is associated with increases in several cancers, as well as increased risk of heart disease. Clearly, arsenic is not a substance to which children should be exposed.

## HOT TOPIC

### The rice and arsenic conundrum

Contaminated well water is the main route of arsenic exposure, but arsenic in rice is an increasing concern. As just described, arsenic is a natural element in the soil found in higher levels in certain areas including those contaminated from high pesticide use or from mining and smelting. The more dangerous form of arsenic found in the soil, contaminated water, and rice is known as inorganic arsenic, and is toxic to the human body.

Because of the nature of the plant and the way in which it is grown, rice tends to absorb and retain more arsenic than other plants. Unfortunately, brown rice, typically viewed as healthier, is higher in arsenic than white rice because arsenic is concentrated in the fibrous husk. The arsenic content of rice and rice-based products depends on many factors, including the rice variety,[74] where and how it is grown, and how it is cooked and processed.[75,76]

Studies have shown a consistent association with rice consumption and arsenic levels; 1-year-old infants who regularly consumed rice products had double the arsenic detected in their urine.[77-79] Common foods of concern are rice, rice crackers, rice cereal, rice noodles/pasta, rice cakes, and rice milk.

Studies, including a Consumer Reports review in 2012, have shown considerable variation in the quantity of arsenic in rice and rice products. Based on the research, to reduce exposure to this toxic metal, consider the following:

- Cut back on specific brown rice-based products that are known to be higher in arsenic.
- Look for lower arsenic rice varieties. Rice grown in the southern US is reportedly higher in arsenic than white Basmati or Jasmine rice grown in certain areas of California, India, and the Himalayas.
- Limit the intake of rice crackers and rice cakes for young children because the arsenic levels in these may be higher than plain rice.
- Be cautious about rice milk.
- Use cooking methods that reduce the level of arsenic in the rice. Rice should be soaked in filtered water overnight, or at a minimum rinsed well prior to cooking.

*Mercury*

Mercury, another potent neurotoxic metal, is known to damage brain cells. There is increasing concern about the developmental effects of common low-level mercury exposures.[6,81-83] The main route of mercury exposure is through contaminated food, namely fish. *Two thousand tons* of mercury per year rain down on us worldwide, mostly from coal burning, and an estimated third of the world's total environmental mercury comes from coal burning in Asia. As this mercury rains down into the oceans, it is taken up by plankton, which then get eaten by small fish, which then get eaten by bigger fish, in a process known as bioaccumulation. The larger the fish, the more mercury they have accumulated in their tissues, and the more mercury a mother and her baby will take in if consuming these fish. This is why avoiding consumption of large fish like swordfish, grouper, shark, or even most tuna is important during pregnancy.

Unfortunately, we also know that the unborn child accumulates mercury from its mother, and levels in the baby can far exceed that of the mother.[84] The National Academy of Science has found evidence of mercury toxicity to the growing baby brain at even very low doses, so being strict about avoiding mercury during pregnancy is crucial. Not only is seafood becoming contaminated, but foods including vegetables and rice grown overseas in high coal-burning areas are increasingly found to be contaminated.[85] Be cautious of where food is grown, not only for the potential pesticide exposures, but also the mercury content. To see which fish are safe to eat during pregnancy, go to the Natural Resources Defense Council (NRDC) website and download their mercury wallet card that has listings of low, moderate, and high mercury fish. A partial list is available in the preceding chapter in Table 6.11. Smaller fish are a safer bet, and herring, sardines, trout, salmon are generally still considered safe and beneficial to eat.

## Water

Filter water to avoid lead and arsenic. Most grocery stores have DIY (do it yourself) filter stations where purified drinking water is available for 25 to 40 cents per gallon. If it is in the budget, people can have purified water delivered or home **reverse osmosis (RO)** filters installed. RO filters use a semi-permeable membrane to remove 99% of dissolved substances and bacteria. Popular pitcher filters remove some toxic substances, but arsenic removal was found inadequate in the majority of brands tested in one study. RO filters are more effective.[80] Additionally, when using pitcher filters, it is essential that charcoal filters are changed as recommended, or pollutants will not be properly filtered.

Do not gamble with water quality during pregnancy or childhood. Play it safe, and if you use well water, get it tested. Consider using RO filtered water, given that, in addition to arsenic, lead pipes are still in use all over the US. Schools should be routinely testing their water and installing RO filters if their water is contaminated. The health of the child's brain depends on healthy water.

## Electromagnetic fields and radiofrequency exposure and the child

The International Agency for Research on Cancer (IARC) and the World Health Organization (WHO) are among the institutions that have expressed ongoing concerns about exposure to **electromagnetic fields (EMF)** and **radiofrequency (RF) emissions** and their potential harm to the unborn or young child. All electronic devices give off EMFs but in our modern world of cell phones, laptops, and Wi-Fi our exposure to EMF and RF has steadily increased. While no *definitive* adverse health effects have been shown in the *adult* population using cell phones or electronics, there have been some concerning findings in recent research. However, research into the effects on the pediatric population and especially the unborn child is sparse.

The child in the womb and early in development may be more sensitive to effects of EMF and RF from electronics and cell phones for several reasons. Babies and young children have a high number of *stem cells*, which are cells that have not yet fully developed and may be more vulnerable to radiation. The brain of the fetus, baby, or child is more vulnerable during early critical periods of growth and development when such exposures may cause harmful effects that can be seen decades later. The baby's skull bones are also thinner than adults, providing less protection to the brain from these emissions. Studies in this area have raised serious interest and concern for the effects on children.[86-88]

EMFs have been shown in numerous studies to alter the body's immune system, but the long-term effects this could have on the unborn or young child are currently unknown.[89-91] In a study done by Kaiser Permanente, they found a **linear dose-response** relationship, showing association between EMF exposure in pregnant mothers and risk of developing asthma in children.[92] Some animal studies have shown unfavorable brain changes in young animals when they or their pregnant mother were exposed to EMF and RF from mobile phones.[93-95] Studies have shown that laptops, when placed in the lap of a pregnant mother expose the unborn child to EMF above safety standard levels.[96]

There is enough preliminary data to warrant caution and further research. The BabySafe Project is a collaborative comprised of physicians and researchers around the world who have concerns about the effects of radiation on young brains. The WHO has an ongoing initiative called the International EMF Project to support ongoing research. The EMF produced by mobile phones are classified by the International Agency for Research on Cancer as possibly carcinogenic to humans. *In France and several other European countries, Wi-Fi has been banned in preschools and kindergartens because of concerns for the possible adverse effects on young children.*

I am not advising that mothers move to a cave while pregnant or for the first thousand days of a child's life. The research may still be sparse and inconclusive that EMF are harmful to children, but let's not automatically assume that these exposures are safe for the youngest and most vulnerable members of our world. It's all about awareness and precaution.

When it comes to our children's health, let's apply the "precautionary principle" which asserts that "the burden of proof for potentially harmful actions by industry or government rests on the *assurance of safety* and that when there are threats of serious damage, scientific uncertainty must be resolved in favor of prevention." [97]

Although definitive harm has not been proven, be aware that electronics, cell phones, and laptops could have negative effects on infants and young children. Consider taking some steps to decrease this exposure:

+ Don't use a laptop in your lap when pregnant or use one of the EMF shields on the market.
+ Don't leave cell phones right next to the developing baby for prolonged periods.
+ Don't let young children hold cell phones up to their heads for prolonged periods.
+ Evaluate the home Wi-Fi system and the location of routers in relation to a pregnant mother or infant.
+ Review if your baby monitor could be a source of high levels of RF radiation.
+ Check out www.babysafeproject.org for more resources on this topic.

# NUTRITION R$_X$

We covered a lot in this chapter, and this new information may seem overwhelming. Try to keep in mind that even a series of small improvements can decrease the risks of cumulative toxic exposures and give our babies a better start in life.

**1** Drink filtered water to avoid contamination by lead, arsenic, or harmful organic compounds (PFAS). Pitcher-type filters are okay, but reverse osmosis (RO) is better.

**2** Consider getting tap or well water tested for lead and arsenic if there is any chance of contamination (as there is a *significant* chance of contamination in many households).

**3** Eat organic whenever possible, especially the Dirty Dozen foods, to avoid harmful pesticide residues. Costco, Sam's Club and Walmart now carry organic frozen foods, which make them more affordable.

**4** Support local organic farms and Community Supported Agriculture (CSAs) that do not use harmful pesticides; many accept food stamps now making them accessible to more people.

**5** Eat real, unprocessed foods as much as possible during pregnancy, and avoid the highly processed packaged foods that contain multiple additives, preservatives, hidden sugar, and endocrine disrupting chemicals.

**6** Shop, prepare, and cook your own food as much as possible—it is the best way to control what mom and baby are getting in their bodies.

**7** When selecting fish, use caution and verify that mercury levels are safe for mom and baby.

**8** Never microwave foods in plastic containers; store foods in glass or ceramic as much as possible.

**9** Drink out of stainless steel or glass water bottles or find BPA/BPS free containers; eliminate plastic baby bottles and use glass.

**10** Read the labels on cosmetics and avoid phthalates and other harmful compounds.

**11** Do your research and select cosmetics and household products that are safe for infants and pregnant mothers. Several Apps exist to help select products that do not contain phthalates and other potentially harmful chemicals.

## RECOMMENDED READING

1.  Leo Trasande, Sicker, Fatter, Poorer: The Urgent Threat of Hormone-Disrupting Chemicals to Our Health and Future. . . and What We Can Do About It (Mariner Books, 2019).

2.  Phillipe Grandjean, Only One Chance: How Environmental Pollution Impairs Brain Development -- and How to Protect the Brains of the Next Generation (Oxford University Press, 2015).

3.  The Environmental Working Group: www.ewg.org

4.  Natural Resources Defense Council: www.nrdc.org

5.  The National Institute of Environmental Health Sciences research on EDCs: https://www.niehs.nih.gov/research/programs/endocrine/index.cfm

6.  The NYU Division of Environmental Pediatrics: https://med.nyu.edu/departments-institutes/pediatrics/divisions/environmental-pediatrics/

7.  For more information on the HELIX exposome project: http://projecthelix.eu/

8.  For more information on the dangers of PFAS: https://www.reuters.com/article/us-usa-water-foreverchemicals-idUSKBN1ZL0F8 https://www.nationalgeographic.com/science/2020/01/pfas-contamination-safe-drinking-water-study/ https://www.ewg.org/research/national-pfas-testing/ https://factor.niehs.nih.gov/2019/5/feature/1-feature-pfas/index.htm

9.  US Geological Survey on Arsenic in Drinking Water: https://www.usgs.gov/mission-areas/water-resources/science/arsenic-and-drinking-water

10. For more information on EMF and potential health effects: www.babysafeproject.org https://ehtrust.org/

# CHAPTER EIGHT

# BREASTFEEDING

There is no argument. For the infant, breast milk really is nature's most perfect food. The contents and composition of breast milk have been perfectly designed over millions of years to provide all the essential calories and nutrients in the optimal levels and ratios. Yet breast milk is so much more than just calories, vitamins, and minerals; it is a dynamic interactive system of communication from the mother's immune system to the baby's, helping to prevent infection and allergies. It perfectly supports the development of the baby's **microbiome** and the digestive system and is the superior food for maximizing brain and nervous system growth. Furthermore, it promotes vital infant-mother bonding.

However, the reality is that not all mothers can breastfeed for physical, social, or psychological reasons. There are also situations when the infant does not have access to breast milk because of illness, adoption, or foster care. This chapter is not meant to be a "guilt trip" for mothers who have to formula feed. Rather, if you are formula feeding, it is important to know not all formulas are created equal. In the next chapter I will give you the knowledge and tools to pick the best one possible for your child. In these cases, choose a formula that mimics breast milk as described in this chapter, to provide nutrition as close to nature as modern science can get us.

Remember, the ultimate goal in feeding our children is to optimize the growth and development of their brain and body, support a healthy microbiome, and minimize epigenetic programing for future disease. One of the best ways to help accomplish these goals is to breastfeed our infants. Breast milk is truly a miracle of evolution, and the incredible properties and benefits are still being uncovered by modern science.

In this chapter we will take a deeper look into what it is that makes mother's milk such a superfood, and how we are using this knowledge to continually improve infant formula to more closely mirror the real thing.

I feel it is important to educate and inform *everyone* of the significant benefits of breastfeeding. Becoming armed with the most updated information about how breast milk benefits the infant should encourage us all to improve social and systemic support structures for new mothers. Breastfeeding can be *hard*, especially with your first child. It can be frustrating, painful, and demoralizing but support is available (several resources are listed at the end of the chapter). However, the breastfeeding mother still needs more systemic support. We need to convince partners, spouses and families, healthcare professionals, employers, and the general public to support the breastfeeding mom any way they can. We hope to convince more mothers to start breastfeeding, and if possible, stick with it to the one-year mark or beyond. The benefits for children are potentially lifelong, and everyone in society wins when children are healthier.

## Breastfeeding by the Numbers

The American Academy of Pediatrics (AAP)[1] recommends that infants be exclusively breastfed for the first six months, with continued breastfeeding alongside the introduction of appropriate complementary foods until the age of one year or longer. The Canadian Paediatric Society and the WHO extends this recommendation internationally to 2 years of age.[2]

There are clear health benefits to breastfeeding for both the infant and the mother, and yet

Only 44% of babies are exclusively breastfed until 6 months worldwide.

1 in 5 babies in the US are never breastfed at all.

Less than 50% of infants in the US are breastfed exclusively without use of formula by 3 months of age.

Young mothers less than 20 are much less likely to initiate any breastfeeding.

Only 25% of US babies are breastfed exclusively without use of formula for the first 6 months.

75%–90% of mothers start out breastfeeding in the US and Canada, but many stop because of challenges.

Only 25% of infants are still being breastfed at 12 months of age.

60% of women do not breastfeed as long as they intended initially.

Barriers to breastfeeding and a lack of support for many mothers influence the duration of breastfeeding. According to the **CDC** and the Surgeon General, the top obstacles include

+ Issues with lactation and latching
+ Concerns about infant nutrition and weight gain
+ Mother's concern about taking medications while breastfeeding
+ Unsupportive work policies and lack of parental leave
+ Cultural norms and/or lack of family support
+ Unsupportive hospital practices and policies
+ Lack of knowledge about proper breastfeeding technique and the health benefits to the baby

Nearly a quarter of US hospital maternity wards used to give babies formula as a general practice. Hospitals also used to supply formula samples to new moms as a marketing technique, but this practice is currently being phased out. This had been occurring in over 65% of the US hospitals as of 2012, according to the AAP. Thanks to the Baby Friendly Hospital Initiative, fewer hospitals are giving out free samples of infant formula to new moms and are dedicating resources to encourage breastfeeding and supply lactation support. There are now more than six hundred Baby-Friendly designated hospitals in the USA, where close to a third of babies are born.

## TEN STEPS TO PROMOTE SUCCESSFUL BREASTFEEDING-
## WHO AND THE BABY FRIENDLY HOSPITAL INITIATIVE

+ Communicate a written breastfeeding policy to all healthcare staff.
+ Train all healthcare staff in the skills necessary to implement this policy.
+ Inform all pregnant women about the benefits and management of breastfeeding.
+ Help mothers initiate breastfeeding within one hour of birth.
+ Show mothers how to breastfeed and maintain lactation, even if they are separated from their infants.
+ Give infants no food or drink other than breast milk unless medically indicated.
+ Practice rooming in; allow mothers and infants to remain together 24 hours a day.
+ Encourage breastfeeding on demand.
+ Give no pacifiers or artificial nipples to breastfeeding infants.
+ Establish breastfeeding support groups for assistance after discharge from the hospital or birth center.[1,3]

## STATISTICAL HEALTH BENEFITS OF BREASTFEEDING
## FOR THE INFANT AND YOUNG CHILD

There are many health benefits for breastfeeding babies.[1,2,4] Studies on breastfed babies show numerous reductions in health risks as compared to those who are formula fed.

3-fold reduction in the risk of being hospitalized for respiratory infections

74% reduction in the severity of respiratory syncytial virus (RSV), a serious viral lung infection that can hit newborns the hardest

50% lower chance of ear infections

63% reduction in overall ear and throat infections

64% reduction in gastrointestinal infections

77% reduction in necrotizing enterocolitis (NEC), a life-threatening intestinal disease of the newborn

36% lower chance of sudden infant death syndrome (SIDS)

27%–42% reduction in the occurrence of asthma and eczema (depending on family history)

52% reduction in rates of celiac disease

31% reduction in incidence of childhood Crohn's disease and colitis

15%–30% reduction in the rates of becoming obese

30% reduction in incidence of type 1 diabetes

40% reduction in incidence of type 2 diabetes

20% reduction in risk for childhood leukemia

In addition, some studies indicate that the exclusive breastfeeding of infants results in higher intelligence scores and academic performance ratings in school age children. The beneficial cognitive effect was even larger for premature infants who were breast versus formula-fed. Breastfeeding also protects the mother, with reduction in the risk of breast and ovarian cancer by 28% if the mom has breastfed for a year.[1,2]

The benefits of breastfeeding are clear and profound enough that the Centers for Disease Control (CDC), the Surgeon General's office, the **American Academy of Pediatrics** (AAP) and the **World Health Organization** (WHO) are all working hard to change policies and improve support for the breastfeeding mother. The bottom line is that not enough mothers are breastfeeding or not breastfeeding long enough to maximize the health benefits to the child. We need to encourage breastfeeding as the optimum choice for all moms, not set them up for failure from the get go. By educating all mothers about the benefits of breastfeeding, we can empower them to make a fully informed decision. Access to support groups and skilled lactation consultants should be a part of perinatal care for every mother. Offering more support to both new and experienced mothers is vital for feeding our children in the early stages.

## WHAT IS IN BREAST MILK?

Lots of important things![5-8] Let's take a brief look at the ingredients in breast milk and how they benefit the baby. The three main ingredients in breast milk are lactose (milk sugar), lipids (fats) that supply energy for the baby and building blocks for their brain, and a special ingredient called **human milk oligosaccharides (HMO)** that feeds the infant microbiome. Breast milk also contains proteins for the growth of the infant as well as immune proteins that help the infant fight off disease and "teaches" the immature immune system of the baby. It contains all the vitamins and minerals needed for the growth of a term infant up until roughly six months of life when it is time to add complementary foods. (See the next chapter, Baby's First Foods.).

Previously thought to be very stable in content, it is now known that *breast milk composition is variable, and that the mother's diet can impact the content of her breast milk for better or worse.* Nutrients like vitamin $B_6$, $B_{12}$, choline, and the type of fat in breast milk all vary with the mother's diet. The body does not "filter out" the undesirable things a mother may be eating, so it is important for the breastfeeding mother to eat a healthy diet, continue her prenatal vitamin And consider other supplements that may be needed to optimize breast milk content, depending on her diet. We will go into these factors more later in this chapter.

### Carbohydrates in breast milk

Breast milk has its calories primarily from fat (50%) and lactose (40%). The fact that human milk contains lactose should probably tell you that it is the best carbohydrate source for the infant, NOT sucrose (table sugar) or fructose (fruit sugar or high fructose corn syrup) or even glucose. The amount of lactose in breast milk is thought to be stable and not dependent on the mother's diet, but lactose content decreases and fat content increases the longer a mother breastfeeds.

*What if my baby is lactose intolerant?*
A commonly circulated myth is that infants are often lactose intolerant, which is patently false. True deficiency in the ability to digest lactose in an infant is *very* rare, maybe one in a million children (with the exception of Finland, where it is slightly more common). Why would mother nature make a baby intolerant to the source of almost half its calories? She wouldn't. Whereas 70%–80% of adults in the world are lactose intolerant, babies, except in rare cases, are not.[9]

In reality, babies are commonly intolerant or allergic to the cow's milk or soy proteins contained in formula or being expressed through mom's breast milk but are unlikely to be lactose intolerant unless there has been some damage to their intestines from a viral infection or from an allergic process. When you remove the offending allergen (milk or soy), and allow the gut to heal, often any transient **lactose intolerance** will disappear.

Lactose (known as a disaccharide) is made of two sugars and is broken down by the intestinal enzyme lactase into the individual sugars, glucose and galactose, prior to absorption. Glucose and specialized energy molecules called **ketones** (derived from fat) are the primary fuel source for the infant brain. The baby's brain consumes 70% of the total calories they eat over the first year of life, versus the adult brain, which consumes only 20%.[10,11] No wonder babies get so hangry! (hungry + angry = hangry) Adequate calories (glucose and ketones) are obviously very important to keep this supply chain going. Galactose from lactose can be used for energy but is also a component of important structural compounds in the brain called sphingolipids. Sphingolipids are an important part of the nerve insulation **myelin,** which is vital for the growing and developing brain.[12] Lactose also helps promote a proper microbiome in the infant gut by acting as a prebiotic, and provides some fuel to the developing microbiome.[13] Formulas with lactose have resulted in higher counts of the **probiotic** *Bifidobacteria* in the infant and decreased counts of harmful bacteria.[14-16] It is also felt that lactose helps with the absorption of calcium and other minerals.[9,13]

*Maternal high fructose diet and breast milk "secondhand" sugar*
Human milk does not naturally contain much, if any, fructose. Fructose will be explored in more detail in Chapter 17. Fructose is a sugar only meant to be eaten in small amounts and never in significant amounts by infants. Small amounts of fructose are found naturally in the context of a fruit or vegetable, but not in the massive amounts people are getting

in modern society thanks to added sugar in our foods and sweetened drinks like soda. It has recently been discovered that a mother consuming considerable amounts of sugar and high fructose corn syrup will have detectable levels of fructose in her breast milk, essentially "sweetening it up." Another recent study showed that breast milk fructose remains elevated for five hours after the mother drinks a standard sized soda beverage with a meal.[17] The infant is not designed to metabolize fructose and researchers are becoming concerned about potential negative consequences and long-term health implications, including increased risk for future obesity and **type 2 diabetes** due to epigenetic programming.[18] This is yet another reason for the pregnant and lactating mother to minimize consumption of sweetened drinks such as soda and other high-sugar foods and drinks.

### Fat content of breast milk

Healthy human breast milk contains a considerable amount of fat. If you have ever seen a bottle of pumped breast milk, the cream truly rises to the top. This fat not only supplies the bulk of the necessary calories for the infant, but also is the major component by weight of the developing baby brain. Don't forget that the infant brain *doubles* in weight by 6 months, then grows another 40% by age 1. Most of this brain weight gain is actually fat! Consequently, babies' brains need lots and lots of fat to grow and develop, which is why breast milk is so high in fat.

During this period of life, infant brain development could be negatively impacted by inadequate or improper fat intake by the mother. Fat is the most variable component of breast milk, depending on the mother's diet, and human milk contains dozens of types of fat.[19-22] The amount of fat is also higher in the hindmilk, the milk at the end of the feed, as compared to the early milk. The fat composition of breast milk of women in one European study was found to have 35%–40% **saturated fat** such as palmitic acid, 50% monounsaturated fat (think olive oil), and 15% **polyunsaturated fats (PUFAs)**.[20,23,24] The fat in breast milk will quickly conform to the type of fat in the mother's diet within two to three days, reflecting her intake.[7] This conformity is a good thing if her diet contains healthy amounts of **omega-3** (EPA/DHA) from fish or supplements, monounsaturated fat from sources like olive and avocado oil, some (but not excessive) saturated fat (meat, coconut oil), and not too much vegetable oil. High **omega-6** vegetable oils in the Western diet have been crowding out other healthy fats for the last forty years and are easily damaged (**oxidized**) when heated, representing a potential health threat. Omega-3 and omega-6 fats need to be in balance in the diet to avoid displacing those vital omega-3 in breast milk. Healthy amounts of omega-6 fats are found in vegetables, nuts, and seeds, as well as the long chain omega-6 **ARA** in meat, poultry, and eggs. Moms need to avoid the dangerous trans and hydrogenated fats and minimize her intake of deep-fried foods during pregnancy and lactation to protect the growing baby brain.[25]

Breast milk levels of the vital omega-3 DHA are the most dependent on mom's diet, but amounts of omega-6 ARA are more stable. DHA and ARA are crucial to baby's brain and eye development in the first thousand days. During this period, 40,000 **synapses** (brain connections) are formed *every second*, and proper formation of these synapses depend on omega-3 DHA. As discussed in the last chapter, most moms are not getting enough omega-3 DHA in their diet. Moms who eat fish or take fish oil supplements when they breastfeed have measurably higher DHA in their breast milk, and their children are found to have higher amounts of DHA in their brains, which may improve cognitive performance later in life. Vegetarian and vegan moms have been found to have lower omega-3 LCPUFA in their breast milk (up to seven times lower), so this is a population who really needs to supplement this important nutrient. Intake of roughly 200 to 300mg of DHA a day or combined 500 mg of EPA + DHA has been recommended by some expert committees for breastfeeding moms. There is limited conversion of plant-based omega-3 (**ALA** from flax seed oil, nuts, canola, or soybean oil) into EPA and even less to vital DHA in the breast milk, so DHA should optimally be supplied in the diet pre-formed. That being said, consuming foods rich in ALA during breastfeeding (nuts, flax, green leafy vegetables) will help produce some EPA and help balance out the omega-6 in the diet.[7,20,21,24,26]

One fat used for energy production is called **medium chain triglyceride** (MCT), which is a short chain saturated fat with numerous potential health benefits. MCTs are getting a lot of press lately as they support a process called **ketosis**, where fats are processed in the liver to form clean burning energy molecules called ketones. Ketones can be burned for energy by many tissues and are the only other fuel source besides glucose that the brain can use. High levels of ketones, which can develop in diabetics and in a few other health conditions, leads to a dangerous condition called **ketoacidosis**. Having lower levels of ketones in the body is called *nutritional ketosis* and is not dangerous and is the *normal state of health* for the breastfed infant! The newborn breastfed infant is continuously in a state of nutritional ketosis, supported by the MCT in breast milk, which can constitute anywhere between 4% to 27% of breast milk fat and represent up to 10% of their calorie intake.[27-29]

Interestingly, ALA, the shorter chain omega-3 fat found in oils such as flaxseed and canola, is largely used for the production of ketones in the infant, rather than being converted to the brain-friendly DHA, which indicates that ketones also have a high level of importance in the developing human brain. As it is now known, the brain loves ketones, especially in the infant, and the steady supply of ketones likely has some neurological and developmental benefit to the infant. More in-depth studies on this are needed to thoroughly understand this process. Ketogenic diets are known to treat certain seizure disorders and potentially help delay the cognitive decline in conditions such as Alzheimer's, so there is an established link with brain function and ketones in both children and adults. That being said, I would not advise a breastfeeding mom to be on a ketogenic diet or taking high doses of MCT oil, as we don't really know what this might do to her breast milk or to the baby.

*Milk Fat Globule Membrane (MFGM)*[30-32]
Breast milk delivers healthy fats in a triple wrapped bundle called **Milk Fat Globule Membrane** (MFGM). This molecule is being researched for its importance in the development of the human gut and brain. It is made up of a mix that includes close to 200 different proteins and a variety of specialized fats including phospholipids (such as phosphatidylcholine), sphingomyelin and gangliosides (important for nerve development and insulation), and cholesterol. Preliminary studies on supplementing MFGM in formula-fed infants suggest improved **neurodevelopment**, intestinal growth and maturation, immune system function, and a healthier microbiome. Currently only a few commercially available formulas contain MFGM.

## Breast milk proteins
Mother's milk contains a variety of proteins, both for infant growth and protection against infections. The main proteins in animal milk are divided into **casein** and **whey**. Interestingly, human milk has the *lowest concentration of casein* of any animal milk.[20] Human milk is much higher in whey, and ranges from only 20% to 50% casein over the course of lactation, which is quite different from cow's milk protein which is close to 80% casein and only 18% whey. Essentially the whey and casein ratios in

these two milks are *opposite,* especially earlier in lactation. Casein proteins are much larger and less soluble in the infant stomach compared to whey, and can be potentially harder to digest and more allergenic.[51] This can be clinically important in the infant with an immature digestive system; it may be beneficial to have more easily digestible proteins (whey) available. Several infant formulas now manipulate their proteins to more closely resemble the whey and casein ratios found in human milk to decrease the chance of the infant developing an allergic response and improve digestibility to mitigate infant reflux.

Other proteins in human milk help fight off infections. A large number of white blood cells found in breast milk attack bacteria and viruses directly, but these cells also teach the infant's own immune cells how to work properly, increasing the maturity level of the child's immune system. These immune cells found in breast milk include both macrophages (the "seek and destroy" immune cells), as well as T-cells and other lymphocytes (white blood cells).[6] Lactoferrin is found in high amounts in mother's milk, which is a protein that inhibits many infectious organisms like bacteria, viruses, and fungal invaders. Antibodies from the mother, the highest concentration of which is known as secretory IgA, help to bind and destroy bacteria and viruses adding additional protection for the infant.

Numerous proteins that act as *growth factors* to help with development and maturation of the intestines are also found in breast milk. These proteins (including TGF-b, epidermal growth factor, and brain derived neurotrophic factor) have been identified to promote proper development of the gut nervous system. The human gut lining includes more than 100 million nerve cells—acting in some ways like a brain, and in fact, the gut "talks" to the brain and the baby's microbiome. This communication in the infant gut helps to stimulate proper intestinal motility as well as preventing excessive inflammation and "leaky gut" described earlier. Given these factors it is easy to see why breastfed children are known to have lower risk for infection, as well as lower risk of allergies and **autoimmune diseases** later in life; their immune system gets a significant boost right from the beginning.

### Human Milk Oligosaccharides (HMOs)[33–36]
Breast milk contains the ultimate baby prebiotic called human milk oligosaccharides (HMOs). Oligosaccharides are carbohydrates produced in the breast milk that are not digestible by babies but travel intact to the colon where they feed the beneficial probiotic bacteria and "talk" to the immune

system of the gut. HMOs are the third largest component of breast milk, so they must be very important to the growing infant and their gut bacteria. There are more than 200 different types of HMOs produced by the mother that have been identified, and each mother's composition of HMOs is different and may in some ways mirror her blood type.

HMOs have several important roles in the infant that have been recently discovered that involve protection against infection, development of the immune system and supporting the infant microbiome. HMOs directly feed the microbiome, especially an important species called *Bifidobacterium infantis* (*B. infantis*). *B. infantis* is an early colonizer of the infant gut and sets up camp in the intestine of the baby, helping boost the immune function, decrease inflammation, and promote proper intestinal motility. This is more evidence that there is no better way to support the proper colonization of the infant intestine with healthy probiotic bacteria than to breastfeed.

HMOs have also been found to decrease the ability of bad bacteria to bind to the intestine, making the bad bacteria easier to destroy and eliminate. This class of molecules directly communicate with immune cells in the baby's intestines and regulates the inflammatory response and activity of the gut immune system. There is some evidence that HMOs help prevent both diarrheal and respiratory illnesses in the infant.

HMOs also directly increase the production of **short chain fatty acids (SCFA)** by probiotic bacteria. Recall from the microbiome chapter that SCFA are fuel for the intestinal cells, help to decrease intestinal inflammation, and may have a role in neurodevelopment, potentially acting as **epigenetic modifiers** turning off harmful genes.[37] Synthesized HMOs are now being added to some infant formulas because of increasing recognition of their importance to the microbiome. While not identical to human HMOs, synthetic HMOs still appear to hold some of the same health benefits. Breastfeeding and HMO intake both have been shown to reduce the number of harmful bacteria in the infant gut such as *Klebsiella* and *Enterobacter*, as well as *E. coli*. Supplementation of HMOs in formula improves stool frequency and helps formula-fed infants to develop stool patterns that more closely resemble those of breastfed infants.[38]

## Other vital nutrients

*Choline*

Another vital nutrient for the growing baby brain is choline. Choline was discussed earlier in the context of important nutrients for the pregnant mother, but the importance doesn't stop at birth. It is also equally important for the growing infant to receive this nutrient throughout early life. Choline is considered a B vitamin that is involved with nerve growth and function; it is an important part of the nerve cell membrane as well as one of the main **neurotransmitters** called **acetylcholine**. It is also a key player in **methylation** pathways that can help with detoxification and epigenetic signaling. Breast milk contains a significant amount of choline in several forms, but mostly as water soluble *phosphocholine* and *glycerophosphocholine (GPC)*.

To some degree, the choline content of breast milk may be variable and dependent on the mother's diet and the mother's genetics.[39] Prior studies have shown an increase in breast milk concentration of choline with a higher choline diet or choline supplementation. However, baseline breast milk choline was found to be similar in two very different ethnic populations given sufficient choline in the maternal diet.[40] The current recommendation is for infants to receive 125 mg of choline per day. This amount was determined by prior estimates of healthy breast milk intake by a term infant (born at a gestational age of 37 to 42 weeks).

It is worth noting that many mothers worldwide are getting less than the recommended maternal dietary choline intake of 550 mg per day. This deficit could result in suboptimal choline content of breast milk, leaving the infant with less than they need for optimal brain development. What long-term effects this may have on the baby are currently being studied.

There is an apparent relationship between choline and folate, and mothers carrying an **MTHFR** mutation (discussed in the chapter on maternal nutrition) may be at increased risk for lower than optimal choline levels. Inadequate maternal intake of folate may lower choline levels in the body and breast milk.[41,42] There is evidence that choline works synergistically with the omega-3 DHA and lutein, two nutrients in breast milk that may promote optimal brain and memory function.[43,44] Prior recommendations for pregnant women carry over to lactating mothers, including a diet with sufficient choline rich foods (meat, fish, and eggs and clean sourced liver if available—refer to the list in chapter 6). If quantities of these foods are not consumed at sufficient levels, breastfeeding mothers should consider taking a choline supplement of 500 mg daily to ensure that the breast milk has enough of this crucial nutrient.

### Lutein and Other Phytonutrients

Lutein is an antioxidant found in green leafy plants and egg yolks. It is a relative of beta-carotene that is concentrated in breast milk. It is found in the baby's eyes and brain and is felt to be important in infant eye and brain development and protection. Breast milk levels are highly dependent on maternal intake, so this is yet another reason to make sure that mothers are eating a lot of fresh vegetables when pregnant and lactating.[45] Countries with a higher average vegetable intake than the US have 2- to 3-fold higher lutein levels in their breast milk.[46] A high vegetable diet will ensure that breast milk has optimal levels of lutein to support the baby's eyes and brain. Remember that lutein may work synergistically with choline and omega-3 DHA.

Lutein is just one of many protective plant compounds called phytonutrients found in fruits and vegetables. Recent studies have shown that a significant number of these **antioxidant** phytonutrients are found in mothers' milk, likely acting to protect the baby from **oxidative stress** and toxic chemicals in the environment. These compounds (other than lutein) are not found in formula; they will also be in lower supply in the milk of a mother who eats fewer fruits and vegetables. Breastfeeding mothers should continue "eating the rainbow" of colorful fruits and vegetables to maximize the delivery of these phytonutrients to the baby.[47,48]

### Breast Milk Microbiome

Breast milk is *not* sterile, nor should it be! Over *two hundred species of bacteria, possibly up to one thousand, have been identified in the human breast milk microbiome.*[35,49,50] These organisms reflect the intestinal microbiome of the mother. There is a process by which probiotic bacteria are transported from the mom's intestine and delivered intact to the breast for secretion into the milk, which is then consumed by the baby. This is another route by which mother nature continues to support the microbiome of the infant after the initial inoculum of bacteria from the birthing process (unless they were a C-section delivery). An estimated 800,000 bacteria daily are delivered to the infant through the breast milk. This would suggest several things:

+ It is important for the mother to maintain a healthy microbiome during pregnancy *and* lactation.

+ These probiotic bacteria are extremely important, as there are duplicate means of introduction into the infant's gut from the mother. When you take into consideration the HMOs and other milk oligosaccharides that are powerful **prebiotics**, it is obvious that mother nature is not messing around when it comes to supporting these healthy intestinal bacteria.

+ Adding one or two probiotic species to a formula may not be sufficient to perform the job mother nature intended.

## COLIC AND REFLUX: WHEN TO CONSIDER ELIMINATION DIETS

Infant colic, which refers to excessive fussiness and crying (greater than three hours per day for more than three days per week) can push a parent to the brink. Anyone who has had a colicky infant knows the stress that this puts on the entire household, and unfortunately can be a trigger for "non-accidental trauma" to the baby, such as shaken baby syndrome. The combination of a colicky infant and sleep deprived parent can be dangerous, so it should be taken seriously. These parents must get help and support!

Criteria of "Classic" Infant Colic

+ Crying lasting 3 hours or more per day
+ Crying episodes at least 3 or more days per week
+ Begins in first 3 weeks of life
+ Peaks at 6-8 weeks of age
+ Episodes start to decrease after 12 weeks of age
+ Perceived to be more than normal amount of crying for age
+ Baby is healthy and behaves normally between episodes
+ Happens at predictable times during the day
+ Fussy episodes are not relieved by normal consoling activities (rocking, soothing)

People in the field of pediatrics, especially those that have their own children, understand how soul crushing this phase of parenthood can be. The good news is that this phase only lasts a few months, and there may be ways to help a colicky baby. Recent research provides good evidence that infant colic is associated with intestinal and systemic inflammation, as well as intestinal **dysbiosis** that includes an altered microbiome with lower amounts of probiotic *Bifidobacteria* and *Lactobacillus* and higher amounts of some unfriendly bacteria.[52] This provides some direction for therapeutic options to correct the dysbiosis and decrease the inflammation, and thereby improve symptoms.

*Trigger Foods*
Although extensive medical research has not been performed on the numerous possible trigger foods for fussiness and colic in mother's diets, anecdotal evidence suggests that garlic, cruciferous vegetables such as brussels sprouts, cabbage, broccoli, and cauliflower (especially raw), and certain spices and spicy foods can make some babies gassy and potentially fussy. If a baby is experiencing this discomfort, mothers should reduce these foods and make sure the vegetables are eaten cooked and not raw to see if that makes a difference. Other trigger foods for some babies may include potential allergens.

*Allergens in the Mother's Diet*
The link between cow's milk protein intolerance and infant colic has been known for over thirty years, but is still somewhat under recognized by many parents and primary care providers.[53,54] This adverse reaction has been shown to take place not only in infants fed cow's milk-based formulas, but also in infants exposed to cow's milk protein *coming through mom's breast milk*.[55] The delivery of intact dietary proteins consumed by the mother and transferred to the infant through breast milk is a phenomenon that is thought to have evolved in order to decrease the chances a child will be allergic to certain foods (in a process known as **immune tolerance**). However, this process can backfire and do the opposite, causing an allergic response in the infant known as **non-IgE mediated** milk protein intolerance described in Chapter 13.

Other foods have been shown to trigger this response in some infants as well, including soy, wheat, and egg. This intolerance has a spectrum of severity, from fussiness, colic, and reflux to mucus and bloody stools on the more extreme end (called milk-protein colitis). Some research studies have shown mixed results with maternal "elimination diets" and use of **hypoallergenic** formulas. However, in a 2005 study published in *Pediatrics*, a top medical journal, the authors found that maternal elimination of milk, soy, wheat, eggs, nuts and fish significantly reduced colic behavior in the infants in their study.[56]

What this tells us is that these **food sensitivities** may not be the cause of colic in all colicky babies, but certainly do contribute in many cases. Unfortunately, no blood test or skin test is going to tell you if your child is reacting to one or several of these foods in your diet or in their formula. Diagnosis is based on dietary elimination and symptom tracking. Will eliminating milk products, soy, wheat, or eggs make a difference in your colicky baby? You won't know unless you try.

Colic is rarely caused by **primary lactose intolerance**. **Secondary lactose intolerance** is typically caused by an inflamed intestine and is reversed when the intestine is healed after recovery from an infection or after removal of an allergen. Typically, any component of *secondary* lactose intolerance is eliminated by removing the offending allergen (often cow's milk protein) from mom's diet or formula, allowing the infant's intestines to heal. Remember that lactose is the primary carbohydrate in breast milk. Chances are good that your child is not the one in a million with a primary lactose intolerance.

> **Primary lactose intolerance:** When a baby lacks the ability to produce the enzyme lactase for digesting milk sugar. This is very rare in infants, common in adults.
>
> **Secondary lactose intolerance:** When there is *reversible* loss of the lactase enzyme due to irritation/inflammation of the infant intestines.

It is also exceedingly unlikely that an infant is reacting to the human whey and casein proteins in the mother's breast milk. Taking a child off breast milk should be the absolute last resort for a fussy baby after *everything* else has been tried. This could include eliminating the most likely allergens and trigger foods in mom's diet for at least a four-week trial, as well as considering a probiotic for both mom and baby.

## HOT TOPIC

## COLIC AND PROBIOTICS

Parents of colicky infants could discuss with the pediatrician a trial of a multispecies probiotic and could consider taking one themselves if breastfeeding. As stated elsewhere, studies are showing an association between colic, inflammation, and dysbiosis in the infant intestine.[52,59,60] Correcting that dysbiosis may have beneficial effects on colic. Studies have shown that maternal supplementation of a multispecies probiotic can reduce the inflammatory chemicals in her breast milk while increasing probiotic counts, in addition to potentially relieving symptoms of colic and reflux in the infant's intestines.[57] A large **meta-analysis** showed that supplementing infants with a specific probiotic called *Lactobacillus reuteri (L. reuteri)* reduces symptoms of colic in a significant number of infants.[58] Studies using a probiotic containing several species of *Lactobacillus* and *Bifidobacteria* showed significant improvement in colic in addition to decreased inflammation in the intestines.[59,60] Probiotic supplementation may be especially important for colicky C-section babies who have a disturbed microbiome, but can be effective in vaginally born breastfed infants as well. Currently, the data is not as strong for formula-fed babies receiving *L. reuteri* or other probiotics and more research is needed, but probiotic therapy for this group of colicky infants also holds much promise. Overall, published evidence would indicate that taking a good quality probiotic while breastfeeding or given to infants is safe. Given that *L. reuteri* and *Bifidobacteria animalis* as well as multispecies probiotic strains are *all* showing safety and potential effectiveness for infant colic, a trial of a good multispecies probiotic for the colicky infant should be considered and discussed with the pediatrician.

## Infant Reflux

Infant reflux is often a major preoccupation for parents, but reflux may not always be a cause for medical concern. Infant reflux is fairly common, with up to 70% of normal healthy infants having a degree of daily reflux or "spitting up" in the first months of life. Infant reflux is also known to get better with time, lessening markedly after 6 months of age as the infant's digestive system matures.[61]

To clarify, most infants have a degree of normal Gastroesophageal Reflux (GER), meaning they spit up some of their feeds but they are otherwise healthy and have no significant medical issues. A smaller population of infants are afflicted with chronic Gastroesophageal Reflux Disease (GERD) that requires intervention. Unfortunately, the excessive concern over infant reflux has caused a phenomenon of overprescribing acid blocking medications for infants such as ranitidine and omeprazole over the past decade, with potential negative consequences on the infant microbiome.[62–65] Both the American Academy of Pediatrics (APP) and the North American Society For Pediatric Gastroenterology, Hepatology & Nutrition (NASPGHAN) *do not generally recommend automatically starting acid blocking medicines* for fussy babies suspected of having reflux.[66–68] In fact, acid blocking medications have been shown not to help with most reflux or fussiness in multiple studies.[67,69–72]

The primary recommendations for the infant with excessive reflux by pediatric academic groups are[68,69,73]

+ Limit overfeeding the infant; use smaller more frequent feeds as directed by PCP or dietician
+ Consider thickened formula using rice or oat cereal or other thickener in breast milk under guidance from a pediatric dietician or PCP
+ Try switching to a hypoallergenic formula if already formula fed
+ Try an elimination diet for the breastfeeding mother

Acid blocking medications are considered a *last line of therapy* after other therapies have been tried. Discontinuation of breastfeeding *is not recommended* except in extreme cases because of the myriad health benefits to the baby from drinking the mother's milk.

A word of caution: too much rice cereal added to thicken formula or breast milk can potentially boost the caloric concentration to unsafe levels for younger infants. One teaspoon per two ounces of formula or milk is the absolute maximum, which still brings the caloric density of the milk to about 27 calories per ounce, compared with 20 calories per ounce in regular formula or breast milk.

There is concern about arsenic levels in many rice products; the AAP recommends oat cereal instead of rice to thicken formula. Any possible effects on the microbiome and **epigenetics** in a young infant consuming a significant amount of rice or other processed starch has not been well researched. In addition, rice and other cereal may not work as a thickening agent with breast milk because of certain enzymes present in the mother's milk.[74] There are other commercial thickeners available for formula and breast milk, but should only be used under guidance from the PCP and a qualified pediatric dietician.

### Probiotics, Food Allergies and Reflux

Compared to colic, less research has been done on the effects of probiotics and infant reflux, but there is some positive data. A study in 2011 showed improved stomach emptying and decreased spitting up in infants given *L. reuteri*, the same probiotic used to treat infant colic.[75] A 2014 study on *L. reuteri* by these authors showed decreased colic and reflux in infants given the probiotic in early infancy.[76] In addition, a 2017 study showed reduction in both colic and reflux in a set of infants given a multi-species probiotic.[77] Overall, these studies suggest the potential benefits and good safety profile of probiotic supplements for the refluxing baby; these supplements could be considered before trying an acid blocking medication. Similar to colic, a link between an allergic immune response (to cow's milk proteins and other potential allergens in breast milk and infant formula) and reflux and vomiting in some infants may exist.[55,69,78]

Below is a list of alarming symptoms that can be associated with reflux that should prompt evaluation by a medical provider.

+ Vomiting green/yellow bile
+ Vomiting blood
+ Forceful projectile vomiting
+ Losing or not gaining weight
+ Refusing the breast or bottle
+ Excessively fussy; screaming and arching
+ Onset of reflux *after* 6 months of age
+ Association with significant constipation
+ Association with significant distention
+ Association with breathing issues

My advice to the mother of a colicky or refluxing infant is remove all dairy and soy from the diet if breastfeeding, while working with the primary medical provider or a pediatric gastroenterologist. (Don't worry about removing soybean oil or soy lecithin, which are common food ingredients, as these typically do not cause a reaction because they contain very little of the offending protein.) Discuss a trial with a good probiotic supplement for your baby.

Occasionally in my practice, I recommend that mothers remove eggs and wheat from the diet as well as dairy and soy to settle things down in the baby's GI tract if the infant is not doing well. I suggest giving this approach a minimum of three to four weeks to see if this has a positive effect, but you should start seeing improvements within two weeks.

Because of the profound health benefits of breast milk, the mother should not stop breastfeeding for colic or reflux unless she has exhausted all other approaches, and it is determined that the child may be in danger. Remember that time is on your side, and that this too shall pass.

Typically, by four months colic improves, and after six to nine months reflux improves regardless of the changes we make.

Make sure to discuss concerns with the pediatrician before making any major dietary change. Removing dairy, soy and other potential allergens from a mother's diet is possible and safe while maintaining adequate calories; many mothers have done this with positive results. With education and planning these eliminations are easily implemented without suffering nutrient deficiencies, but these mothers may need to pay special attention to their diet to maintain adequate calcium, vitamin D, and choline if dairy and eggs are both removed.

Reintroducing foods into mom's diet that were problematic in earlier infancy is a bit of an art form and is best worked through with the pediatrician or pediatric gastroenterologist and a knowledgeable dietician if possible. The hope is that the infant's immune system will mature and develop a tolerance to these food proteins, which can be re-introduced potentially between six and nine months, first through breast milk and with several weeks between each re-introduced food.

In my practice, I usually have a breastfeeding mother try eating eggs first (because of the choline content) and watch for negative reactions prior to giving the infant eggs directly. After several weeks, wheat would be the next reintroduction; soy and dairy should be the last of the eliminated foods to be reintroduced into mom's diet in later infancy. Negative reactions in the infant including vomiting and major reflux, rash, blood in the stool, or blowout diarrhea, should be discussed promptly with their provider. These symptoms may indicate that the infant's immune system is not yet tolerating these foods.

# NUTRITION Rₓ

**1** Given the clear health benefits, we all need to be supporting the practice of breastfeeding as much as possible. Families, spouses, employers, healthcare providers, hospitals, and the government should all work toward promoting successful breastfeeding.

**2** Know that breastfeeding can be difficult, painful, and stressful at times but is very important for the health of your baby; the advantages for the rest of their life are considerable. Please get the support you need and don't give up—it gets better with time!

**3** If you are a new mom, get support anywhere you can: other moms, relatives, your OB, midwives and OB nurses, your PCP and pediatrician, but especially lactation consultants and the La Leche League. Feeding therapists such as **speech-language pathologists** are sometimes trained in breastfeeding and can be a valuable resource. Demand a consult with a lactation consultant after giving birth prior to discharge. Consider getting plugged into a breastfeeding support group prior to giving birth.

**4** The tide is turning. Be aware that employers are legally mandated to allow for breastfeeding or pumping at work, and must supply a clean quiet, private area (not a bathroom stall!) to pump or feed.

**5** Breastfeed on demand, letting the baby set the schedule. Younger infants feed more frequently

**6** Find a quiet comfortable place to nurse to minimize distractions

**7** Allow baby to completely drain one breast before switching sides. Hindmilk is nutrient rich!

**8**     Breastfed infants may grow slower than formula-fed infants, but this is the healthy norm.

**9**     Proper nutrition is important for mothers during breastfeeding and affects the quality of breast milk. Minimize added sugar, deep fried foods, and highly processed foods during lactation.

**10**     Moms need an extra 200 to 500 calories a day during breastfeeding, but make sure they are from healthy, protein rich foods as protein requirements also increase!

**11**     Continue a good prenatal or multivitamin during breastfeeding as insurance that you are meeting nutrient requirements.

**12**     Calcium requirements are the same as during pregnancy, so you do not need to take high doses.

**13**     Optimize breast milk quantities of vital omega-3 for the baby brain. Continue to eat salmon, trout, sardines, or herring several times per week, or consider a fish oil supplement with 500 to 1000 mg EPA/DHA. Vegetarian/vegan moms could consider 1 to 2 tbsp of high-quality flaxseed oil daily plus an algae source DHA of 200 to 500 mg daily to optimize their breast milk supply of omega-3.

**14**     Non-vegetarian moms should eat meat and eggs regularly while breastfeeding, to supply valuable protein but also to increase the important brain nutrient choline in their milk. Consider a choline supplement of about 500 mg daily if not eating eggs and meat regularly.

**15**     Continue to eat a lot of vegetables for the antioxidants and **phytonutrients** like lutein, and for the fiber to promote a healthy maternal microbiome.

**16**  Mom's probiotic bacteria continue to be delivered to the baby after they are born through breast milk. Eat plenty of fiber as well as probiotic rich foods such as unsweetened yogurt (mixed with fruit) or sauerkraut and other fermented vegetables. Consider a good multi-species probiotic if there have been any recent antibiotics to ensure transfer of good bacteria through your breast milk.

**17**  Minimize concentrated sources of sugar and fructose in your diet to avoid excessive fructose delivery to the baby through your breast milk. Fructose is not good for the baby.

**18**  It is recommended that all infants receive 400 IU of vitamin $D_3$ daily. I prefer drops that have just coconut oil and vitamin D without all the other additives. One drop daily does the trick.

**19**  Avoid alcohol, tobacco, and illicit drugs while breastfeeding.

**20**  There is no current evidence that small amounts of caffeine in mom's diet are harmful to the baby but try to limit intake to one cup of coffee daily.

## RECOMMENDED READING

1.  La Leche League International: https://www.llli.org
2.  Baby Friendly USA: https://www.babyfriendlyusa.org/for-parents/resources-for-parents

# CHAPTER NINE

# INFANT FORMULA

Not all mothers are able to breastfeed or breastfeed as long as they would like, even in the best of circumstances. I recognize that this can cause an incredible amount of guilt and angst for the parent that wants to breast-feed but is unable. Choosing a formula can be daunting. This section is meant to educate parents and providers on making good formula choices, and hopefully decrease some of the stress surrounding these decisions.

Breakthroughs in science are still unlocking some of the "secret ingredients" contained in breast milk, which is helping formula companies close the gap and more closely mimic the benefits of breastfeeding. To be clear, breast milk will always be superior to formula and is the unquestionable top choice for the baby. However, for the parent that has to formula feed, it is good to know that your choices are improving as the science advances.

Parents can be bombarded with the plethora of formula choices available on the market. What are the differences, and what is the best choice for a particular child? Essentially, the same basic components are found in infant formula and breast milk: proteins, fats, carbohydrates as well as the essential vitamins and minerals needed for infant development. Most formula vitamin and mineral profiles that are approved by the FDA are similar and standardized to meet the **RDA** of the developing infant.

To make an informed decision about which formula is best, ask the following questions:

+ What is the protein source?
+ What type of carbohydrate do they use?

+ What types of fat do they put in the formula?
+ What effects could these choices have on the growing infant?

Formula has come a long way in the past thirty years as we learn more about breast milk, infant digestion, and nutrient requirements. The formula companies would be the first to admit that formula will never be as good for the baby as breast milk, but they are trying to close the gap. I applaud the formula companies for continuing to research the many components of breast milk to adjust their ingredients and manufacturing techniques to more closely mimic breast milk.

Some of the more recent formula advancements include

+ The addition of DHA **omega-3** and the **omega-6 Arachidonic acid (ARA)** to almost all formulas for the baby's brain development.
+ The addition of **oligosaccharides** and synthesized HMO to feed the baby's **microbiome** and enhance their immune system.
+ The new exploration of using **milk fat globule membrane (MFGM)** as a fat delivery system for its developmental and immune benefits.
+ The return to the use of lactose as the carbohydrate source, rather than corn syrup solids. (Corn syrup supplies glucose to the baby but may not have the same health benefits to the baby as lactose.)
+ The adjustment of the **whey** to **casein** protein ratio to more closely mirror breast milk (human milk is 60%–80% whey and 20%–40% casein).
+ The addition of **medium chain triglycerides (MCT)** to stimulate mild ketone production in the infant.
+ The addition of some **probiotic** bacteria to promote the infant microbiome.
+ Increased amounts of choline based on data showing the benefit to the baby's brain development.
+ The addition of lutein to mimic the increased amounts found in healthy breast milk.
+ Several companies have removed any genetically modified organisms (GMOs) from the formula as well as removing recombinant bovine growth hormone (rBGH) produced milk based on consumer concerns.

However, with so many formulas on the market it is hard to figure out which ones contain the most beneficial compounds. We will try to help make your selection process a little clearer.

## PREMATURE INFANTS

A full review of nutrition for premature infants is beyond the scope of this book, but we should highlight a few important points. Babies born early miss out on a good portion of the third trimester, a crucial window of nutrient accumulation. Because of this, preterm infants require special formula or breast milk fortifiers for catch up growth and nutrient storage. Even "late preterm" infants born between 34- and 37-weeks gestation may have increased needs that are just now being discovered.

Key nutrients that may need to be increased for the premature infant include iron, zinc, calcium, phosphorus, vitamin D, choline, and omega-3 DHA. Premature infants need to be followed closely by a pediatrician and pediatric dietician even after discharge from the NICU (Newborn Intensive Care Unit) to monitor growth and iron levels. Monitoring iron levels with a **ferritin** test is especially important for this group to ensure adequate but not excessive iron levels.

### Protein in Infant Formulas

The main category choices available in infant formulas are typically based on the protein source. Below are listed the main types of formulas found on the market.

+ Cow's milk protein-based formulas
+ Soy protein-based formulas
+ Partially or extensively **hydrolyzed** (pre-digested) **proteins** in milk-based formula
+ Elemental hypoallergenic formula
+ Specialty formulas based on goat milk, rice, and A2 casein (non-US only)

**Hydrolyzed proteins** in formula are at least partially broken down prior to ingestion, making them potentially less likely to cause allergies and more easily digested by the infant. *Partially hydrolyzed* are not broken down as much as *extensively hydrolyzed* formulas, so are not officially considered hypoallergenic, but may be helpful in some cases.

## INFANT FORMULAS

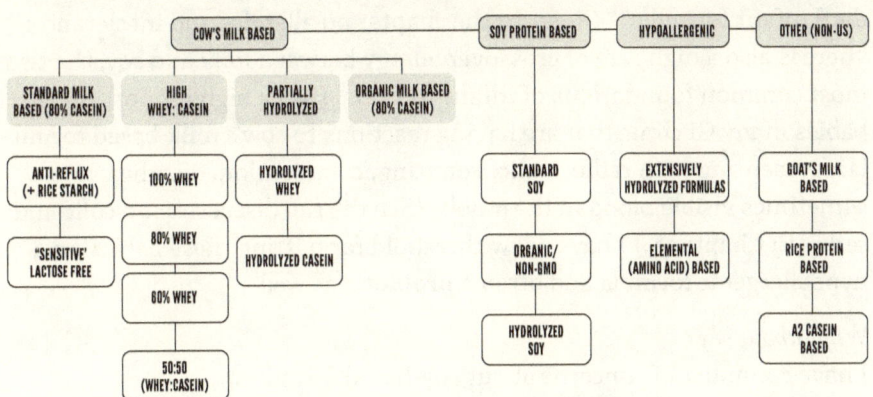

For updated list of formulas under each category refer to book/author website

Standard infant formula is based on intact cow's milk protein. The protein from milk is purified and added to the formula in the proper amounts for infant growth. Recall that cow's milk is 20% whey and 80% casein, which is the *opposite* of human breast milk (which is up to 80% whey and only 20% casein).[1-4] This high casein content in standard milk protein-based formula makes it potentially problematic for an infant. Remember that casein is harder to digest, which could make it more likely to stimulate reflux and potentially more allergenic as compared to whey, so there may be an advantage to having a higher whey/casein ratio in the formula for many infants. Ratios in infant formula can vary from 100% standard milk protein (80% casein) to 100% whey protein (no casein) depending on the formula. Given that early breast milk typically has an 80:20 ratio of whey to casein, when choosing an initial formula, I prefer one that approximates this with increased whey content to improve digestibility and decrease the likelihood of an allergic reaction.

Formulas that contain partially broken down (hydrolyzed) milk protein in addition to whey protein further reduce the risk of allergic reaction to the formula but are not technically classified as **hypoallergenic.** These may be a good first choice if there are concerns about an infant with high potential for reacting to standard cow's milk formula. If adverse reactions to this type of formula occurs, then a trial of a truly hypoallergenic formula may be warranted and should be discussed with the child's PCP.

Despite formula advances, the fact remains that up to 15% of babies may have an adverse reaction to cow milk proteins and may not tolerate standard infant formula.[5,6] (Refer to the chapter on allergies and intolerances.) There is also a high rate of crossover allergy between milk and soy, the two most common foundations of infant formula. I see a high proportion of babies in my GI clinic that are having reactions to cow's milk-based formulas, presenting with reflux, colic, vomiting, constipation, diarrhea, and sometimes visible blood in the stools. (See the full discussion on colic and reflux in Chapter 8.) I have a low threshold for putting these babies on a hypoallergenic formula and often a **probiotic** as well.

*What about soy?*
I have a number of concerns about soy-based formulas.

First, there is a high rate of crossover *allergy* between cow's milk and soy protein; up to 15% of infants with a *cow's milk allergy* will also react to soy. There is an even higher crossover rate with gastrointestinal *milk protein* **hypersensitivity**/*cow's milk protein* **intolerance** in infants, with up to 60% of milk sensitive infants with GI symptoms also reacting to soy, according to the AAP.[7] We will clarify the difference between an allergy and an intolerance in Chapter 13. While some infants seem to tolerate soy-based formulas without any issues, I avoid recommending these formulas given their associated risks for allergies and allergic reactions.[8]

Second, unless the formula is made from organic soy (which a few infant formula companies are using) there have been concerns voiced by the general public about elevated levels of the herbicide/pesticide glyphosate in soy formula.

I cannot find much published medical literature supporting or refuting the claim that the levels of glyphosate in soy formula definitively pose a health risk to infants. The same goes for genetically modified soy in the diet of the pregnant mother or infant—it has never been studied or tested in these populations. In fact, despite that glyphosate is the most commonly used pesticide in the US, the USDA Pesticide Data Program apparently does not routinely test levels in the food supply as they do with other pesticides.[9] The wary consumer may opt to avoid of these potential exposures in our youngest and most vulnerable population.

Third, there is growing concern in the medical literature about the high levels of phytoestrogens (plant hormones called isoflavones) that are contained in soy. These plant estrogens are found in concentrations thousands of times higher in soy formula compared to cow's milk-based formulas or in breast milk. Subsequently, the levels of these isoflavones are found to be *thousands of times higher* in the bloodstream of babies fed these formulas, having the potential to interfere with hormone balance in the developing infant and possibly acting as an **endocrine disrupting chemical** and **epigenetic modifier**.[10] A 2017 study confirmed epigenetic changes in vaginal cells of girls raised on soy formula, adding fuel to concerns voiced about soy formula feeding and later risk of uterine fibroids, endometriosis, and early puberty.[11] This is an area in need of further investigation.

Fourth, high amounts of aluminum have been found in soy formula, the highest of any formula tested. There is no role for aluminum in the human body and it is listed as a potential neurotoxin. This has raised concerns about unwittingly exposing the baby with immature detoxification systems to an increased level of a potentially neurotoxic metal.

Fifth, soy contains high amounts of **anti-nutrients**, which are compounds in the plants that block the digestion and absorption of certain nutrients. Soy contains several of these anti-nutrients. Phytic acid blocks iron and zinc absorption and also blocks absorption of iodine, which is crucial for thyroid function. Soy also contains trypsin inhibitors, which block protein digestion. Extra nutrients, including zinc and iron, are supplemented in these formulas, but this brings into question whether soy protein and soy formula are an optimal source of nutrition for a baby with immature digestion.

Taking all these concerns together, one can see why many nutrition experts and researchers are not fans of soy formula or high amounts of soy in children's diets.[8,9,12] While in past research soy formula use has not been shown to be associated with any major increased health risks to infants, questions remain as researchers are continuing to look deeper into some of the potential effects. In 2006, the European Society for Gastroenterology, Hepatology, and Nutrition (ESPGHAN) Committee on Nutrition made a position statement regarding soy formulas indicating that they "should only be used in specified circumstances because they have nutritional disadvantages and contain high amounts of phytate, aluminum, and phytoestrogens, the long-term effects of which are unknown."[8] I agree with this statement. If a baby can't be on breast milk and does not tolerate cow's milk-based formula, I recommend a hypoallergenic formula.

*Hypoallergenic formulas*

Hypoallergenic formulas contain proteins that are partially or completely digested, which makes them less likely to stimulate an allergic reaction. They are used in cases of milk protein allergy or intolerance in infants. I do not consider soy formula hypoallergenic for the reasons listed earlier. There are partially hydrolyzed (digested) whey or milk-based formulas on the market that are less allergenic and may be a good starter choice for concerned parents even though they are not pre-digested enough to be considered officially hypoallergenic. Also, hydrolyzed rice-based formulas available in Europe are considered hypoallergenic and suitable for a milk-protein allergy but these are not available in the US.

True hypoallergenic formulas fall into two types: the extensively hydrolyzed formulas and the **elemental formulas**.

*Extensively hydrolyzed formulas* (Alimentum, Pregestimil, Nutramigen) start with cow's milk proteins and add enzymes to break these proteins down to smaller units called peptides. These smaller units of milk proteins are much less likely to cause a reaction, but a proportion of infants can still react to these formulas.

The *elemental formulas (Neocate, EleCare, Alfamino, PurAmino)* are broken all the way down to amino acids, the single building blocks of proteins. Technically it is impossible for an infant to be allergic to any components of these elemental formulas, as the immune system cannot react to single amino acids. In my practice, if I have evidence that an infant is having a serious reaction to a standard formula, especially with gastrointestinal bleeding, weight loss, and recurrent vomiting, I choose the elemental formula to stop the reaction before it can cause any more damage.

If a baby is formula fed and extremely fussy, colicky, or has great deal of vomiting or gastroesophageal reflux, switching to a hypoallergenic or elemental formula with broken down proteins has been shown to help many infants. If your formula-fed child is excessively fussy or has extensive reflux or blood in their stools, talk to their PCP about considering hypoallergenic formula (rather than a lactose free, "anti-reflux," or soy formula).

I generally recommend a dairy elimination diet for breastfeeding moms or switching to a hypoallergenic formula for baby, and possibly adding a probiotic supplement *before* trying reflux medications like ranitidine, famotidine or omeprazole for a colicky (or refluxing) baby. As discussed previously, according to the AAP, there is very little evidence to support giving a fussy infant one of these acid blockers despite their widespread use. However, they can be helpful in certain circumstances.

Unfortunately, hypoallergenic specialty formulas are quite expensive. Unless parents qualify for WIC or Medicaid, they may be paying out of pocket because insurance companies increasingly deny coverage for hypoallergenic formula. Because of the effectiveness of hypoallergenic formula as a *medical treatment for milk protein intolerance, infant colitis, and colic,* and evidence of harm to the child if we withhold these treatments, I hope this policy changes soon. It is not ethical to deny coverage for an effective medical treatment, compromising the care of infants whose families can't afford the needed formula.

### Carbohydrate content of formula

Remember that lactose is the natural carbohydrate source for the breastfed infant and may have health benefits for the baby and their microbiome. The myth of the lactose intolerant baby is widespread, but mostly inaccurate, with true infant **lactose intolerance** being extremely rare. Some formula companies have gone back to using lactose as their carbohydrate source, but many of them still use corn syrup solids, especially in their "sensitive" formulas. An international expert group on infant nutrition "considers it prudent to include lactose in infant formula" because of potential health benefits to the baby and recommends against the use of glucose.[13,14] It is worth noting that the European Commission mandates at least 30% of the carbohydrate in infant formula sold in Europe be from lactose unless the formula is designated lactose free.

To clarify a point made previously about sugar, no formula that I have seen uses *high fructose corn syrup* (a highly suspect ingredient), but instead these formulas use corn syrup or corn syrup solids instead of lactose as an alternate carbohydrate source. Corn syrup (as opposed to high fructose corn syrup) is essentially 100% glucose (with no fructose).

Science is still evaluating the metabolic and microbiome effect of feeding an infant glucose versus lactose. If mother nature put lactose in her formula (breast milk), logic would dictate that is the best form of carbohydrate for the baby, and perhaps should be included in a formula if you are unable to breastfeed. Unfortunately, at present all the hypoallergenic formulas have removed lactose as their carbohydrate source, so a child will get glucose by default if they need a hypoallergenic formula. To clarify, glucose may not be directly harmful to the baby, but there is evidence that lactose is better for them and their microbiome.

The formula-fed infant definitely should not get fructose or regular sugar (sucrose) as a carbohydrate source because of the increasing concerns about alterations of their microbiome and programming for future obesity. Evidence suggests that the increased sweetness alters future taste preferences and feeding behaviors leading to epigenetic programming for future disease such as obesity and **type 2 diabetes**.[14] There is also evidence that sucrose-containing formula is worse for the baby's teeth and promotes cavities more than lactose-containing formula.[15] The international Codex Alimentarius (www.codexalimentarius.org) that sets international standards for infant formula has recommended that formula contain no sucrose or fructose. The European Union (EU) has subsequently *banned* the use of sucrose in any European infant formula, but the US is not there yet. I advise against using a formula with sugar (sucrose) for any infant and feel this needs to be banned in the US as well.

### Fat content of formula

Fat in breast milk has two purposes: 1) fuel for energy either by direct fat burning or creation of **ketones**, and 2) structural uses to build the growing baby brain. There are literally dozens of different types of fat in breast milk, and the content will vary depending on the mother's diet.[16,17] We do know that breast milk contains significant amounts of **saturated fat** and some cholesterol, medium chain triglycerides (MCT) for ketone production, the essential fatty acids LA and **ALA**, and the **long chain polyunsaturated fats (PUFAs)** including DHA and ARA.

Logic dictates that these fats be contained in infant formula as well, and currently they are included in most formulas in varying amounts. One of the areas of advancement in formula production has been an adjustment in the fat content to include these important classes of fats for the baby. Most formulas now contain some mix of palm, soy, coconut, sunflower, or safflower oil to provide a mix of saturated and unsaturated fats. Coconut and palm oil which provide saturated fat also have some MCT which can be used for ketone production, and most formulas these days seem to contain the important long chain PUFAs (DHA and ARA). Experts feel it is important to have balanced DHA and ARA in the formula, as they are both present in breastmilk and are needed for brain and eye development; having one without the other could create an imbalance. Amounts may be variable, but DHA is found in a range of 0.3 to 0.5% of total fat in formula, although it can be as high as 0.7 to 1% in the breast milk of mothers who eat a lot of fish.

Many formulas still contain standard palm oil, which has been shown in research to actually inhibit fat and calcium absorption in the baby, cause harder stools, alter the microbiome, and decrease the absorption of the essential DHA oil.[18-22] The inclusion of higher amounts of palm oil in infant formula (as well as the high amounts of casein protein) are some of the main reasons that formula-fed babies tend to be more constipated compared to breastfed babies. It has been found that the form in which the palm oil is included in formula makes a big difference. There is a type of palm oil called b-palmitate that more closely mimics breast milk fat, is better absorbed, and is less likely to cause constipation by improving fat and calcium absorption as well as increased numbers of the beneficial probiotic *Bifidobacteria*. Based on the current evidence, some parents may choose to find a formula that does not contain standard palm oil, and either has the beta-palmitate or an alternative form of saturated fat.

## Additional Formula Ingredients

*Choline*
We reviewed the importance of choline for the infant in both the pregnancy and breastfeeding chapters. Given what we now know about the importance of choline in the developing brain, most formula companies include it in adequate amounts in their infant formulas. Estimated adequate intakes for choline are 125 mg per day for infants 0 to 6 months and 150 mg per day for infants 7 to 12 months. Federal code requires US *non-milk-based* formula to have a minimum of 7 mg choline per 100 calories of formula, but there are apparently no requirements for milk-based formula. Based on the recommended choline intake for infants, I would make sure your formula is supplying at least 24 mg choline per 100 calories which should get your baby to the recommended levels. Lower amounts may fall short of requirements, potentially impacting brain development.[23]

*Lutein*
Lutein is an **antioxidant** from green leafy vegetables that is concentrated in breast milk and the baby's eyes and brain. The amount in breast milk is highly variable depending on the mother's diet, so it is difficult to say what a true "normal" level is. However, research studies show average levels of 21 to 25 mcg/liter of lutein in breast milk.[24,25] Given the potential

synergistic effect with DHA and choline, some companies are improving their formulas with lutein.

*Iron*

This is another area where breast milk and formula differ significantly. Iron content of formula is becoming more of a hot topic.

A healthy term infant, especially one who is born to an **omnivorous** mother (vaginally), should have iron stores to last them until about 6 months of life. The endorsed policy of delayed umbilical cord clamping at birth by obstetricians and midwives further maximizes the baby's iron stores and is associated with better infant outcomes. As discussed earlier, iron is vital for infant brain development, but as with many nutrients there is a sweet spot: too little as well as too much iron has negative effects.

## HOT TOPIC

Breast milk is low in iron by design; however, the iron is highly bioavailable (easier for the infant to absorb). Breast milk contains iron concentrations of 0.2 to 0.4 mg/liter, which is estimated to be 50% absorbed.[26] Infant formula in the US has *much* higher iron content, containing 12 mg/liter, which is estimated to be 10% absorbed. Compared to US formulas, European infant formulas are significantly lower in iron, generally containing 4 to 8 mg/liter. In addition, Europe has two types of formula: one for 0 to 6 month-old infants with lower iron content and one for 6 to 12 month old infants with slightly higher iron content to reflect the increased iron needs of the older infant.[26] US formulas do not make this distinction, but rather have a one size fits all approach.[26-28] This means that *a formula-fed infant in the US is receiving 30 to 60 times the amount of iron compared to a breastfed infant*, and double the amount of the European formula-fed infant.

Why is this a potential concern? In large part because the extra unabsorbed iron passing through the infant gut may negatively affect the microbiome, which is in the process of becoming established during infancy. The infant microbiome will in many ways guide this infant's immune system and brain development through the critical first thousand days. Some scientists think that the extra iron found in many formulas may shift these intestinal bacteria to a less desirable balance and increase potentially harmful bacteria with unknown consequences. Higher iron formulas may have the potential to increase unhealthy bacteria such as *E. coli* in the intestines of the formula-fed infant.[29] Excessive iron is also theoretically a pro-oxidant, meaning that excessive iron has the potential to damage the body unless quenched by antioxidants. A 2012 study using a randomized controlled trial showed better cognitive outcomes in every measure tested on term infants with adequate iron stores receiving a low-iron formula that more closely matched breast milk as opposed to a high iron formula that matched the US standard.[30] The results of this study remain somewhat controversial, and to date this study has not been replicated. This is an area that needs further research.

European formulas for infants 0-6 months generally do not exceed 4 to 8 mg iron per liter, but optimal amounts for most infants could actually be lower according to some experts.[26,29] The flip side of this is that many infants are born iron deficient. If an infant is iron deficient, their body would benefit from higher iron amounts in formula, up to a point. However, if excessive iron is given to infants who already have adequate iron stores, there could be concerns including *increased* risk of infections and impaired growth, as well as an altered microbiome.

Whether a potential need exists to lower the standard iron content of US formula and emulate the variable approach Europe uses would be a worthy discussion. Should we stop using a "one-size-fits-all" high-iron approach for all infants from birth to 12 months in the US?

More adequate testing of iron stores in early infancy in *high-risk infants* (premature, infants of anemic, iron deficient, obese, or diabetic mothers or mothers who smoke) may also be warranted. Early screening using an umbilical cord ferritin or serum ferritin level has been suggested by leaders in the field, thereby identifying which babies may need higher iron content in their formula and diet.[29,34,35]

## European Formulas

There is a growing trend of parents who import European formulas into the US for their babies. HiPP and Holle are the two main non-FDA-regulated formulas from Europe in use in the US. There are several reasons why increasing numbers of parents are choosing to go this non-sanctioned route, some of which are valid concerns. While I do not advocate the importation of non-FDA regulated formulas, I will address this briefly.

In a poll of women who import formula, 85% said they chose a European formula because they believed that these formulas were held to stricter standards than formulas in the US.[31] The main formula companies in Europe are highly regulated, in some ways more so than formula companies in the US. They have stricter and more updated laws and quality standards in place to protect the infant. This was briefly outlined in a recent review in the *Journal of Pediatric Gastroenterology and Nutrition* (*JPGN*), the top pediatric gastroenterology journal.[31]

According to this review, US formula regulations have not been significantly updated since 1980, whereas the European infant formula laws have been frequently updated with the most recent revision in 2014. The largest concerns by the authors in this review were not the quality or nutrient content of European formula, but rather the lack of mixing instructions in English and differences in the labeling of hypoallergenic formulas. This is a legitimate concern. An improperly mixed formula can be dangerous for the baby, either if it is too diluted or too concentrated. An equally valid concern was also that if there were a product recall in Europe, this would not reach the American consumer who had imported the product through alternate channels. The unregulated manner of importing these products also allows for less quality control in shipping and storage, and increased risk of tampering.

However, to denigrate these products or insinuate that they are inferior or dangerous is misleading and disrespectful to our European colleagues in science and medicine. Germany, Switzerland, and the UK have the highest scientific standards that match or exceed our own, and if these formulas are approved for use by the EU regulatory commission, they have been scrutinized as well as any US product.

On further examination of EU formula regulations, there are interesting distinctions.

+ They do not allow genetically modified products into formula.
+ They test for pesticide residue with strict limitations, thereby ensuring that European formulas are essentially free of pesticides.
+ The use of sucrose in infant formula is strictly banned and they have strict limitations on additives, some of which may have the potential for harm, such as carrageenan.
+ As stated previously, European formulas also have a lower iron content, which may be more desirable in the younger term infant at low risk for iron deficiency.

Many of these factors are obviously appealing to the discerning American parent who wants to do best by their child. These are not uneducated anarchists who have decided to go rogue. Rather than try to punish these parents, we should examine the reasons why this practice is increasing. Should the US consider updating and adopting some of the formula standards in place in Europe?

## SAY NO TO THE GOAT

Feeding a baby goats milk is an exceedingly *bad idea*, and several of the sickest, most anemic infants I have ever admitted to the hospital were being fed goats milk by parents that thought they were doing the right thing and avoiding cow's milk. Goats milk is too low in several nutrients and binds folate making it unavailable to the infant. In addition, the protein/carbohydrate ratios are wrong and very different from breast milk. There are goat milk-based formulas that are approved in Europe that add the missing nutrients to make this *potentially* an acceptable alternative for European parents. But *anyone who suggests that you feed your baby straight goat milk is not someone you should be taking health advice from*.

I would also heavily advise against trying to make your own "homemade" infant formula from goat milk with other ingredients added in to try to make it less damaging to the baby. This is dangerous and no parent should take this risk with their infant. Granted, the type of protein in goat and sheep products, called A2 beta casein, is different than that of cow's milk, and in some cases may *possibly* be less allergenic compared to standard cow's milk protein, but this does not make it acceptable for an infant to drink straight goat's milk.[32,33]

There are now A2 infant formulas available to consumers, using milk from cows that only produce the A2 casein. There is a high crossover allergy between cow and goat milk, so typically an infant showing signs of having an allergic reaction to milk-based formula should go on to a truly hypoallergenic formula.

### Colic and Reflux in Formula-Fed Infants

For the formula-fed infant with significant colic or reflux, discuss the use of a good probiotic and hydrolyzed or hypoallergenic formula with the child's PCP. "Gentle" formulas containing hydrolyzed whey or combined hydrolyzed whey and milk protein are commonly available and easier to digest. Although not officially hypoallergenic, these formulas can improve symptoms in some babies. Truly hypoallergenic formulas may include either extensively hydrolyzed or amino acid-based formula. Soy formulas are not hypoallergenic and are not recommended for use in these situations. I don't generally see the point of using an "anti-reflux" formula that adds a thickener but still contains intact cow's milk protein with high amounts of casein (the protein that may be causing the issue). I also don't see the point of "sensitive" formulas that contain intact milk proteins but remove the lactose. See a complete discussion on reflux and colic in Chapter 8 for more details. Be sure to avoid overfeeding and make sure that the formula is mixed correctly and not too concentrated. Continue to work with your pediatrician or gastroenterologist so that they can monitor symptoms and growth.

### TYPICAL FEEDING VOLUMES FOR INFANTS

| Age (months) | Ounces of formula per feed |
| --- | --- |
| Newborn | 1-2 oz (30-60ml) every 2-3 hours |
| 0-1 | 2-3 oz (60-90ml) every 3 hours |
| 1-3 | 3-5 oz (90-120 ml) every 3-4 hours |
| 3-6 | 4-6 oz (120-180ml) every 3-4 hours |
| 6-9 | 6-8 oz (180-240 ml) every 4-5 hours |
| 9-12 | 8 oz (240 ml) 3-4 times per day |

# NUTRITION R$_X$

**1**   If you are formula feeding, consider choosing a starter formula that contains lactose, more whey than casein (80% whey) to mimic breastmilk, or perhaps hydrolyzed casein and whey to improve digestion and decrease risk of allergic reaction if there is a strong family history of allergies.

**2**   Look for a formula containing prebiotic oligosaccharides optimally including HMO to support the microbiome.

**3**   Make sure the formula contains the important fatty acids DHA and ARA for brain and eye development, with at least 0.3% of fats as DHA but typically not more than 0.5%.

**4**   Especially if your baby is constipated, talk to your PCP and consider a formula that does not contain standard palm oil, which can cause hard stools in babies and inhibits absorption of crucial DHA and calcium. The b-palmitate version is better tolerated.

**5**   If your baby is having serious issues with vomiting and reflux, colic, eczema, or poor weight gain, talk to their healthcare provider about a trial of hypoallergenic formula, and possibly a good probiotic.

**6**   Because of increasing evidence of risks from exposures to endocrine disrupting chemicals (EDCs) found in many plastics, choose bottles that are BPA and phthalate free, or glass bottles that do not contain these chemicals.

**7**   Do not microwave any baby bottles, but certainly not plastic ones, which increases the release of EDCs.

**8**   Go off hunger and fullness cues and don't overfeed. Every baby is different!

**9**   Don't force baby to finish the bottle.

**10**   The pediatrician will track infant growth and make sure feedings are adequate.

**11**   Infants must be held during feedings until they can hold the bottle; avoid bottle propping.

**12**   No juice or cereal in the bottle unless advised by pediatrician. Never put soda or sweetened drinks in the baby bottle.

**13**   Do not give cow's milk, goat's milk, or milk substitutes to an infant; breastmilk or formula only

**14**   Never give an infant honey because it may cause botulism, a severe form of food poisoning.

# CHAPTER TEN

# BABY'S FIRST FOODS

When and what to start feeding a baby has been a subject of some debate in recent years. It is the cause of a fair amount of angst among parents. The timing of baby's first foods, which ones to pick, the way to offer these foods, and the setting in which to do so are important choices. We are not just trying to get calories into our children to help them grow, we are trying to create a healthy eater for life. This takes hard work and the right road map.

Remember that the **first thousand days** of our children's lives are incredibly important developmentally, with a high rate of ongoing growth occurring in the brain, creating a heavy nutrient demand.[1] Children's **microbiomes** also start to take on a more adult pattern and are heavily impacted by the foods they are given. Selecting the right foods early on to supply these needs can therefore have powerful effects on their brain as well as their overall health later in life.

First foods should meet the criteria discussed in earlier chapters:

+ They should support growth and development of the child's brain (feed the brain)
+ They should support a healthy microbiome in the infant's gut and thereby support their immune system, brain, and metabolism (feed the gut)
+ They should limit epigenetic programming for future disease (feed the genes)

If first foods follow these guidelines, then the child should be getting adequate but not excessive calories for overall growth and will be getting all the key nutrients in the right levels to optimize their development. Using a template of healthy food choices as well as proven strategies developed by feeding experts, parents can embark on this feeding journey with more confidence. The more parents know, the easier it will be to make informed choices, paving the way for a happier, healthier child and family down the line.

This chapter will provide guidelines for how to start an infant on solid food and the scientific evidence that supports each of these recommendations. As a pediatric physician trained in nutrition and a parent who has gone through this process with my own children, I know the *what*, the *why* and the *when* of feeding an infant. Both personally and professionally I learned a great deal about *how* to feed a child from feeding experts including **speech-language pathologists (SLPs)** trained in feeding children. I incorporate their expertise into this chapter as well and devote a separate chapter to feeding issues and disorders.

> How to feed a child is the domain of SLPs, occupational therapists (OTs), and behavioral/developmental specialists trained to help children who have serious feeding issues. These experts analyze problems with swallowing mechanics, physical and developmental abilities, feeding cues and other behavioral or psychological barriers to eating. When feeding issues arise (and they frequently do) these specialists are gold. They train parents how to overcome food aversions, picky eating, mechanical swallowing issues, and a whole host of feeding disorders. These experts can be a valuable part of a multidisciplinary team to help children with feeding difficulties.

First, let's look at *when* to start solids, *what* the best early foods should be and *why*; then we will explore *how*.

## WHEN DO I START SOLIDS?

Up to the age of 5 to 6 months, all the baby's nutritional needs are typically met by breast milk or formula. With the exception of vitamin D drops for the majority of babies without adequate sun exposure, and iron supplements for some premature infants, babies typically do not need anything else for their nutrition. By the age of 5 to 6 months, most infants are ready to start eating some solid foods in addition to breast milk or formula, and there is a biological need for this extra nutrition as the baby's stores of iron start to run low at this point.[2,3]

The **World Health Organization** (WHO) currently recommends starting solid foods alongside breastfeeding at 6 months of age. Given individual variation, there is no exact "magic moment" for all babies, but somewhere between 5 to 6 months of life most infants are neurologically and physically ready to try solid foods.

Some babies may be ready between 4 and 5 months, but evidence would show that feeding solid foods before 4 months of age is unnecessary and perhaps unwise. The infant gut needs to be mature enough to handle the increased work of digestion, and the kidneys need to be able to process the different concentrations of minerals and nutrients that solid food contains.[2] Some research shows an increased risk of obesity in babies fed solid food prior to 4 months of age but this has been challenged and likely depends on whether the infant is formula fed or breastfed.[4,5] There is also evidence that early introduction of foods prior to 4 months alters the infant microbiome in potentially unfavorable ways, altering the immune system and increasing the risk of allergic or **autoimmune disease** in a susceptible infant.[6-8] Because of this, the introduction of solid foods before 4 months of age is not advised. I generally do not recommend introducing solid foods until between 5 and 6 months for all these reasons.

Feeding needs to be safe. Food should not be pushed on a baby who is not able to swallow it without choking, gagging, and potentially aspirating (food into the lungs instead of the stomach). The focus should be on *developmental readiness* to feed instead of chronological age, as is the cornerstone of the **baby-led weaning** concept. Feedings are advanced when *the baby* is ready, not when the parents are ready. Each child is an individual and should be treated as such. Work with your pediatrician to determine if the baby is showing signs of being developmentally ready to start some solid foods, typically somewhere between 5 and 6 months.

**Developmental cues that a baby is ready to accept solid food:**[9]

+ Sits without support for short periods
+ Has good head and neck control
+ Munches/chews and moves pureed food to the back of the mouth
+ Does not automatically push food out of the mouth with the tongue

+ Brings hands and objects to their mouth
+ Shows interest in food, watches food intently, grabs food

However, if the child reaches seven months of age and is still not accepting any solid foods, or is choking and gagging repeatedly with food introduction, they need to be assessed promptly by the pediatrician who may recommend a feeding specialist (see text box p.179). Feeding difficulties in a baby can indicate that something is wrong with their swallowing mechanics, stomach, or esophagus. Delay in getting help with a problem feeder can cause a baby to miss that developmental golden window of opportunity for introducing new foods and textures and can lead to **Pediatric Feeding Disorders (PFD)**. Parents should seek help early (before 9 months) if feeding issues arise in their infant.

## WHAT FOODS SHOULD BE FIRST?

After 6 months, the breast-fed baby needs complementary foods (foods other than breast milk or infant formula) to provide additional nutrients. Otherwise, **neurodevelopment** or immune system impairments can stem from inadequate iron, zinc, and other deficiencies. First foods, also referred to as complementary foods, complement the nutrition found in breast milk by filling in the gaps and supplying the extra nutrients the baby needs to grow. Beyond 5 to 6 months, breast milk is not adequate by itself to supply all the essential nutrients for a developing infant with a rapidly growing brain.

While there are nutritional differences between formula and breastmilk, the goal for babies receiving either is the same: a steady introduction of healthy foods starting at 5 to 6 months, so that by the end of the first year, the child is eating a wide range of minimally processed foods that supports their development. At 12 months, they should not remain overly reliant on breast milk or formula for nutrients and calories.

Choosing the correct foods early on helps to supply key nutrients like iron, zinc, choline, and **omega-3** fats needed by the growing brain. Meat and fish can play an important role in the early weaning diet. Delaying complementary foods that supply important nutrients can have negative consequences on the baby's rapidly growing brain as well as their immune system and overall growth. There is also growing concern that an early diet containing large amounts of highly processed foods and sugar may also be programming children for future disease, damaging their **metabolism,** and their developing microbiome and brain. Several studies in the last decade have shown an association between a weaning diet high in sugar and processed foods and decreased IQ with lower scholastic achievement in later childhood.[2]

An early diet that provides an ongoing supply of prebiotic fiber and **phytonutrients** is important for the development of a healthy microbiome. The infant microbiome continues to develop and evolve over the first thousand days of that child's life, and is shaped by the type of diet that they are fed. As discussed previously, breastfed and formula-fed infants tend to have detectable differences in their intestinal microbiome. These differences could be amplified or corrected depending on the type of weaning diet that is chosen.

Choosing a weaning diet containing real, whole foods with plenty of naturally occurring fiber and phytonutrients and avoiding excessive sugar and highly processed foods will help set their microbiome to one that promotes health versus chronic disease. Recall that a whole host of diseases and disorders are being linked to alterations of the microbiome including everything from constipation to autoimmune diseases such as inflammatory bowel disease, and even brain disorders such as autism (see Chapter 3.) Transitioning from an infant diet that is exclusively breast milk or formula to one that is composed primarily of regular table foods by 12 months of age further shifts the types of bacteria that live in the intestines to more of an "adult" type microbiome, which eventually becomes set for better or worse. Choose a healthy, whole food weaning diet to decrease the risks associated with **dysbiosis**.

### Meat and fish

So, what are the optimum first foods? From an evolutionary perspective, what did our ancestors feed their cave-babies? Rice cereal? More likely, they fed them chewed up meat or mashed up fish and vegetables. This is perfect because breast milk is low in iron (by design) and the baby's iron stores start to run low right about the time that foods are being introduced. The zinc content of breast milk is initially adequate in the first few months of life but drops off markedly as the infant approaches 6 months of age. Animal proteins, especially beef, poultry, game meat, and fish are nutritional powerhouses that contain good amounts of iron and zinc as well as $B_{12}$ and other B vitamins in forms that are readily utilized by the baby. Meat, poultry, fish, and eggs are also sources of high-quality protein that is efficiently used by the baby for growth. While fortified infant cereals have become the weaning standard and still play an important role worldwide, we will explore why this may not be optimal for many children.

*The role of animal-based foods in the early diet*

A growing base of scientists and the **World Health Organization** (WHO) support the importance of including some meat, poultry, and fish products in the early diet. The American Academy of Pediatrics (AAP) recommends two servings per day of iron-rich foods, including meat or iron-fortified cereal, to meet the baby's needs.[10] Despite this, surveys in the US show that less than 5% of babies are regularly consuming meat and the number of parents feeding their infants baby food meat is declining.[11] Traditional weaning practices in the US for breast fed infants often do not contain meat or fish. This may have potential consequences.

These foods supply vital iron, zinc, high quality protein, choline, vitamin $B_{12}$, and long chain omega-3 **polyunsaturated fatty acids (PUFA)**. These nutrients are difficult or impossible to get in adequate amounts for a developing infant brain from a purely plant-based diet, or a **complementary diet** that is mostly dairy and grain based *unless the properly fortified foods and nutritional supplements are included*. Parents choosing not to include animal-based foods in the weaning diet need to make every effort to ensure these vital nutrients are supplied elsewhere in the diet or through supplementation to avoid negative consequences.

Studies show a meat-based complementary diet improves infant growth measured by height (length) of infants without increasing the *weight for height* as compared to infants consuming a grain based or dairy based complementary diet.[68,69] This evidence suggests lower potential risks for developing obesity in infants fed a meat-based complementary diet.

Recent studies also demonstrated that lower dietary protein *quality* is associated with risk of poor growth in early life and that incorporation of animal-based foods in the diets of young children improved growth and decreased risk of growth failure.[67] This seems to indicate that adding some animal-based products early to a breastfed or formula fed baby's diet helps them grow better, get taller, but not overweight.

A meat-based complementary diet is safe, feasible and recommended by top nutrition researchers, including Dr. Nancy Krebs who is the head of Nutrition and Professor of Pediatrics at the University of Colorado.[2,10,18,70] Incorporating some animal-based products in the early diet will help ensure the baby gets adequate zinc, iron, protein, choline, and omega-3 DHA for proper growth and brain development. Beef, dark meat chicken and turkey, or game meat that is pureed or mashed with some olive oil, breast milk or formula are perfect first foods.

*Iron and Zinc-Nutrients at Risk in the Infant Diet*
Worldwide iron deficiency is the leading nutritional problem in childhood. A quarter of all children worldwide are iron deficient, and an estimated 15% of children in the US and Europe do not have adequate iron in their bodies to support optimal brain development. Given the high rates of maternal iron deficiency, obesity, and **gestational diabetes**, all of which increase an infant's risk of iron deficiency, many infants are being born already low in this essential nutrient. This will be worsened by an inadequate weaning diet.

Iron deficiency during the first thousand days can lead to irreversible developmental issues.[3,12] Having adequate iron intake and absorption during this time is crucial for proper brain development. Iron deficiency also impairs the function and development of the infant immune system, opening the door to infections.[13–15] Breastfed babies older than 6 months who do not consume meat or an adequately fortified cereal are at risk for nutritional deficiencies, most notably iron and zinc.

Iron intake recommendations during infant weaning range internationally from 8 to 11 mg daily, based on an estimated low absorption of 10% of iron from non-meat sources.[3,16] Recall that breastmilk only contains about 0.5 mg of highly absorbed iron per day. Zinc requirements for the weaning baby are estimated to be 2.5 mg per day, and breast milk only supplies about 0.5 mg per day.[17] This clearly leaves an iron and zinc gap in the diet that needs to be filled by complementary foods. The inclusion of meat or fortified infant cereals containing both iron and zinc closes this gap.[17,18]

The forms of iron in food and how well they are absorbed influence how much is needed. The type of iron found in animal products (**heme iron**) and the iron found in plant products or added to iron-fortified foods like cereals and formula (**non-heme iron**) are different. For example, up to 40% of heme iron in a meal is absorbed for use by the body compared to a maximum of 15% of non-heme iron.[19,20] Despite being an animal-based product, eggs contain substances that reduce iron absorption and therefore are not a good isolated iron source but should still be part of early food introduction.[20] Vitamin C, breast milk, and the presence of some animal proteins in the diet all help to increase the absorption of non-heme iron. In fact, including a little meat in a vegetable blend increases the absorption of the non-meat iron almost 3-fold.[21]

As discussed earlier, anti-nutrient compounds in certain plants can partially block the absorption of iron and zinc. Two examples of **anti-nutrients** are **phytates** and lectins, which are high in grains, cereals, and legumes (beans and lentils). Soy protein has been shown to independently inhibit iron absorption.[22,23] Infant consumption of cow's milk can also block iron absorption and is not recommended.[39] However, these anti-nutrients are not as concerning if the baby or toddler is getting enough heme-iron from animal products and avoiding over-consumption of grains and beans.

Non-heme iron and zinc need adequate stomach acid to be absorbed, whereas heme iron does not.[28] It is thought that stomach acid in children does not reach adult levels until later in childhood, perhaps by age two.[29,30] This low stomach acid in infants could contribute to inefficient absorption of non-heme iron early in life, further suggesting the utility of animal products in the early diet.

The widespread use of acid blocking medication in infants for reflux and fussiness (which is not often indicated, according to the AAP) may inhibit the absorption of iron and zinc. The long-term effect of acid blocking medications on children and infants is not well researched and needs more data.[31–33] For the sake of brain development, I suggest that all babies on acid blockers for reflux should incorporate some heme-iron containing protein in their diet to insure they are absorbing the iron or take steps to boost the absorption of non-heme iron.

The baby's absorption of iron is therefore affected by multiple factors: the presence or absence of animal protein, the amounts of anti-nutrients, vitamin C, breast milk, the presence or absence of inflammation in the intestines, as well as the overall iron levels in the child's body. Determining and meeting the optimum iron intake for a young child's brain development is more than just meeting the **RDA** and becomes more complicated without heme iron in the diet.

More is not better. If a child who is formula fed eats several servings of high-iron fortified cereal daily, they are getting a fairly high amount of poorly absorbed iron in their diet, considerably more than the recommended intake of 11 mg. This amount helps to prevent deficiency, but excessive iron could have negative effects. The downstream consequences of feeding a high amount of more poorly absorbed iron to a developing child is starting to receive more concern. In the chapter on formula feeding we discussed how unabsorbed iron from high-iron formula may have negative effects on the intestinal microbiome, fostering the growth of some unfavorable bacteria.[24] This was shown to also be the case in infants fed highly iron fortified cereal, where unfriendly bacteria and inflammation in the intestines increased, and beneficial **probiotic** bacteria decreased.[25-27]

In contrast, a few ounces of meat containing heme iron goes a long way, with less unabsorbed iron reaching the intestines. My inclination is that foods containing more highly absorbed heme iron are better for most babies than high amounts of fortified iron that are not well absorbed.

## TABLE 10.1 IRON AND ZINC CONTENT OF FOODS

| Food (per 2.5 oz jar/serving) | Iron (milligrams) | Zinc (milligrams) |
|---|---|---|
| Pureed beef | 0.8 | 1.5 |
| Ground beef | 1.85 | 4.4 |
| Liver (beef) | 4.8 | 4.0 |
| Chicken and gravy | 0.4 | 0.6 |
| Chicken thigh | 1.0 | 2.0 |
| Chicken breast | 0.8 | 0.75 |
| Turkey dark meat | 1.1 | 2.6 |
| Turkey white meat | 0.5-1.0 | 1.3 |
| Salmon | 0.6 | 0.6 |
| Trout | 1.4 | 0.6 |
| Sardines | 2.0 | 1.0 |
| *Fortified rice cereal | 5-6.75 | 0-1.0 |
| *Fortified oat cereal | 6.75 | 1.0 |
| *Black beans | 1.6 | 0.85 |
| *Lentils | 2.3 | 0.9 |
| *Spinach (baby food) | 0.6 | 0.3 |
| *Spinach (cooked/pureed) | 2.0 | 0.6 |
| *Egg (1) | 0.8 | 0.6 |

*non-heme iron sources that are less efficiently absorbed

*The importance of zinc*

Mild zinc deficiency is relatively common in infants and children even in the US and is a huge problem worldwide. The WHO states that one third of children in the world are at risk for zinc deficiency. Zinc is needed for growth, brain development, and a functioning immune system. We want to do everything we can to support the baby's brain and immune system in the first thousand days. Zinc is also crucial for production of digestive enzymes in the pancreas and even mild zinc deficiency could impair the child's ability to digest foods.[34,35] Children in developing nations with a diet low in zinc and high in anti-nutrients are at high risk for infections because their immune systems cannot effectively fight off invaders. They are also at risk for stunted growth because they cannot effectively digest and absorb nutrients. Infections and inflammation of the gut in these children further impair nutrient absorption, creating a vicious cycle.[36,37]

Zinc-rich foods include meat and seafood, but zinc is also found in seeds, nuts, and beans and some fortified infant cereals. Similar to iron, many plant sources of zinc like beans and grains also contain the antinutrient phytate that may partially block absorption. It is currently unclear how much effect this has in infants raised in more economically developed countries but worldwide it is a major concern.[38] A high intake of cow's milk can also block zinc absorption.[39] Given the anti-nutrient factors found in common foods, it is important to note that a child could have seemingly adequate iron or zinc intake on paper, yet not be getting the optimal amounts their body needs because these minerals are blocked from absorption by the anti-nutrients, lack of stomach acid or by excessive milk intake.

It is worth noting that absorption of zinc from animal products is about 55% efficient, versus a diet without animal proteins that is high in grains and legumes where absorption may be as low as only 15%.[19,40,41] If we are not accounting for the digestibility and absorption of key nutrients, we can be misled into thinking a child's intake is adequate when it is not, leading to subtle or not so subtle deficiency. Another point to consider is that zinc is lost through the stool when a child has diarrhea, so extra care is needed in infants or children with chronic diarrhea.

Zinc is vital for the developing baby and growing child so care must be taken to ensure adequate intake. A few ounces a day of meat or seafood should be included in the weaning diet. If not, it is essential to include a zinc fortified cereal or other zinc supplement (5mg/day) to insure the child meets their requirements.[22] Discuss this with their healthcare provider.

*Get those omega-3s!*

Mashed up salmon, trout, sardines, or herring (be careful to remove all the bones!) are also great first foods, and supply lots of brain building omega-3 DHA and other healthy fat, as well as zinc, iron, choline, B12 and high-quality protein. Let's not forget that that the baby brain is more than doubling its weight in the first year, and most of this weight is fat. That little baby brain needs lots and lots of good healthy fat to grow, and a baby should *never* be on a low-fat diet.

As described previously, the rapidly growing baby brain uses lots of omega-3 DHA throughout the first thousand days and cannot use the plant-based **ALA** omega-3 for building new **neurons** and new connections. Recall that the child's body is not efficient at converting the plant-based omega-3 ALA to the long-chain omega-3 DHA needed by the growing brain. There is some conversion of ALA to another long chain omega-3 called EPA, but this is not the primary omega-3 used in the brain. There is evidence this ALA is instead often being used for ketone production to burn for energy. Current evidence would suggest that the conversion of plant-based omega-3 to essential DHA is less than 5% efficient, possibly even lower than 1%, and that several factors can influence this rate including genetic predisposition and background diet. A diet too high in **omega-6** fats from vegetable oils or low in magnesium and zinc may further impair this rate of conversion.[42-46]

The infant receives an average of 60 mg DHA daily from breastmilk. However, a concern arises as an infant makes the transition to a solid food diet; the amounts of DHA supplied by breast milk decrease while rapid brain growth continues to require this nutrient throughout the toddler phase.

Precise DHA requirements and recommendations for the older infant and toddler have yet to be established but given the amounts in healthy breastmilk and the ongoing rapid growth of the brain, **the older baby brain would benefit from at least 100 mg DHA daily**. International research organizations such as the International Society for the Study of Fatty Acids and Lipids (ISSFAL) would echo these recommendations. Therefore, to make sure an optimal amount of DHA is delivered to their brain for those first thousand days, a dietary source of this nutrient should be included early in the diet.

Cold water fish (salmon, herring, sardines, trout, and cod) and omega-3 enriched eggs can all provide an ongoing source of DHA for the baby's brain. Beef and game meat will also contain small amounts. Keep in mind that grass-fed beef has double the amount of DHA compared to grain fed beef.[47] Salmon is one of the best sources because of the high DHA and choline content. When my wife and I were raising our children, we grilled or baked salmon and trout and mashed it up with some avocado and our babies loved it as an early weaning food. As always, when feeding infants fish, make sure there are no bones and avoid the higher mercury fish such as tuna, swordfish, mackerel, and orange roughy, as the mercury can damage their growing brain. See Table 6.9 in the pregnancy nutrition chapter for a high and low mercury seafood list. Vegetarian parents should add omega-3 DHA eggs to their children's diet, and vegan parents should strongly consider incorporating an algae-source DHA supplement.

**Eggs**
Despite eggs being a common allergen, they are a nutritional powerhouse. Eggs should be introduced to a baby by 9 months of age but optimally in the first few months of adding complementary foods. The fat, choline, and $B_{12}$ in the yolks are great for the baby's brain, and the high-quality protein in eggs is excellent for overall growth. There is an ongoing role for dietary choline in both prenatal and postnatal brain development, and this nutrient is low in purely plant-based foods. Adding eggs in early complementary feeding improves choline intake, and may help promote ongoing brain development and growth.[48] As mentioned before, there are also omega-3 DHA enhanced eggs which can be a great source of choline and DHA for those parents wishing to avoid fish.

As with any new food, watch for rashes, eczema, respiratory issues, vomiting or diarrhea as possible signs the child could have a food allergy or sensitivity, and contact a pediatrician or primary care provider if concerns arise. The most recent evidence-based recommendations state that egg introduction early (around 6 months) while breastfeeding may help to *prevent* the development of egg allergies later on. Consider placing eggs on the list of first foods to be introduced. Scrambled eggs are a great soft self-feeding food for baby-led weaning as well. If possible, try to choose cage free or free-range pasture-raised eggs that endorse more ethical treatment of the chickens ("Certified Humane"). Locally produced eggs from small farms or individual households are making a big comeback. These eggs are likely to have better nutritional value and fresher taste than mass produced eggs, but all eggs will have benefits for the baby. From pregnancy right on through childhood, unless there is an allergy or intolerance, eggs should be a staple.

## Vegetables

Vegetables supply important fiber, **antioxidants**, vitamin A (as beta carotene) and phytonutrients that support that developing microbiome as well as turn off genes that code for inflammation and chronic disease. Vegetables can be introduced either by themselves or blended with an animal protein (chicken and carrots being a favorite). Carrots, green beans, peas, squash, spinach, and sweet potatoes are all staples of early food introduction. It is never too early to start "eating the rainbow" of colorful vegetables. The natural green, yellow, orange, and red pigments in vegetables all have important antioxidants and phytonutrients that are missing in processed food. These foods are also rich in soluble fiber to support the ongoing development of the child's microbiome.[49,50]

Any of these vegetables can be steamed or boiled until soft, pureed using a hand blender or food processor with a little olive or avocado oil or breast milk/formula to add some good fat and give them a creamier mouth feel. Veggies may be served in soft finger-sized portions for those choosing to do baby-led weaning. I encourage parents to make their own baby food as much as possible, but if doing a baby-led weaning there is no need for baby foods, as the child weans onto essentially the same foods that adults eat, just cooked a little softer.

> A time saving tip to assure a steady supply of baby food is to make a batch of pureed veggies, or meats, and then freeze them in ice cube trays. When frozen, empty the food cubes into a labeled bag in in the freezer. At mealtime, simply defrost the cubes: one veggie, one meat and voila! Just make sure to cool down the food before putting it into the ice cube trays, as hot foods in plastic potentially releases some of the chemicals such as phthalates that are being linked to a host of health issues in children and adults. Better yet, use the BPA/phthalate free silicone trays to make the cubes.

We should try to feed our young children organic as much as possible, especially with any of the "Dirty Dozen" most contaminated fruits and vegetables, due to the potential dangers of pesticide exposure. (See the section on pesticide dangers in Chapter 4) Several baby food companies make organic baby foods, so it may be wise to choose these products when possible, especially for the Dirty Dozen.

## Fruits

Fruits are great in the early diet, but not as a first food, or even the first five foods. Fruits do not have substantial iron (other than prunes), they are very low in zinc, and have no choline, $B_{12}$, or DHA. Fruits do contain important fiber, antioxidants, and phytonutrients. However, the reason for waiting on fruit introduction is less about nutrition and more about taste preferences. It can take 10 to 30 times of introducing a savory food or naturally bitter food like certain vegetables to children before they will accept it. Persistence pays off! Sweets and fruits only require one taste to get a child "hooked," as we are genetically programmed to respond immediately to sweet tastes.

If children are given sweet foods early in the game, they may come to expect sweet tasting foods and have a harder time eating unsweetened foods later on.[2,51] That being said, apples, peaches, pears, plums, berries, bananas, and other fruits should absolutely be part of the feeding plan after building a base of the other foods that the child is happily willing to eat. Fruits and vegetables fulfill the role of adding prebiotic fiber to the diet to promote a healthy gut microbiome. They are also high in antioxidants and phytonutrients, which play a protective role and epigenetically program against inflammation and chronic disease.

> High sugar foods should NEVER be a part of an infant's diet, as this is one of the influences that is likely programming kids to become obese and get **type 2 diabetes** early in life. The American Heart Association (AHA) and the American Academy of Pediatrics (AAP) both recommend NO added sugar for children age two years or younger.[2,52-54] Frequently eating high sugar foods in the early diet can program children to want excessive amounts of these foods, which is going to damage their dental health, their metabolism and their microbiome early on in life. Avoid giving infants or young toddlers soda, candy, cakes, cookies, or high sugar yogurt. Occasional treats may be added for birthdays and special occasions later in childhood but avoid high-sugar processed foods when a child is weaning to a regular diet.

## Milk

I recommend that infants drink only breast milk or formula during their first year because they need the extra nutrition. Small amounts of water can be given but generally not more than a few ounces. *After* 12 months of age, cow, goat, or alternative milks such as almond milk may be introduced. Recall that feeding cow's milk to an infant has been associated with increased risk of gastrointestinal bleeding and iron deficiency, so definitely hold off until after 12 months of age before introducing it. Also note that there have been concerns about the arsenic content of some rice milk, so this may not be the best choice for a toddler either. Infants should not be getting any fruit juice or sweetened drinks because of the excessive sugar. Occasionally, it may be recommended that a constipated infant drink a few ounces of juice as a stool softener, but this should be minimal and temporary.

The brightly colored "kid" yogurts commonly advertised are almost all loaded with sugar, and many have artificial food coloring (AFC) that may not be great for some children's brains (see the section on AFC in the next chapter). These products have no place in an infant diet. Unsweetened yogurt can be added as a complementary food as babies get to 9-12 months and blended with (organic) berries to make a probiotic and antioxidant rich treat with a fraction of the sugar. My wife and I fed our older infants unsweetened full-fat goat yogurt (because of cow's milk protein intolerance) with defrosted organic frozen berries and they loved it.

### Grains

Despite the fact that infant cereals have been a staple of infant weaning diets for decades, based on increasing evidence, this may not be the best choice for them. Grain products don't need to be among the very first foods for infants because they are high in carbohydrates and relatively low in overall nutritional value unless heavily fortified. They are more of a second line food. They are poor sources of iron and zinc (unless they are fortified), have no omega-3 fats, are very low in choline, and contain those anti-nutrients that block iron and zinc absorption. Yes, there are some B vitamins in grains and beans, but certainly less than is found in animal-based products (except folate which can be found in legumes as well as green veggies).

Many infant cereals are fortified with nutrients including iron and zinc to try to bolster them up nutritionally, but this still does not mean they are the optimal first foods. Some of the most popular infant cereals are heavily fortified with calcium, iron, vitamin C, zinc, vitamin E, vitamins $B_1$, $B_2$, $B_3$, $B_6$ and $B_{12}$, as well as folic acid, and *can be a source of these important nutrients to prevent deficiency in a child not consuming meat products.* However, if we take a step back, we realize that what is being attempted is the fortification of a nutritionally inadequate food with the goal of making it more like a natural product *that already has exactly what that child needs nutritionally.*

Some rice cereal and many other infant and breakfast cereals, unless they are whole grain varieties, can be considered **ultra-processed foods** by the United Nations NOVA classification. Ultra-processed foods are now being linked to increased risk of type 2 diabetes and obesity among other chronic diseases.[55,56] The typical infant cereals remove much of the fiber during processing, thereby giving these foods a high *glycemic index* (meaning they turn to sugar almost instantly in the child's GI tract and will raise blood sugar very quickly). Starchy, highly processed low-fiber foods can also be constipating for some babies. The removal of fiber also potentially negatively affects the baby's microbiome, which needs prebiotic fiber to grow. Some infant cereals are also hydrolyzed, meaning they have been somewhat pre-digested with enzymes as part of the processing, which releases free sugars and further raises the glycemic index.[57] There is mounting evidence that having increased sugar and highly processed, high glycemic index carbs in early life could program the child for later obesity and type 2 diabetes by altering taste preferences, the baby's microbiome and epigenetic programming.[51,58,59] While some important nutrients are often added to these infant cereals after processing, what they don't add in are fiber, phytonutrients, omega-3 DHA, or choline.

When adding grains to an infant's diet, consider those that are less highly processed, such as steel cut or rolled oatmeal instead of instant oatmeal or mashed rice or quinoa instead of highly processed infant cereal. There are whole grain infant cereals available on the market that are less processed and have more fiber.

For the parents feeding their baby meat, consider skipping infant cereal, or at least wait until ample veggies and meat/fish/eggs/poultry are introduced first. Whole grain oats, rice, and quinoa have good amounts of fiber, a lower glycemic index, and **prebiotics** for the child's gut microbiome. Be cautious of instant oatmeal which typically has a high amount of added sugar and should be avoided. Keep in mind that whole grains, while healthier overall do contain anti-nutrients that can block absorption of iron and zinc, so the amounts included in the infant diet should be moderate and in balance with other nutrient rich foods such as vegetables and meat.

### The bottom line on infant cereals
If choosing to use an infant cereal as an early staple in the child's diet *in place of meat*, make sure it is fortified with both iron and zinc, and consider adding in other sources of choline and DHA. Given the current data on arsenic in rice products, it may be better to choose an oat or alternate

grain-based infant cereal. Aside from having much lower arsenic levels, oats also have the advantage of having more prebiotic soluble fiber to feed the microbiome. Use of a heavily fortified infant cereal may be important for those parents trying to raise a vegetarian child, as this may be the main source of iron and zinc in their diet. However, rather than being the "gold standard" for those parents willing to include meat in their baby's weaning diet, it really isn't necessary to add these grains or cereals in the baby's diet until later as a potential second line food if preferred. The child will do just fine without them.

> There had previously been some thought that introducing some **gluten** (wheat) into the diet early during breastfeeding may decrease the chances of getting celiac disease. Unfortunately recent data suggests this is not the case, but in fact, that heavy gluten (wheat) intake during early feeding increases the chances for developing celiac disease.[2]

### Rice and the arsenic conundrum revisited

As described in the **toxin** section, there has been a growing concern about arsenic levels in rice, especially as it relates to infants and small children. To review briefly, elevated levels of arsenic in the body are associated with neurodevelopmental issues, decreased immune system functioning, and increased risk of certain cancers.

Studies have shown a consistent association with rice consumption and level of arsenic exposure, and one-year-old infants who regularly consumed rice products had double the arsenic detected in their urine.[60-62] Common foods of concern in the infant and toddler diet are rice, rice crackers, rice cereal, rice noodles/pasta, rice cakes, and rice milk.[63]

Reduce your child's exposure to arsenic in the following ways:

+ Don't feed your children those rice-based products that are known to be higher in arsenic.
+ Don't rely on infant rice cereal as a diet staple. Use oats, quinoa, or other grain options. Use rice products sparingly and select for products that have tested low in arsenic levels.
+ Look for lower arsenic rice varieties. Much of the rice grown in the southern USA has been reported to be higher in arsenic than Basmati or Jasmine rice grown in certain areas of California or in certain areas of India or the Himalayas.[64,65]

+ There may be a higher arsenic level in rice crackers and rice cakes than in rice, so limit intake.
+ Be cautious about giving children rice milk—some could have elevated levels of arsenic.
+ Cooking methods can reduce the level of arsenic in the rice. Soak the rice in water overnight before cooking, then discard the water and rinse well.

## Beans and Lentils

When to feed babies beans and lentils is a question that warrants further examination. Are they good or bad for the baby? Let's look at this topic a little more closely.

Eating a diet containing both beans and grains can provide "complete" proteins, which means the combination of these foods supply all the amino acids it needs for things like repair and growth. Worldwide, many cultures use beans and lentils as a staple for feeding their infants. The potential benefits and risks of this practice depend on what else is in the diet.

Beans and lentils are a cheap source of protein, folate, and fiber, and they can be dried and stored without refrigeration. In adults, there may be some health benefits to eating these foods, such as improving cardiovascular risk. However, when weaning an infant to a diet using beans, lentils, and grains *instead of* meat, poultry, and fish, the health benefits become more questionable. Are they an optimal staple food for babies? There are a few concerns.

### Anti-nutrients

As previously stated, grains and legumes contain naturally occurring anti-nutrient compounds (**phytates** and lectins), which block the absorption of key nutrients like iron and zinc. These anti-nutrients can be decreased but not eliminated in beans and lentils by proper preparation and cooking techniques like rinsing, soaking, and sprouting, and by prolonged cooking. Does this decrease the anti-nutrients in these foods enough for an infant with an immature digestive tract or are they still going to be nutritionally at risk eating higher amounts of these foods? There are ongoing concerns.

### Protein quality and digestibility

While beans and grains are complementary proteins and contain the essential amino acids required for growth, questions remain. How *bio-available* are they? How well can little bodies use these plant-based proteins for growth and repair? Are the building blocks (amino acids) supplied by these foods optimal for a rapidly developing child?

There are scoring methods for protein quality, telling how well the body can use the protein from certain foods. Using new techniques developed in the past few years, a lower than expected digestibility of legume (bean) protein (less than 60% digestible) was found.[66] By comparison, animal protein was shown to have a much higher score (86-92% digestible). Studies have demonstrated that protein *quality* is associated with risk of stunting (poor growth) and that incorporation of animal foods (including eggs) in the diets of young children who eat mostly grains and legumes improved their growth.[67] This is usually not an issue in developed countries like the US or Europe as a total population, but could be an issue for the individual infant or toddler who is not getting any animal protein in their diet.

I share the opinion of experts in infant nutrition that beans and lentils can be incorporated as a complementary food but should perhaps not be the main source of protein and nutrients for the developing child in the first thousand days.

## VEGETARIAN AND VEGAN DIETS

Increasing numbers of parents are choosing to try to raise their children vegetarian or vegan for moral or ethical reasons. While I don't question the morals behind this decision, I would provide caveats for weaning onto a completely plant-based diet. The ability to provide a nutritionally optimal diet for a child during the most critical developmental period of their life requires that correct steps must be taken to avoid harm. Nutritional difficulties for an infant or young child being weaned onto a strict vegan or vegetarian diet include protein quantity and quality, inadequate zinc, iron, omega-3 fats (EPA/DHA), B vitamins (mainly $B_{12}$), and choline.

It is clearly stated in the medical literature that iron deficiency is the most prevalent nutritional issue worldwide, and that zinc deficiency in developing nations is also a common cause of poor growth and impaired immune system. In fact, the WHO attributes more than 500,000 deaths annually to zinc deficiency from diets lacking zinc rich foods.[71] These same problems are happening in "First World" nations as well, albeit often more subtly and insidiously. Remember that those first thousand days of life are when crucial brain development and immune system functioning are at stake. Please consider the following:

+ The richest and most bioavailable sources of almost all the key nutrients for brain development are found in meat, fish, and eggs.
+ Protein, iron, zinc, DHA, B$_{12}$ and Choline are all vital to the growing brain especially in the first thousand days of a child's life.
+ Suboptimal intakes of these nutrients in the first thousand days may be associated with potentially irreversible downstream effects on the brain.

Weaning the child to a vegetarian or vegan diet has nutritional risks for the deficiencies listed at the beginning of this chapter. Medical and nutritional supervision is advised.[2] If the decision is made to wean the child to a vegetarian or vegan diet, the child should be followed closely by a pediatric trained dietician who can monitor growth and recommend proper supplements, if needed.

### Testing for deficiencies

The primary care provider should consider testing the plant-based child for low iron and B$_{12}$ periodically. When testing for iron deficiency, a **ferritin** level is needed (not just a **hemoglobin**) to accurately check the child's iron levels and iron stores.

+ Testing for omega-3 fatty acids in the body is also possible but can be a little more difficult–RBC fatty acids or Omega-3 Index are two testing methods.
+ Testing for zinc levels in the blood is notoriously inaccurate for detecting mild deficiency and is not recommended except in major deficiency states.

The healthcare provider or dietician may consider starting the vegetarian child empirically on zinc, DHA, B$_{12}$, and choline supplements to supply the growing brain with these missing nutrients.

*Surviving versus Thriving*

This is probably a good time to talk about surviving versus thriving. Many children *survive* without healthy, unprocessed food and without concentrated sources of brain nutrients in their diet. But are they thriving? Thriving not just in the sense of growing adequately, but also in meeting a child's full potential with a thriving body and mind.

Can children develop optimally without concentrated sources of vital nutrients like DHA, iron, zinc, choline, folate, phytonutrients, fiber, and more biologically active forms of the B vitamins? Probably not.

Can children develop optimally with high amounts of sugar and processed foods in their early diet? Probably not.

My purpose in writing this book is to inform parents and health professionals about the optimal way to support the growing child, *based on scientific evidence.* I want every child to thrive not just survive. I don't want any child to miss a critical developmental window and not achieve their full brain potential. Inadequate nutrition during the critical first thousand days is contributing to the epidemic of neurodevelopmental and immune disorders we are seeing in today's kids. Remember that once critical developmental windows are closed, they do not reopen. Why chance it? Be informed and be proactive.

Historically, culturally, and socioeconomically there are populations around the world who either choose to avoid or do not have access to nutrient-dense unprocessed foods. From a scientific standpoint, it is important to highlight the potential health ramifications associated with nutrient deficient diets or those high in processed foods for developing infants and children.

### TABLE 10.2 FOOD INTRODUCTION CHART

| First Line Baby Foods | Second Line Baby Foods |
|---|---|
| Pureed beef | Apple |
| Pureed chicken/turkey (dark meat preferred) | Pear |
| Game meat (for those who have access) | Banana |
| Mashed fish (salmon, trout, sardines) | Peaches/plums/prunes |
| Avocado | Berries |
| Carrots | Whole grain rice (low arsenic variety) |
| Squash/pumpkin | White potato (mashed or cubed) |
| Broccoli/Cauliflower | Quinoa (mashed or cereal) |
| Peas | Beans/lentils (mashed) |
| Green beans | Nut butters (peanut, almond, cashew) |
| Spinach/Greens | Whole grain cereals |
| Sweet potato/Yams | Oats/oatmeal |
| Scrambled eggs | |

*For those avoiding meat products, fortified oat cereal with zinc and iron recommended early
Later infancy consider yogurt, cheese, breads, whole grain pasta/noodles, crackers
**Baby vegetables are typically steamed or boiled until soft and mashed or pureed with a small amount of breast milk or formula added. Fruits can be mashed or pureed depending on the infant ability to tolerate textures.

# HOW TO INTRODUCE FOODS

We discussed the "when" and the "what" of introducing foods. Let's get into the "how" a little bit. This has also become a hot topic, with the advent of baby-led weaning (BLW), which differs from traditional weaning.

Traditional weaning methods start with purees or rice cereal for one to several months before gradually increasing textures and food selections. Mashed and finger foods were recommended to start between 7 and 8 months, with the addition of chopped foods between 8 and 12 months. After 12 months, in the traditional model, the baby should be eating what the family eats, but this expectation may be modified based on a child's developmental readiness.

Here are some basic infant feeding guidelines:

+ Feeding starts with offering a few teaspoons of a new food, and then slowly increasing over time to about ½ cup (4 oz) of solid food per meal in late infancy. During this time, the infant continues to breast or formula feed.

+ Eventually infants should eat about ½ cup (4 oz) of food per sitting, but progression is gradual and individual. Never force infants to eat more than they want. It is important for infants to learn to self-regulate their appetite and intake.

+ Be sure to respect their hunger and fullness cues:

  – Hunger signals include getting excited when food is near, pointing to or reaching for food, opening their mouth for the spoon

  – Signs that they are full or not wanting any more include not opening their mouth in response to the spoon, turning away from the spoon (or breast or bottle), or shaking their head no.

+ Do not feed them in front of the TV or computer. They need to focus on the food.

+ Feed the solids first before offering the breast or a bottle.

+ Encourage self-feeding as much as possible.

+ Add one new food at a time to make sure the infant doesn't have any negative reactions, such as an allergy. If the infant develops rash or hives, vomiting, or blood in their stool after introduction of a new food, hold off on giving it again and talk to their healthcare provider.

**TABLE 10.3 STAGES OF FEEDING**

| Stage of Feeding | Feeding Skills to Develop | Textures To Try |
|---|---|---|
| 5-6 months (early feeding) | Eating small bites off a spoon | Smooth |
| | Moving food around mouth with tongue to be able to swallow | Mashed |
| | | Soft finger foods (see BLW) |
| | "Chewing" thicker purees and mashed foods | |
| 6-9 months | Chewing and swallowing lumpy foods | Mashed with lumps |
| | Self-feeding with whole hand grasping | Soft finger foods |
| | Sipping from a cup | Sippy/360 cup or straw |
| 9-12 months | Chewing smaller chunks of foods | Diced/minced Foods |
| | Self-feeding with pincer grasp or spoon | Less soft finger foods |

## Baby Led Weaning

**Baby Led Weaning** (BLW) advocates letting the baby feed themselves soft table foods from about 6 months. The baby sits with the family at each meal and dictates the pace and selection of which foods they incorporate. The parent simply provides the food selection for the baby. Purists of this method denounce using any purees in the feeding of the child, and no spoons are utilized unless the child is using it to feed themselves later.

Proponents of BLW feel that this method reduces the risk of obesity by teaching the child to listen to their hunger cues early and leads to better food choices and better internal control by the child. It also facilitates family bonding during mealtime and "leadership by example" as everyone is essentially eating the same foods. Advocates of BLW also feel that this method leads to faster development of feeding skills and overall gross motor skills since they are practicing them more regularly with every meal.

Concerns about the BLW feeding model by some healthcare providers have included choking risks, inadequate iron and zinc intake, and inadequate calories leading to growth issues. Until recently, there was almost no peer reviewed research testing the benefits and concerns of BLW. A study in 2016 analyzed the diet of 25 infants using BLW versus their traditionally fed counterparts.[72] They found that the BLW infants did consume less iron and zinc, as well as less $B_{12}$ and vitamin C. BLW infants were more likely to be offered fruits, vegetables, bread and rusks (teething biscuits), and less likely to eat meat or iron fortified foods.

In a 2018 study using a modified BLW protocol called BLISS (Baby Led Introduction of SolidS), the researchers followed 200 mother-infant pairs who were randomly assigned to the modified baby-led weaning protocol, versus standard infant feeding practices.[73] The researchers modified the diet to ensure that high iron food was incorporated (either meat or iron fortified cereal) with each meal. They found that using the *modified* BLW, nutritional intake (including iron and zinc) was adequate at 7 months and 12 months of age, and at 12 months there was no difference in nutrient intake between BLW and spoon-fed infants.

However, BLW infants were noted to still have higher intakes of grains and dairy products compared to traditional feeding infants. On the positive side, modified BLW infants were much more likely to be feeding themselves at 7 months, had less food fussiness at 1 year of age, and were more likely to eat meals with their family. There were no differences in the number of overweight children at 2 years between the feeding groups.

Overall, these studies show that baby-led weaning can be done safely and with adequate nutrition if special care is made to incorporate iron and zinc rich foods with each meal, and not rely too heavily on breads or processed carbs. I think these studies also speak to the utility of a hybrid approach to feeding that may make more nutritional sense. A hybrid approach is what we used with our children. Using a hybrid approach may get more meat, seafood, and vegetables in the child earlier, with less reliance on breads, processed carbs, and excessive dairy products which carry their own nutritional risks. I would rather see a hybrid approach that is able to incorporate a full spectrum of whole, healthy foods that feed the brain and the microbiome, and limit the epigenetic programming and appetite dysregulation that comes with high carb/high sugar diets, especially in infants and toddlers.

Advocates of baby-led weaning would recommend dicing up meat into small soft pieces and skipping the puree phase, but this should be done with some guidance to minimize risk of choking. When our children were infants, we fed them meat and chicken puree early, but progressed to soft slow-cooked chicken and meat that was shredded or cubed when they were able to handle the texture without choking. Introduced early, studies have shown good acceptance of meats by infants and is a good way to get more nutrient dense food in them early on.

*Shouldn't we just feed the child whatever they will eat?*
There have been concerns raised about overly restrictive feeding practices during this period that could lead to feeding issues later in life. My take on the subject is this: It is all about the context of how we choose to limit

foods and what we are restricting. Our job as parents is to protect and nourish our children.

Especially when they are the most vulnerable, it pays to be a little extra vigilant about things like sugar, food additives, pesticides, and **endocrine disrupting chemicals**. Avoiding foods that represent a clear and present danger to our children is not being overly restrictive. Whatever restrictions are imposed by avoiding feeding an infant or young child highly processed food is worth it. I have a problem with giving parents a hall-pass to feed without boundaries just because we don't want to stress them out. It's not OK to feed an infant or young child harmful food.
A poor early diet has consequences that are evident every day when we walk down the street or drop our children off at school and see increasing numbers of sick, overweight, neurodevelopmentally challenged kids. We need to fight back by making the best choices we can for our children right from the start.

## WHERE TO FEED A CHILD

The *where* of feeding is all about creating a healthy eating environment. This is referred to as the "set and setting" of mealtimes. Regardless of the weaning method, the early days of infant feeding are about learning how to move food around in the mouth and getting used to tastes and textures. It should be *fun, family centered, and enjoyable, in a low pressure, low stress* environment. The infant should be with the family at set predetermined mealtimes. They should be sitting in their highchair, facing the family, with a footrest if possible, to help them support themselves.

*Don't stress the mess!* Feeding is messy business but that is okay, and it is normal and healthy to let them play around and get familiar with foods, even if a lot of it ends up on the floor or their face. This is an important part of the sensory developmental process and helps the child integrate all the sights, smells, textures, and tastes of food. Just have a damp washcloth on hand at all times and consider putting a shower curtain under their chair if there isn't a family dog that is available to happily clean up the droppings.

Lastly, don't underestimate the importance of family eating. Studies show that eating as a family reduces the risk of obesity as well as disordered eating behaviors.[78,79]

## Parental stress and the development of feeding issues

Outside of digestive or neurological disorders causing feeding problems, the most common contributor to poor infant eating is parental stress and a high stress feeding environment. Infants are unbelievably tuned in to the mood and energy of their parents. A stressed parent automatically leads to a stressed infant, and stressed infants tend not to feed very well. This is difficult, as we are living in a stressed-out frenetic world, often in a single parent or dual earner household. Time is often short, and patience is often shorter. Despite this, it is tremendously important to find a way not to bring it to the table.

This crazy lifestyle is leading us to slip into the default mode of grabbing fast food or highly processed foods that we quickly feed to our children in the car or in as little time as possible at home while everyone is on their phone texting or on social media. This has to stop. Especially early on, mealtimes should not be rushed and mom and/or dad should be paying attention to the feeding cues and fullness signals from their child. There should not be pressure to eat quickly or finish everything that is offered. Infant and toddler portions are small. Don't try to feed them too much. (See Table 10.4 for portion sizes.)

Remember, we are the example for our children, as well as the moderator and director of their feedings. We need to provide healthy food in the right portion sizes for their age. We need to eat our veggies as well and *avoid any negative talk surrounding the act of eating vegetables.*

If they make a face, do not respond with a negative comment like "That was yucky, huh!" Instead, deflect and reframe: "That was a new taste, good job!" Be persistent without pressuring.

Keep offering a steady pitching rotation of veggies with every meal, in a warm nurturing, loving environment without threats, bribery, or coercion. The more times and greater variety of foods that are offered, the more likely they are to accept them. *It can take 6-36 times of introduction before they fully accept some veggies* but remember that neophobia (fear of new food) increases with age. Don't miss out on the window of opportunity to add a number of healthy foods into the child's diet. Children are programmed to want the sweet taste, but *don't fall victim to the trap of offering sugar-laden foods because these foods will be more readily consumed.* Being persistent with healthy foods will help them develop a strong intake of veggies before 18 months of age, after which they become less likely to accept them if introduced for the first time.[74–76]

Feeding a family, especially an infant and toddler takes planning. The old adage rings true: failing to plan means planning to fail. Meal planning and scheduled shopping minimizes parental stress and last-minute mealtime panics that result in junk-eating mode. Having a plan and a good stock of healthy food in the pantry, refrigerator, and freezer makes good choices easier.

### TABLE 10. 4 QUANTITY OF FOOD TYPICALLY OFFERED IN COMPLEMENTARY FEEDING

| Age | Frequency | Amounts per meal |
|---|---|---|
| 6-8 months | 2-3 meals per day | Initially 2-3 tbsp/feed, gradually increase to ½ cup (4oz) |
| 9-12 months | 3-4 meals per day | ½ cup (4 oz) per meal |
| 1-2 years | 3 meals, 2 snacks | ¾-1 cup per meal |

Data from World Health Organization. *Infant and Young Child Feeding*, 2009.[77]

### TABLE 10. 5 HUNGER/FULLNESS SIGNALS DURING THE FIRST THOUSAND DAYS[9]

| Age | Hunger Signals | Full Signals |
|---|---|---|
| 0-4 months | Wakes up and fusses | Turns away from feed |
| | Sucking on hand | Won't open mouth |
| | Opens mouth while feeding to get more | Stops sucking or spits out nipple |
| 4-6 months | Crying/fussing | Stops sucking or spits out nipple |
| | Happy sounds when feeding | Turns away from food |
| | Turns and moves toward food | Stops paying attention to food |
| 6-9 months | Reaching/pointing toward food | Turns away/pushes food away |
| | Signs of excitement when sees food | Won't open mouth |
| 10-12 months | Asks for food with words or sounds | Says "no" or shakes head |
| 1-2 years | Asks for food by name | Says or signs "all done" or "no more" |
| | Gestures or brings food to parent | Throws food or pushes away |

Data from Pérez-Escamilla R, Segura-Pérez S, Lott M. *Feeding Guidelines for Infants and Young Toddlers: A Responsive Parenting Approach.* Healthy Eating Research Building Evidence to Prevent Childhood Obesity; 2017.

# NUTRITION R$_X$

**1** Meat and fish should be baby's first foods because these contain iron, zinc, choline, protein, B$_{12}$ and omega-3 fats essential for that baby's brain and overall growth. Vegetables and eggs should also be included early.

**2** Vegetarian or vegan weaning diets without the proper planning are not nutritionally adequate for a rapidly developing child during the first thousand days. If choosing a plant-only diet, make sure the baby is getting adequate fortified foods and may need supplemental zinc, iron, B$_{12}$, DHA, and choline. It is essential to work with the PCP and a registered dietician specializing in pediatric nutrition to prevent nutritional gaps.

**3** Solid foods should be started around 5-6 months of age; these can sometimes (but not often) be started between 4-5 months if the baby is developmentally ready.

**4** Based on ongoing concerns about arsenic levels, do not feed infants rice cereal, rice cakes or rice crackers as a staple of their early diet.

**5** For baby-led weaning, skip the purees and begin with soft, self-fed foods starting at 6 months.

**6** Modify baby-led weaning to provide iron and zinc rich foods with each meal; don't rely too heavily on dairy or grain products. A hybrid approach can also be used to make sure those nutrient needs are being met. Guidance and support are recommended when choosing baby-led weaning.

7　Make feeding family centered at set predictable times. Meals should take place at the table with the family. No phones, no tablets, and no TV.

8　If the baby is not advancing their diet and not tolerating some solids by 7-8 months, it is really important to see the child's PCP and a qualified pediatric speech-language pathologist or feeding therapist for a feeding evaluation. They may also need evaluation by a pediatric gastroenterologist.

9　Make sure not to microwave any baby food in plastic and try to use as little plastic as possible when storing or serving food to avoid the phthalates and other plasticizer chemicals that can interfere with baby's hormones and brain development.

## RECOMMENDED READING

1.　Nimali Fernando and Melanie Potock, *Raising a Healthy, Happy Eater: A Stage-by-Stage Guide to Setting our Child on the Path to Adventurous Eating (Experiment LLC, 2015)* This book is a step-by-step guide on how to feed the child at developmental stages.

2.　"Feeding Guidelines for Infants and Young Toddlers: A Responsive Parenting Approach" by the Healthy Eating Research panel of experts at http://www.healthyeatingresearch.org

3.　Infant and Toddler Forum CIC: A not-for-profit organization comprised of experts in pediatrics, neonatology and nutrition. www.infantandtoddlerforum.org

4.　1,000 Days Organization: https://thousanddays.org/for-parents/baby/

# CHAPTER ELEVEN

# FEEDING OUR TODDLERS AND YOUNG CHILDREN

Did you know that more than two billion dollars are spent each year by food companies trying to start your child eating highly processed high-sugar food? Almost half the calories in our children's diet are "empty calories" from added sugar and fat that offer almost no nutritional value. The road that leads to future diabetes and heart disease starts early in life. Being proactive and aware of what you feed your little ones will pay dividends down the road with better health and better behavior.

From ages 1 to 3, a child enters the fun phase of toddlerhood, a time of so many new experiences and exploration of their world. This goes for food as well. We want to make sure that we are exposing our toddlers to foods that nurture their growth and appeal to their senses. Colors, shapes, textures, tastes, and smells are new and exciting for young children but can be used to "get them hooked" on unhealthy, highly processed foods if we are not paying attention.

Remember that the early toddler phase falls within the critical **first thousand days** of **neurodevelopment** and **epigenetic** programming. Proper nutrition is especially important during this time when great numbers of **synapses** are forming, resulting in rapid brain growth. Children at this age are also still within the window when their **microbiome** is being shaped and their bodies are more vulnerable to epigenetic programming that can set adult patterns for chronic disease. Because of these developmental changes, toddlerhood is still a vitally important time to protect and feed the brain with the right foods. This is a critical period when healthy eating can turn off the genes for chronic disease and foster a healthy microbiome that can benefit a child over a lifetime.

Optimally, between 6 and 12 months of age, the child should have been introduced to the first and second-line foods and have a healthy diet consisting of a good base of meat and poultry, fish, multiple vegetables, eggs, nut butters (peanut, almond, cashew), fruits, and some whole grain products. As described in the upcoming chapter, imbalances in the diet, omission of important food groups, and over-reliance on processed foods can leave a child open to nutrient deficiencies. Food allergies or intolerances may have arisen that also limit introduction of some foods. (Refer to Chapter 13 if there are concerns about food allergies.)

The 12-month mark is when many mothers are weaning their children off breast milk or formula; or perhaps they are still nursing or giving bottles a few times a day. For the formula-fed child, if they are a good eater, they may not need the added nutrition from the formula after one year of age. However, if possible, it is recommended for the breastfeeding mother to try and maintain some breastfeeding beyond the first birthday, even though the child has a decreasing nutritional need for the milk. For those fall and winter babies, extending breastfeeding until the spring could help protect them from serious respiratory infections because of the significant immune system benefits from the antibodies and immune proteins in breast milk.

After 1 year of age, the bulk of a child's calories should be coming from food, not formula, cow's milk, or breast milk. They should be mostly eating what the family eats, with modifications for their smaller size, and should be sitting down to regular mealtimes with the family. New healthy foods and textures should be steadily introduced at a pace that they can handle. However, feeding often does not go as planned for a whole host of reasons.

This early toddler phase from 1 to 2 years is when many feeding issues show up. If a one-year-old does not tolerate solid foods, chokes, and gags frequently, or refuses a great many foods that are offered, they need to be evaluated by their primary care provider and referred for evaluation for a possible pediatric feeding disorder. If a child is excessively picky and refusing a lot of foods, adding healthy foods into their diet may be a challenge. Chapter 16 will go into more detail, both on strategies for feeding the young child, as well as some things to look out for that may indicate a pediatric feeding disorder which are increasingly common, but treatable.

Once a child is school age, this brings with it a new set of challenges. The child is more independent, and they are likely to be eating more meals outside of the home. They are beginning to develop a peer group, many of whom may be unhealthy eaters. This makes the job of parenting more difficult as peer pressure and social conformance become an issue. Fast food, soda, candy, and sugary breakfast cereals are marketed heavily toward this age group, leading to the "I wants" at the grocery store. Schools and daycares may be complicit in feeding children candy and highly processed junk foods, further undermining efforts to feed them healthy foods. Between work, school, and extracurricular activities, many parents are hitting warp speed, enter survival mode, and feel more like chauffeurs than parents. Unfortunately, due to a combination of all these factors, this is often the time when the diet begins to deteriorate as reliance on fast food and highly processed packaged meals take over.

Conversely, many children in America are growing up in food insecure households that are strapped for cash, just scraping by and not sure where the next meal is coming from. They may live in a "food desert," where the nearest grocery store with decent produce is miles away, forcing these folks to rely on fast food or convenience store food that is calorie rich but nutrient poor. Many of these communities are more accurately being described as "food swamps," offering only mini-markets stocked with junk foods, soda, alcohol, and tobacco. "Food swamps" are being linked strongly to risk of obesity in the US and worldwide.[1,2]

Food subsidy programs may fail to emphasize healthy foods and have loopholes allowing many at-risk children to still fall short on healthy foods in their diet. Many folks are not choosing healthy food options due to lack of access, affordability, transparency, and reliable information that are necessary for anyone to have or maintain a proper diet. Survival mode does not breed optimal nutrition. It is in these instances especially that government "safety net" programs, and school nutrition programs really need to work harder to provide better access to healthy food, instead of sugar rich, highly processed food for our children.[3,4]

Optimal nutrition not only requires access to the right foods but also an understanding of the importance of preparing healthy meals. Parents see themselves as too busy during these times, feeling too stressed and too pressed for time and prioritize other activities over shopping for and preparing healthy food. The end result is the same—our children and our families become victims of the food industry and our health suffers from being exposed to ultra-processed food that undermines our health. This leads to a state of **high calorie malnutrition,** which in the Western world is far more common than historical starvation that is caused by overall shortage of food and calories in other nations. I will state this again even though it is not popular or politically correct. *To have a truly healthy family, it is imperative to shop, prepare, and cook the food for a significant proportion of meals, minimizing processed foods as much as possible.* There are relatively simple, not overly time-consuming ways to cook healthy meals that won't break the bank.

Developing a healthy eating plan early on in childhood will help create a healthy eater for life, rather than leaving the child vulnerable to nutrient deficiencies and caloric excesses that can impair their health and brain performance and open the door for chronic disease. Most parents want the best for their kids. They want them to be healthy and happy and to perform well academically. By being more conscious about what we are feeding them we are much more likely to achieve these goals. Our efforts in feeding them well in every phase of childhood will pay dividends down the road in the way that they feel, perform, and behave.

In this chapter we will go over some basics about what to feed a toddler, how to avoid the unhealthiest "kids' menu" food items, and ways to feed them yummy, healthier substitutes. We will go over some ways to increase their vegetable intake and some toddler-friendly sample menus.

## FOOD "PROGRAMMING" BY THE FOOD INDUSTRY

Anyone who has seen *Fast Food Nation, Fed Up,* or similar documentaries is becoming aware of the tactics used by some companies to get us "hooked" on their products early in life. These calculated maneuvers start programming our children to want their products from their early toddler years. Bright colorful packaging is designed to mimic the vibrant colors of fruits and vegetables in nature and attract the child's visual attention. Foods with lots of added sugar for a sweet "sugar rush," and snack foods with crunchy textures and salty tastes are known as **hyperpalatable foods.** These foods are being investigated for addictive qualities that may ensnare the brains of our children as well as adults.

A lot of science has gone into marketing tactics for foods that have the potential to damage our kids.

> I recently came across an advertisement from the 1960s stating that physicians recommended starting a child on cola early in life. This was advised for children's social development—not to do so would cause them harm! Hard to believe, but then again so is the fact that up until the 1970s certain cigarette brands were touting that they were the #1 doctor recommended cigarettes.

Despite attempts at regulation and alarms raised by watchdog organizations, as well as the **American Academy of Pediatrics** and the **World Health Organization**, a great many unregulated marketing dollars are spent to attract young consumers to high sugar, highly processed, and fast foods. Advertising on social media has now taken the place of some of the TV advertisements. Food marketing comes at us and our children so frequently and from so many angles that we may not notice it anymore, but it can still have powerful effects on food choices. If advertising didn't work, these companies wouldn't be spending more than two billion dollars annually on heavy marketing to children.[5-9] Be aware that our children are targets of these persuasive advertisements.

For many parents, knowing that our children are targeted for profit at the expense of their health should awaken the protective Mama Bear or Papa Bear. One of our main jobs as parents is to protect our children from a multitude of dangers, but we may not realize that one of the biggest threats to their health and well-being could be a diet of harmful foods marketed to them through a variety of media platforms. The less we feed them processed foods, and the more we provide nutritious whole foods we prepare ourselves, the more control we take back. We can reduce the negative programming and poor diet choices that may cause them harm.

## THE DANGERS OF PROCESSED FOODS

Just as there is no healthy diet without vegetables, conversely there is no healthy diet that contains lots of highly processed, packaged, and fast food. Highly processed foods are *calorie dense* and *nutrient poor*. They are filled with refined high glycemic carbohydrates such as refined flour, food starch and hidden sugar. Processed food is where the majority of high fructose corn syrup ends up. They often contain **oxidized** (damaged) refined vegetable oils and historically contained **trans fats** that promote inflammation in the body and brain. Processed foods are typically lacking in **omega-3** fats since these brain friendly fats are not shelf stable enough to survive processing and long-term storage. Unless the manufacturers throw in a few vitamins and minerals to try to make the product look healthier, most highly processed food is fairly devoid of vitamins and **phytonutrients**. Processed foods and the packaging they come in often contain endocrine-disrupting chemicals and additives that may adversely affect hormonal responses as well as brain function and the health of the gut microbiome – especially in children who may be more sensitive.[10] Processed food is the main source of excessive salt in today's diet, which leaches important minerals like magnesium and calcium from our bodies and contributes to high blood pressure and heart disease. The shift in American's diet after the 1970's to one heavy in highly palatable, highly processed food is being directly linked to the obesity and **type 2 diabetes** epidemics, as well as a host of other diseases.[10-14]

> *The Food and Agriculture Organization of the United Nations defines* **ultra-processed foods** *as "formulations of ingredients... typically created by a series of industrial techniques and processes." They are often created by extracting and chemically modifying substances from whole foods with little to no amount of the whole food remaining, and include additives "that are of no or rare culinary use." Examples listed by the United Nations include sweetened beverages, many breakfast cereals, energy bars, packaged snack foods.*

Unfortunately, processed and fast food are the default mode for many parents. What are the hallmark signs of highly processed foods? Does it have more than a few basic identifiable ingredients? Is it delivered through a drive through window? What type of packaging does it come in? If a food product has more than a short list of ingredients and comes in a box, bag, or can, it is probably highly processed. If it contains descriptors that don't sound like food, such as "refined, bleached, extract, corn syrup, hydrogenated, etc." chances are it is highly processed. A highly processed food diet is being implicated in health issues ranging from constipation to metabolic dysfunction and development of type 2 diabetes, and leaves children at risk for nutritional shortcomings that may negatively affect their brain and immune system. Today's modern world is increasingly dominated by the highly-processed **Standard American Diet (SAD)**. This chapter outlines some basics to start our children on a better food journey. The next chapter will explore what nutrient *deficiencies* our children are actually at risk of, and how could this affect their health.

In the Dietary Guidelines for Americans published in 2010, the top 25 sources of calories for kids ages 2 to 18 were listed in decreasing order. This is a horrifying list and should be a wake-up call for parents. Chicken (mostly from nuggets and chicken strips no doubt) and maybe pasta (likely macaroni and cheese unfortunately) were the only things on the top ten that might even be remotely call "real food" other than milk, and we already discussed that milk should be *optional* – not a main source of calories. All other items are sugars, refined grain and sugar sweetened products that are calorie rich and nutrient poor. In total, only seven or eight of the 25 items on this list would I consider real food, and four out of those seven are near the bottom of the list. Sugar sweetened drinks sit as the third highest source of calories.

## TOP 25 SOURCES OF CALORIES IN US CHILDREN AGED 2 TO 18 YEARS (NHANES DATA 2005-2006)

1. grain-based desserts
2. pizza
3. soda, sports drinks, energy drinks
4. yeast breads
5. chicken and chicken dishes
6. pasta and pasta dishes
7. reduced-fat milk
8. dairy desserts
9. potato and corn chips, other chips
10. ready to eat cereals (breakfast cereal)
11. tortillas, burritos, tacos
12. whole milk
13. candy
14. fruit drinks
15. burgers
16. French fries
17. sausage, hot dogs, bacon and ribs
18. cheese
19. beef and beef dishes
20. 100% fruit juice
21. eggs
22. pancakes, waffles and French toast
23. crackers
24. nuts and seeds
25. cold cuts

According to the Department of Health and Human Services "empty calories from added sugars and solid fats contribute to *40% of total daily calories* for children 2 to 18 years of age and half of these empty calories come from six sources: soda, fruit drinks, dairy desserts, grain desserts, pizza, and whole milk."[15] It is easy to see what this diet is doing to our children, but unfortunately too many turn a blind eye to this epidemic.

## FOOD ADDITIVES OF CONCERN

*Antibiotics and hormones*
It may be wise to minimize potential **EDCs (endocrine disrupting chemicals)** and **MDCs (microbiome disrupting chemicals)** in the young child's diet. Two of the main ones include antibiotic and hormone residues in meats. Choose meat raised without these chemicals.

*Preservatives*
Not all preservatives are bad, and some preservatives are necessary to prevent food spoilage. However, certain additives and preservatives in processed foods, such as processed meat, may be associated with negative health effects. Nitrates and nitrites are preservatives commonly used to preserve lunchmeat and other processed meats. These chemicals are potentially linked to increased risk of cancer and possibly thyroid disruption. Although not allowed in foods specifically produced for infants and young children, exposure in young children is common after weaning onto table foods.[16,17] If possible, look for products without nitrates or nitrites in foods fed to a young child. There are also many sodium-based preservatives that add to the excessive sodium load of processed foods, but salt as a preservative is not inherently bad unless it is excessive.

*Carrageenan*
Carrageenan is a thickener used for decades in the food industry and is labeled GRAS–generally recognized as safe for use in foods. There have been more concerns raised recently about the effect of long-term consumption of this additive. Carrageenan may be a MDC and alter the normal gut bacteria; other concerns focus on potential damage to the protective lining of the intestines, contributing to inflammation and "leaky gut." This chemical has been used for decades to give colitis to laboratory animals and is now being shown in animal models to contribute to **insulin resistance** and development of diabetes. Different forms of carrageenan

exist, some having higher toxic potential than others, which further adds to the controversy. Investigation of the biologic effects of carrageenan is ongoing.[18-21]

Two recent studies give pause to the notion that the types and amounts in our diet are safe for all people. A small pilot study just published showed significantly improved insulin resistance in pre-diabetic adults fed a carrageenan-free diet for 3 months.[22] Another small pilot study in adults with ulcerative colitis showed improved inflammatory markers and no relapses on a carrageenan-free diet versus those receiving carrageenan.[23] The EU has banned its use in infant formula but not in other foods. Based on the premise of "first do no harm," some researchers feel this additive may be better limited or avoided in children.

*Titanium Dioxide (E171)*
This food additive falls under the category of "nanoparticles," which are microscopic particles added to food and pharmaceuticals to improve their appearance. Increasing evidence is linking these nanoparticles with intestinal inflammation and disruption of the intestinal barrier.[24-27] Some gastroenterologists are becoming concerned for the role titanium dioxide could be playing in the intestinal inflammation found in Crohn's and colitis. It has also been found that these particles may cross into the bloodstream and become lodged in certain organs. A recent expert panel review concluded that "the existing body of evidence raises concern for human health regarding long-term ingestion of E171."[27]

*Emulsifiers: Carboxymethylcellulose (CMC) and Polysorbate 80*
These products are used to stabilize the consistency of foods and give them a smoother texture. Also listed as GRAS, recent research is raising concerns about these products being linked with alterations of the gut microbiome, promoting intestinal inflammation, and insulin resistance and pre-diabetes. These are additives of concern for those with or pre-disposed to **inflammatory bowel disease (IBD)** and caution may be warranted.[28-30]

*Sodium*
A high amount of salt is added to processed foods. Due to worries about excessive salt intake on our health, choosing varieties lower in sodium makes sense. Added salt (sodium chloride and other sodium salts) may increase blood pressure in some individuals and potentially increases appetite and our production of stress hormones (cortisol).[31] Excessive salt

may also increase losses of calcium and possibly magnesium in the urine. The average sodium intake in US children is more than 3,100 mg per day while the recommended intake is less than 2,000 mg per day for younger children.[32] The main sources of excessive salt in the diet are the highly processed hyperpalatable foods our kids are gorging on.

*Sugar*

Listed by many different names, added sugar now invades 70% of the processed foods in our food supply. This subject is explored in detail in Chapter 17. Briefly, added sugar is a key driver of increasing risk of diabetes and obesity. It pays to read labels and choose products with the least added sugar. The Hypoglycemia Support Foundation provides a comprehensive list of over 200 added sugars currently being used in food and beverage products. (https://hypoglycemia.org/added-sugar-repository/).

*Artificial Food Coloring*

There has been interest and controversy regarding the role of diet and artificial food coloring (AFC) in hyperactivity and behavioral issues since the 1970's when pediatrician Dr. Ben Feingold brought this issue to the forefront with the Feingold diet. This diet removed most of the AFC and a naturally occurring chemical called salicylates and was reported to improve the behavior of a significant number of children with ADHD. However, this diet and the food coloring theory were attacked and then largely discredited. Or was it? Let's revisit the AFC issue briefly.

Far from being "put to rest," the AFC issue has had a resurgence. Recent double-blind placebo-controlled studies (the gold standard for research) have been published showing the high amounts of AFC consumed by US kids (100 mg per day) **or** lower amounts mixed with a common food additive called sodium benzoate cause *hyperactivity and behavioral changes in the general population, not just kids with ADHD.*[33-35]

Consumption of AFC has increased 500% since the 1950s, from an average of 12 mg/day to 62 mg/day in the 2000s. Intakes of over 100 mg a day are not unheard of in kids eating a highly processed food diet. AFC appears on the label as Red #40, Yellow #5 and #6, Blue #1, and are coloring agents made from petroleum (Yum!). AFC is often found in high sugar foods such as candy, cereals, pastries, and sweetened beverages.[36] Food companies know that kids are attracted to bright colors and will use this to make food items more appealing to younger kids. The foods highest in

AFC were listed in a recent medical journal and include foods targeted to children, such as brightly colored candy, slushies, sweetened drinks, macaroni and cheese, cupcakes, and toaster pastries. It is worth noting that several food companies recently removed AFC from all their macaroni and cheese products.

When consumed by children, these substances are partially metabolized by the gut bacteria but can also be absorbed if the intestine is hyperpermeable ("leaky gut," which is common in autism, autoimmune disease, and other conditions). Several of these AFC metabolites, including sulfanilic acid, may damage nerve cells by causing toxicity and **oxidative stress**. Theoretically these effects on the brain could contribute to hyperactivity, ADHD symptoms, and learning disabilities. It is also thought that in some children, a possible allergic-type reaction can occur to AFC with **histamine** release in the blood leading to behavioral changes.[37] This would indicate there may be a more vulnerable population of children who react negatively to higher amounts of AFC in the diet.

If there is nothing to this, why does the European Union version of the Food and Drug Administration require all products with AFC to carry warning labels stating, "this product may have an adverse effect on activity and attention in children"? The dirty little secret is that food products sold in Europe often do not have the same chemicals and additives as their US equivalent, including AFC. The European products instead use natural colorings that are approved by their regulatory agencies. Unfortunately, the US FDA balked when asked to regulate AFC in America, stating a lack of evidence of harm.[35] It seems that this decision is being called into question.

## WHAT SHOULD A TODDLER EAT?

This is a bit of a loaded question, given the state of most people's diets filled with sugar and highly processed food. There is typically no reason why a toddler physically cannot eat the same meal that has been prepared for the rest of the family, and the goal should be to get the *entire family* eating healthy, real food. Set a schedule as much as possible with three meals (breakfast, lunch, and dinner) and two snacks (midmorning and midafternoon). Limit constant snacking or "grazing" in between mealtimes.

Each toddler meal should include

+ a protein (an ounce or two of meat, poultry, fish, or eggs),
+ a vegetable or two (½ cup or so)
+ a carbohydrate (potato, sweet potato, *whole grain* noodles or bread, quinoa or rice—¼ to ½ cup).

As much as possible, try to minimize the "kid menu" items, which are filled with highly processed food. We will go into this in more detail and provide a few ideas for healthy meals and snacks that will feed their brain and microbiome without programming them for chronic disease.

## Components of a healthy diet

Whole, *real* foods are the foundation of health. Unfortunately, *"real food"* seems to be lacking in a great many of our diets, as we increasingly rely on highly processed convenience foods for feeding ourselves and our children. What are the main components of a healthy diet?

### Vegetables

There is no healthy diet without significant amounts of vegetables. Period. With the exception of Inuit people following the traditional Inuit diet, vegetables should be plentiful in the diet. Vegetables contain a host of important nutrients and are referred to as a nutrient dense, low-caloric density food. This means we get a lot of nutritional bang for the buck without a lot of calories rolled in. Without regular intake of vegetables, a child is missing a host of important nutrients including vitamins like folate and **antioxidants** such as beta carotene and the carotenoids as well as other phytonutrients. Vegetables are also an important source of Vitamin K, fiber, magnesium, potassium and calcium. The fiber in vegetables is one of the main foods for the microbiome, and a lack of vegetable fiber in the diet is likely starving our good bacteria. Phytonutrients as described later in this chapter are plant compounds that are being found to have significant health benefits including strong antioxidant activity and the ability to act as **epigenetic modifiers.** Phytonutrients from vegetables and fruits shut off genes related to inflammation and chronic disease as well as turning on genes that enhance the body's innate protection and detoxification mechanisms and even potentially enhance brain function. Phytonutrients are also being found to support and interact with the intestinal microbiome in ways that support proper immune system function and decreased inflammation in the body, helping to prevent chronic disease.[38-41] Based on the phytonutrient content, vegetables can be classified by their color and used to determine if children are "eating the rainbow" and getting healthy amounts of the protective nutrients in their diet.

## TABLE 11.1 EATING THE RAINBOW WITH VEGETABLES

| Color | Examples | Phytonutrients |
|-------|----------|----------------|
| Red | tomato, beets, peppers | lycopene, anthocyanins, carotenoids |
| Orange/Yellow | yam, squash, carrot, peppers, sweet potato | carotenoids, bioflavonoids, lutein |
| Green | spinach, kale, greens, broccoli, peppers | folate, flavonoids, isoflavones, indoles |
| Blue/Purple | red cabbage, purple potatoes, purple cauliflower and carrots | anthocyanidins, flavonoids |
| White | onion, cauliflower, garlic, leeks | allicin, flavonoids |

It is a somewhat inconvenient truth for many people that vegetables, (not processed grains) should be the basis of any healthy human diet. Perhaps they did not grow up liking or eating vegetables, and subsequently have a hard time feeding them to their children. Fresh vegetables are viewed by many as too labor-intensive to buy, prepare, and cook on a busy schedule, and they are not typically offered as a fast-food option, so they are the first food group to take a back seat. This is a good time for a reminder of the difference between *surviving* and *thriving*. Can a child *survive* on a grain-based diet with very few vegetables? Yes, of course. Can they *thrive* on this diet? Unlikely. They can get by for a while, but sooner or later a bad diet will catch up to the best of us, and often when it does, the end result is not pretty. No one can outrun a bad diet forever.

According to the CDC, in order to meet their nutrient requirements, children ages 2 to 8 years need to eat 1 ½ cups of vegetables daily. Older children need to eat the equivalent of around 3 cups of vegetables daily. Every parent should evaluate whether their children are consuming their required minimum vegetable intake.

The most commonly eaten vegetables by children in the US were potatoes (French fries), tomatoes (ketchup and pizza sauce), onion, lettuce, corn, then carrots. In the US, *9 out of 10 children* do not meet their vegetable requirements. This despite the fact that French fries and ketchup are considered by the USDA to be vegetables, even though they are not considered by most educated nutrition professionals to be vegetables. A third of the vegetables eaten in 2010 were white potatoes and 63% of these potatoes were fried, making this statistic even more disturbing. While standard white potatoes can be a source of vitamin C and potassium, the colorful potato varieties that contain the highest phytonutrient and overall nutritional value are not the kind commonly used for most French fries or consumed in the average diet.

Depending on how it is processed and eaten, corn could be considered a grain or a vegetable. Ground into flour and used for making tortillas, chips and other baked items, corn classifies as a grain. Eaten as a whole kernel (fresh, frozen or canned), corn classifies as a vegetable. In the past, I had a somewhat low opinion of corn nutritionally. However, a recent review from Cornell University illustrates that *whole corn* can contain some important phytonutrients as well as fiber for the microbiome.[42] Just like potatoes, the more colorful the corn, the more nutrients it has. Yellow, red and blue corn are going to have more nutrients than white corn, although none of them take the place of eating a variety of other vegetables like broccoli, cauliflower and green leafy vegetables. Variety is key, and so is eating a food in its least processed form. *On any given day in America, one in three kids are not eating a single real vegetable.* Is it any wonder why our nation's health is taking a nosedive?[43-45]

An important narrative that should be addressed is the idea that we should all be eating "plant-based" diets. While this sounds good on the surface, knowing the importance of vegetables to human health, this term has been warped to become the newest marketing mantra of the processed food industry and other groups with a hidden agenda. What exactly is meant by a "plant-based" diet? The truth is that many "plant-based" foods are what brought us here to the current global pandemic of metabolic disease that is spiraling out of control. Sugar and high fructose corn syrup are plant-based. Most highly processed grain-based snacks are plant-based. To imply that a diet that avoids meat, poultry, fish, and eggs but contains highly processed and sugar-added foods is somehow health-ier than one that contains unprocessed meat, fish and poultry alongside lots of fresh fruits and vegetables is misleading at best. Not all plants are healthy, and many healthy plants are processed into metabolically damag-ing forms. Just saying "plant-based" isn't enough. It isn't simply what is in the food, *but what is done to the food and its metabolic impact.* This logic applies to *all* foods, plant- and animal-based. What "plant-based" *should* mean is a diet containing lots of unprocessed vegetables and fresh fruit *with or without* the presence of unprocessed meat, poultry, eggs and fish. That is the type of "plant-based diet" that I endorse.

*Unprocessed Animal Protein*

Beef, game meat, pork and poultry contain protein that is complete (all the amino acids for growth), B vitamins (in their enzymatic & more bioavailable forms), vitamin $B_{12}$ (the only viable food source other than possibly one type of seaweed) and also contain the most bioavailable sources of iron and zinc. Meat is a great source of choline which has important roles in brain function and development. Because of the high nutrient density including the vitally important nutrients iron, zinc, $B_{12}$ and choline, I do believe that sustainably raised meat and poultry are an important part of a child's diet, especially during weaning and early stages of growth and development. Meat has gotten a bad rap because of factory farms and concern for unethical and inhumane practices, and for manufacturing the highly processed meat products that are often associated with fast food diets. When examining healthy diets that are high in vegetables, but also containing unprocessed sustainably raised beef and poultry, or wild game, most of the anti-meat arguments fall apart.[46-52] This subject is more controversial than it should be, given the heavily politicized anti-meat movement taking place in the US currently. My fear is that this anti-meat movement will carry over to our children whose immune systems, neurodevelopment and growth may potentially be adversely affected if these nutrient dense foods are withheld from their diet.

*Fish and Seafood*

These foods are good sources of complete protein, one of the best sources of iodine (important for the body's ability to make thyroid hormones) and the key brain nutrients, omega-3 fats and choline. Cold water fish are the best source of the vital long chain omega-3 fats EPA and DHA, crucial for controlling inflammation, proper brain development and brain function. Remember Sardines, Mackerel, Anchovies, Salmon and Herring (SMASH) are high omega-3 but so are Trout (SMASHT). Fish and shellfish can also be good sources of highly bioavailable iron and zinc. Avoid the high mercury fish for the most part, listed by the **NRDC**. In my opinion, and based on the research it is difficult to get adequate omega-3 fats for a child with a growing brain without having some fish or an omega-3 supplement in the diet.

*Eggs*
A great source of complete protein and choline, eggs also have $B_{12}$ and lutein; some also contain a moderate amount of omega-3 fats in them. Eggs can therefore be considered brain food for our children and can be used as a weaning food as well as a breakfast staple for the growing child. Choose free range/pasture-raised locally grown eggs whenever possible for both ethical and nutritional reasons. The cholesterol scare surrounding eggs was not founded in science. Eggs are healthy and great for kids.

*Healthy fats*
Olive oil (especially extra virgin), avocados and avocado oil, nuts/seeds and nut/seed butters contain the essential **omega-6** fatty acid (linoleic acid) as well as the healthy omega-9 fatty acid (oleic acid) in addition to the antioxidant Vitamin E. I feel that butter, ghee, and coconut oil used in moderate but not excessive amounts can be healthy as well, and that some **saturated fat** in limited amounts is not harmful to the growing child. Recall that most of the saturated fat in our blood is not from our diets, it is made in our own bodies. The growing child needs healthy fat for growth of their body and brain. The only true dangerous fats are the hydrogenated trans fats and oxidized polyunsaturated fats found in highly processed and fried foods. See the primer on dietary fat in chapter 6 for more details. Unless specifically prescribed by a medical provider, no child should be on a low-fat diet.

*Fruits (NOT juice)*
The phytonutrients and antioxidants contained in fruits and vegetables are important in reducing inflammation in the body, supporting the immune system and can help protect against many chronic diseases. The fiber and phytonutrients found in whole fruits also help fuel a healthy microbiome. Choose organic, if possible, and avoid the conventionally grown Dirty Dozen fruits and vegetables known for being prone to harmful levels of pesticide residues. (Listed on pg 122 or at EWG.org. )

The Dirty Dozen are the fruits and vegetables to focus on buying organic when possible. The Clean Fifteen are the fruits and vegetables found to have the lowest pesticide residues, making them safer to buy conventionally grown.

Berries especially are packed with phytonutrients and antioxidants, soluble fiber, and vitamin C, but all whole fruit can have health benefits for the child. "Eating the rainbow" also applies to having a variety of colorful fruits as well as vegetables in the diet.

### TABLE 11.2 EATING THE RAINBOW WITH FRUITS

| Color | Examples | Phytonutrients |
|---|---|---|
| Red | strawberries, cherries, plums | lycopene, anthocyanins, carotenoids |
| Orange/Yellow | oranges, cantaloupe, mango, lemon | carotenoids, bioflavonoids, lutein |
| Green | avocado, green apple, pears | flavonoids, isoflavones |
| Blue/Purple | blackberries, blueberries, grapes | anthocyanidins, flavonoids |

According to the **CDC**, in order to meet their nutrient requirements, children ages 2 to 8 years need to eat 1 to 1 ½ cups of fruit and older children need to eat the equivalent of 1.5 to 2 cups of fruit daily. Because of the high sugar content and lack of fiber, juice should be avoided for the most part, and the AAP advises a *maximum* of 4 ounces daily for younger children up to school age, and maximum of 8 ounces daily for older children.[53] Dried fruit still contains phytonutrients and fiber but also has more concentrated natural sugar, so it should be eaten in smaller amounts. Give kids whole fruit instead whenever possible.

*Nuts and Seeds*

Almonds, walnuts, cashews, and other nuts, as well as seeds such as pumpkin and sunflower contain the short chain omega-3 **ALA** and omega-6 fat LA as well as monounsaturated fats. They are rich in certain micronutrients such as zinc, calcium, and magnesium, and vitamin E. They also contain prebiotic fiber and important protective phytonutrients such as resveratrol, as well as other polyphenols and flavonoids. Incorporated into a healthy eating plan such as the Mediterranean diet, nuts can be a nutritional powerhouse. Technically, peanuts are a legume and not a nut although in their less processed form also contain many of the same healthy nutrients. While a younger child should not be given nuts due to the choking risk, nut and seed butters can be incorporated early on during the weaning and toddler phases and can be a great source of calories and these nutrients. However, it is important to read labels and choose the nut and seed butters with no added sugar and avoid those with partially hydrogenated oils.

*Whole grains*

Brown/wild rice, quinoa, amaranth, buckwheat, barley, millet, oats, 100% whole grain breads and pastas contain carbohydrates for energy, fiber (insoluble and soluble) for the microbiome and proper bowel movements, some B vitamins and a few phytonutrients. Although grains are the main source of carbohydrate calories (other than sugar) in the American diet, and in moderation can be incorporated as part of a healthy diet, grains actually do not contain any nutrients that cannot be obtained from other sources. *Processed (refined)* grains in the form of flour-based products are one of the leaders of the nutrient-poor calorie-dense food category. *Whole* grains can be incorporated in a healthier manner because they have the fiber matrix still intact, which feeds the microbiome and lowers the **glycemic index** and **glycemic load** (how quickly they turn to sugar in the body) and consequently how rapidly the body will have to pump out insulin to metabolize them. (See Chapter 17 for more information on glycemic index and the effect on the body.) The outer part of the grain (removed during processing) is also where most of the vitamins and phytonutrients are found. Hello processing, goodbye to fiber and vitamins. Increasingly, there is evidence that diets high in refined grains disturb the microbiome and may epigenetically program us for chronic disease, while whole grains do not.[54-56] In fact, whole grains are being found to have some protective qualities likely due to the increased fiber and phytonutrients. It can be difficult to consistently choose whole grain options, but cutting down on children's intake of highly processed, bleached flour will benefit them in the long run. Select healthy whole grains whenever they are available: examples include steel cut or rolled oats, quinoa, brown or wild rice. Look for *100% whole grain* on the label of products including breads, cereals and pastas to avoid being duped by deceptive marketing. If it doesn't say 100%, it is not a truly whole grain product and will likely contain a large amount of refined flour. Keep in mind that while many people have no issue with **gluten**-containing grains, there is mounting evidence that a significant number of people have adverse reactions to wheat, barley and rye in their diet. We will go into the topic of celiac disease and gluten sensitivity in detail in chapter 14.

*Full-fat dairy*
Examples include whole milk, and whole-milk products such as yogurt, kefir, and cheeses. Dairy products contain calcium, protein (**whey** and **casein**), a special fat called **conjugated linoleic acid** (CLA) that may hold some health benefits, vitamin D (if fortified), and iodine. Grass-fed cows that are allowed to graze on open pastures produce products with more omega-3 and CLA (a potentially protective fat) which improves their health profile. There has been a more recent emphasis on substituting

reduced-fat dairy products in the diets of children to try to reduce the risk of obesity, which I think is unfounded. I am a believer that it is the processed carbohydrates and sugar that are the main issue in the obesity epidemic, not the fat in a child's diet. If dairy is included in a child's diet, I would advocate for full-fat products. I don't feel there is a need for low-fat dairy products in the diets of most young children.[57]

While it is a staple and well tolerated in many children's diets, dairy could be considered an optional food because of the high rates of dairy allergies and intolerances in children, explained in detail in Chapter 13. Dairy can be part of a healthy diet in those children without allergies and sensitivities, however it is not an absolute *necessity,* and a child can be weaned onto a dairy free diet without risk of nutritional deficiency if done correctly. We do not need large amounts of dairy or calcium in our diets to support our bones, but we do need to meet basic calcium, phosphorus, magnesium, vitamin D requirements. Dairy products can fill that calcium need, but there are also alternatives for those with allergies and sensitivities. I also remain cautious about dairy because of the heavy reliance on dairy calories (milk) in many children's diets that leaves them lacking in other important foods and nutrients. Drinking lots of milk (more than 16 oz) at the expense of other foods like meats and vegetables puts the developing child at high risk for iron deficiency and anemia, zinc insufficiency, and a lack of fiber and phytonutrients that impair their microbiome and contribute to constipation, anemia, and a dysfunctional immune system.

As an aside, some children tolerate goat and sheep milk products even if they have a *sensitivity (intolerance)* to cow's milk leading to gastrointestinal symptoms. However, children should not consume these products if diagnosed with an actual IgE mediated (anaphylactic) allergy to cow's milk. There is a slightly different protein structure (A2 casein) in goat and sheep products that may not cause the same reaction as cow's milk casein (A1 casein). Goat yogurt and goat and sheep cheese can then be incorporated into the diets of *some* children with cow's milk intolerance without issue.[58-61] See the chapter on food allergies and intolerances for more information.

*Beans and Lentils (Legumes and Pulses)*
Beans, peas, lentils, etc. are rich in fiber, protein, phytonutrients and folate. Children consuming legumes in high amounts as the *only* main protein source could leave them at risk for iron and zinc deficiency. As part of a balanced diet, these foods can provide health benefits. Adequate

soaking, rinsing and slow cooking can reduce the level of the **anti-nutrients** in beans and lentils, but not eliminate them. These foods are staples of a plant-based diet, and provide an important protein source for these folks, but the impact on iron and zinc status in a developing child must be accounted for.

Below are listed some major categories of common foods, the key nutrients they contain, and the systems in the body they support. Antioxidant and phytonutrient rich foods support the body's internal antioxidant and *Detoxification* systems that protect our cells from damage. Fiber and phytonutrient rich foods support the *Microbiome*. Other nutrients like magnesium and omega-3 protect the *Cardiovascular* system. Iron, zinc, DHA, and choline support a growing *Brain*. Quality protein supports proper *Growth*, and carbohydrates and fats supply *Energy*. Iron, B12 and folate are important for making *Blood*, and iron, zinc, vitamin A and C are needed for a functioning *Immune* system.

## TABLE 11.3 KEY NUTRIENTS FOR BODY SYSTEMS SUPPORT

| Food Category | Key Nutrients Contained | Biological Systems Supported |
|---|---|---|
| Green leafy vegetables | folate, carotenoids (Vitamin A), fiber, phytonutrients, vitamin K, Mg, Ca, Iron*, Zn* | All |
| Cruciferous vegetables | antioxidant phytonutrients, folate, fiber | Detoxification, Microbiome, Immune |
| Squash/sweet potato | carotenoids (Vit A), fiber, carbohydrate | Detoxification, Microbiome, Immune, Energy |
| White/red/purple potato | vitamin C, potassium, phytonutrients (color based), carbohydrate | Energy, Detoxification (color based) |
| Berries | fiber, vitamin C, phytonutrients | Detoxification, Microbiome, Immune |
| Apples/pears/citrus fruits | fiber. vitamin C, phytonutrients | Detoxification, Microbiome, Immune |
| Avocado | fiber, MUFA, Mg | Microbiome, Cardiovascular, Energy |
| Nuts & seeds and nut/seed butters | MUFA, omega-6 PUFA, Mg, Zn, Ca, Vit E | Cardiovascular, Energy |
| Fish (SMASHT) | omega-3 EPA/DHA, protein, Zn, choline | Brain, Cardiovascular, Immune |
| Shellfish | Zn, iodine, protein | Endocrine(thyroid), Immune, Growth |
| Eggs | choline, protein, B12 | Brain, Growth |

| Food Category | Key Nutrients Contained | Biological Systems Supported |
|---|---|---|
| Poultry | protein, Fe, Zn, B vitamins/B12 | Blood, Brain, Growth, Immune |
| Meat/wild game | protein, Fe, Zn, B vitamins/B12, choline | Blood, Brain, Growth, Immune |
| Whole grains | fiber, carbohydrates, phytonutrients | Microbiome, Energy |
| Beans and lentils | fiber, folate, Fe*, Zn, Mg, protein | Microbiome, Energy, Cardiovascular |
| Olive/avocado oil | MUFA, phytonutrients (EVOO) | Energy, Cardiovascular (EVOO) |
| Full-fat dairy | Ca, CLA(protective fat), protein | Bones, Growth |

Ca- calcium, Fe-iron, Mg-magnesium, Zn-zinc, MUFA-monounsaturated fatty acids, **PUFA-polyunsaturated fatty acids**, EVOO- extra virgin olive oil, CLA-conjugated linoleic acid (a potentially metabolically protective fat). * denotes **non-heme iron** source.

## QUICK TIPS FOR CHILD NUTRITION

*1. Feed children real food*
Believe it or not, we survived for millions of years without premade lunch packs, microwavable noodles, and processed fruit snacks. Cooking and preparing our own food using basic healthy ingredients gives us back immense power in determining our own health and the health of our children. As much as possible, we should try to minimize feeding our young children fast food or pre-packaged, highly processed "convenience foods" that have labels that read like charts of chemicals. Feeding them healthy snacks can be simple, using fruit, nuts or nut butters, and whole grain crackers.

And yes, real food may cost a bit more in the short term. But what really costs more, spending a few extra dollars and a few more minutes on healthy unprocessed food, or diabetes, cancer, heart disease, or a neuro-behavioral disorder? The ROI—return on investment—of feeding our children real, healthy foods is profound. Everyone benefits in a society when children are healthier. Did you ever stop and wonder how some companies are offering "food" at such a low price? Do you think they may be cutting corners on quality? That being said, there are ways to feed our children healthy food on a budget.

*2. Reduce sugar*
The American Heart Association (AHA) and American Academy of Pediatrics (AAP) are now recommending a *maximum* of 25 grams of added

sugar in children's daily diets and *no added sugar for children less than 2 years of age.*[62] This refers to the sugar that is added to foods to make them sweeter, not naturally occurring sugar in foods like fruit, or the lactose that is present naturally in milk. Most kids are far exceeding the 25-gram limit because of added sugar in so many of their foods and drinks. Breakfast cereals and bars, snacks, condiments, and most packaged foods contain added sugar. *It is vitally important for parents to read labels.*

Get rid of the soda, sports drinks, juice boxes, and fruit juice (or just don't start drinking them in the first place). These are the number one sources of sugar in the child's diet and a suspected driver for fatty liver disease and childhood obesity. These drinks may be the gateway to early onset type 2 diabetes. The AAP recommends a *maximum* of 4 ounces of juice daily, but skipping it entirely is not a bad idea.

Minimize feeding a toddler high sugar treats like cookies, cakes, sugary snack foods, sweetened breakfast bars, pastries, cereal, and candy. These foods should be for rare *special occasions in older children*, not an every-day staple in a toddler's diet. Aside from the devastating effects on their dental health, excessive sugar drives inflammation, which is the root of all modern diseases as well as promoting excessive weight gain and type 2 diabetes (See the chapter on metabolic health). Watch out for hidden sugar in products like cereals, oatmeal, salad dressings, yogurts, condiments (ketchup), pasta sauce, and packaged foods, and try to opt for the "no sugar added" or lowest sugar options. Read labels and ingredient lists!

### 3. Better breakfasts

A lower carbohydrate or lower glycemic index breakfast may be better for brain function and future school performance. It is more satiating and keeps a child's blood sugar levels more stable and may help decrease the toddler meltdowns. Scrap the breakfast cereals and breakfast bars—most are loaded with sugar and processed flour. Instead, try scrambled eggs with veggies; breakfast scrambles or breakfast burrito with eggs, sausage and avocado or cheese; full-fat unsweetened yogurt with fruit added; turkey and avocado rolled up in an easy-to-bite finger food; sweet potato and sausage home fries; even a protein shake or smoothie. If looking for a cereal-based breakfast, use steel cut and rolled oats, which are high fiber and much healthier than instant (high-sugar) oatmeal.

### 4. Give them clean water

The toddler should mostly be drinking plain water as they get older, from a cup or water bottle. Recommended total liquid intake guidelines vary, but the Institute of Medicine provides simple recommendations. For children ages one to three offer them 4 cups (about a liter) of fluid (mostly water) daily. Thereafter, give them 1 cup (8 oz) of water per year of age up to 64 to 88 oz per day for older teens. A four-year old should then be getting about 32 oz of water daily, not 32 oz of juice, milk, and certainly not soda or sports drinks. Make sure they are getting *clean (filtered) water.*

### 5. Protect the probiotic bacteria in their microbiome

Avoid antimicrobial soaps that kill good bacteria. Ensure that they have good dietary fiber intake, especially soluble fiber from fruits, vegetables and, if needed, fiber supplements like inulin and psyllium. Remember that without dietary fiber, their healthy gut bacteria will starve. Incorporate fermented foods that contain significant amounts of **probiotic** bacteria. Examples include yogurt, kefir, sauerkraut, probiotic pickles, and fermented/pickled veggies.

### 6. Reduce chemical exposures

Try to avoid the "dirty dozen," high-pesticide fruits and vegetables and eat organic when possible. Organic does matter, as certain pesticides are being linked to birth defects and behavioral and learning issues. Be cautious of mercury in seafood (See Table 6.9 for high and low mercury seafood lists). Don't heat or microwave in plastic packaging, dishes, or containers. Don't pour hot liquids into plastic cups. This can cause harmful chemicals to leach into food that can affect learning, behavior, and hormone levels. Store and heat foods in glass or ceramic dishes and containers. Cook in stainless steel or cast iron. Be wary of non-stick coatings, flame retardants, and stain-resistant coatings as they are potentially toxic to our children. Examine all sunscreens, lotions, and cosmetics for phthalates, which are chemicals that can alter a child's hormones or possibly contribute to early onset of puberty. Try to avoid artificial colorings – especially if a child has ADHD or behavioral issues. Wash their hands with soap and water before every meal and snack, so chemicals from house dust don't get into their mouths.

### 7. Be Predictable

Feed children at predictable times. Aim for three set meals and two or three snacks daily. Mealtimes should involve the whole family seated at the table as much as possible. Try to not allow grazing (constant snacking between meals) as this decreases their intake of healthy real food and disturbs their appetite regulation. Do not allow TV, tablets, or smartphones at the table, as the distractions will draw their attention away from parents and the meal and alter their ability to regulate their food intake. Let them feed themselves, despite the mess. Toddlers typically eat small portions, so always be mindful of their hunger and fullness signals. Don't pressure them to "clean their plate." Their little appetites are variable, so if they give signals they are full, respect that. The same goes for the (sometimes) fickle nature of toddler tastes–they may love or refuse the same food within a short timespan. Keep offering healthy foods consistently in a predictable, positive setting.

### 8. Minimize choking risks

Avoid high choking-hazard foods for young toddlers, such as nuts, popcorn, hard candy, large pieces of hot dog or sausage, meatballs, and whole grapes. Cut grapes, meatballs, or hot dogs and sausage into smaller bite-sized pieces. Avoid whole nuts until they are older, but it is fine and recommended to feed them nut butters. Do not let them walk or run around while eating, as this also increases the risk of choking.

## AVOIDING THE DANGERS OF POPULAR "KID MENU" FOODS

Below we will look at some of the most popular "kids' menu" food items that are unfortunate mainstays for children today. What's wrong with these foods? These foods are highly processed, have little to no fiber to feed the probiotic bacteria, minimal vitamins and nutrients, and lots of salt, hidden sugar, and food additives. Many of these foods are considered "hyperpalatable" meaning they are designed to be addictive and stimulate the brain more than other foods. Unfortunately, as a result they are more appealing to even the most finicky children.

Hyperpalatable foods have recently been defined by obesity researchers as ones where "key ingredients in a food creates an artificially enhanced palatability experience that is greater than any key ingredient would produce alone."[63] They are usually combinations of fat and salt (chicken nuggets, French fries, chips, macaroni and cheese), fat and sweet (ice cream), or even just hyper-sweet foods with high fructose content (fructose is the sweetest of the sugars).

The concern with hyperpalatable foods (especially in kids) is their addiction potential combined with a lack of health value.[64] There is growing concern over the contribution of hyperpalatable foods in the obesity epidemic. Unfortunately, there are increasing numbers of children, especially those with autism or developmental issues, whose diet consists *only* of these hyperpalatable foods. This can have serious downstream effects on health.

## TOP TEN KIDS' FOODS—HOW TO IMPROVE THE NUTRITIONAL QUALITY

### Chicken nuggets

There are restaurant and fast-food varieties of chicken nuggets and strips, as well as frozen varieties that can be cooked at home. Both are going to have a lot of variability in their ingredients and health quality, so be choosy. Depending on the source, these can be made from either chicken breast or chicken parts (which parts?) and combined with fillers, such as flours and food starch, and various preservatives and then compressed into a nugget shape.

The method of cooking has a significant impact on the nutritional makeup of these products. The restaurant varieties may be grilled, but many, if not most, are deep fried in oil that may have been in the fryer for days or weeks. Refer back to the section on fats and oils but remember that deep fried foods containing **oxidized oils** may be almost as bad as partially hydrogenated trans fats for damaging children's cells, and causing inflammation.[65,66] When comparing the nutrition information from two leading fast-food chains for their 6-piece chicken nugget entree, one grilled and the other deep fried, the difference is shocking. The grilled nuggets have 100 calories, only 20 are from fat. In contrast, the deep-fried variety contains 270 calories, over half of which are from fat. This would not be a big deal if the fat were olive oil instead of potentially highly oxidized vegetable oils. The deep-fried variety also has almost 25% of its calories from refined carbs in the form of added starchy fillers and a little bit of sugar, versus the grilled version, which has only 1 gram of carbohydrate. The sodium content increases from 330 mg in the grilled version, to over 500 mg in the deep-fried nugget, largely due to several sodium-based preservatives. None of this is a big deal if they are consumed once in a while, but I have treated patients who eat chicken nuggets almost daily. I am concerned about the long-term effects this is having on their bodies.

*Healthier alternative*

There are healthier versions of chicken nuggets and strips, but you need to ask questions and read labels. When going out to eat, look for baked or grilled chicken strips or nuggets (not deep fried) that kids can still eat and dip like other nuggets. If buying a frozen nugget, look for brands that contain the fewest, most simple ingredients, such as chicken breast or thighs (not parts) raised without antibiotics, do not use preservatives (or only natural preservatives like rosemary extract), and do not contain a bunch of fillers like food starch, flour and soy protein. Or just bake, grill, or air fry some chicken thighs or breasts and cut them into bite size or dippable strips instead.

## French fries

Take the innocent potato, add some processed starch and preservatives, maybe some breading, and dunk it in that same nasty old cooking oil discussed earlier. Recall that this is the top "vegetable" consumed by children today. Giving a child French fries occasionally when eating out is no big deal, but for some kids eating fries is a near daily occurrence. Typical French fries are high in unhealthy oxidized fats, starchy carbs, and salt; they should not be a staple of any child's diet, especially one in a critical window of brain development. Fries also tend to be dunked in ketchup, which may contain a lot of added sugar. There are healthier, simpler alternatives to this favorite fast food.

*Healthier alternative*

When eating out, most of the fries are going to be cooked in potentially damaged oil in deep fryers. Sometimes restaurants offer baked fries which may be a better option, especially if you can avoid the added starches and additives. Some restaurants may change the oil in their fryers frequently and use oils that are less likely to get oxidized, but don't count on it. Consider choosing an alternative side order of veggies, baked potato, or rice, depending on the restaurant, for a healthier choice.

At home there are several options for healthier French fries. All you really need for a French fry are potatoes, oil, and salt and seasoning. We bought one of those French fry cutters online and use that to cut potatoes, sweet potatoes, and zucchini into fries. Coat the potato or veggie strips in olive or avocado oil, add some seasoning, and bake in the oven or air fryer for a toddler friendly and dippable side with no preservatives or oxidized oils. When looking for a frozen French fry variety, look for simple ingredients with the least additives and preservatives. One healthier brand of frozen

French fries contains potatoes, canola and olive oil, sea salt, apple juice concentrate, and citric acid (a non-harmful preservative). Consider the baked sweet potato fries that have a bit higher nutritional value that kids still love. When looking for a dipping sauce, opt for ketchup or other dip with lower amounts of added sugar.

## Mac and cheese

The mainstay of the "kids' menu." The ingredients of the out-of-the-box mac and cheese products are basically processed (enriched) white flour, salt, powdered "cheese sauce mix," and natural or artificial coloring with variable amounts of food additives. Thankfully, several of the main manufacturers of this food recently removed the artificial coloring agents used in their products sold in the US to match products sold in Europe (which has more restrictions on food additives). However, some brands may still have artificial colors, so read the labels. Regardless, this is not a health-food by any measure; it is high in salt and highly refined carbohydrates and lacking in significant nutrients other than the iron and vitamins added to the enriched white flour. Prepared per instructions with butter and milk, it contains a considerable 600 to 700 mg sodium per serving, only 1 to 2 grams of fiber, and 50 grams of highly processed carbohydrate. Parents should reconsider whether this food should be a regular staple in a young child's diet.

*Healthier alternative*

Even some of the "health food" varieties of this food are still highly processed and not exactly a health food. They may actually contain more refined carbohydrate per serving (57 grams of refined carbs per serving in the rice/quinoa variety mac and cheese) but contain more fiber (4 grams) and less sodium (500 mg).

Consider making macaroni and cheese at home with real, whole food ingredients. Some restaurants offer whole grain macaroni mixed with real cheese, a little salt, and seasoning, without the artificial food coloring or preservatives. This version can easily be made at home as well. Again, the simpler the ingredients, the better. 100% whole grain pasta means more fiber, reduced **glycemic load,** and is better for the microbiome and our **metabolism.** There is a chickpea-based mac and cheese that has only 38 grams of carbohydrates with 5 grams fiber and 18 grams of protein, which is twice as much as the standard mac and cheese. (And while more balanced, it is still somewhat high in sodium.) Try making the switch to a healthier version of macaroni and cheese–cumulative changes like this add up over time for a healthier child.

## Sugar-laden "kids" yogurt

Poor yogurt, look what they've done to you! Dressed you up with artificial flavors and colors and pumped you full of sugar and preservatives.

Recall that the AAP and the AHA recommend no added sugar for children under two. The leading kids' yogurt variety contains 18 grams of added sugar (already approaching the daily limit of 25 grams for older kids set by the AHA) as well as modified corn starch as a thickener, which boosts the carb content to 29 total grams per serving with only 6 grams of protein. Two popular brands of supposedly "healthy" yogurt and fruit post between 13 and 17 grams of added sugar per container, a modest 5 to 6 grams of protein, along with modified corn starch and carrageenan. Why turn a healthy product into an unhealthy dessert? There are better options for children. Buyer beware!

*Healthier alternative*

Some food companies are starting to improve their products by removing the high fructose corn syrup and the artificial colors. There has also been some effort by several companies to minimize added sugar and offer organic varieties. Thank you to the food companies who are trying to make a difference. Look for yogurts that have the lowest sugar and don't contain high fructose corn syrup or artificial colors and flavors. Full-fat yogurt is better for kids; dairy fat is metabolically protective, so avoid the low-fat varieties. The best option is full-fat unsweetened yogurt with no additives.

To dress it up, add a touch of natural vanilla extract, fresh or frozen berries, and maybe a small drizzle of honey or maple syrup if needed. A local brand of plain Greek yogurt boasts 20 grams of protein per serving, no added sugar, with milk and probiotics as the only two ingredients. This is how yogurt was meant to be. There will always be naturally occurring sugar in plain yogurt (from lactose), around 7 grams per serving, which is totally fine. Couple this with the naturally occurring sugar from berries, and perhaps an optional small drizzle of honey or maple syrup, and you may have a few grams of added sugar and still be significantly below the 13 to 18 grams of added sugar found in the commercial favorites. I encourage all parents to reevaluate the yogurt they are feeding their children.

## Breakfast Bars

These bars are simply another sugar vehicle in the guise of a "healthy breakfast alternative." Some of these popular bars are about as healthy as eating a candy bar for breakfast, with *five to seven different kinds of added sugar* contained in one bar! Common sugars in these breakfast bars include cane sugar, wheat syrup, invert sugar, agave nectar, molasses, honey, dextrose, fructose, corn syrup, fruit juices and extracts. The worst of these bars contain processed flour and sugar, with only 1 to 2 grams of protein, 1 gram of fiber, and *12 to 15 grams of added sugar per bar*. Most of these bars have low or no real nutritional value and are not balanced nutritionally. They are not appropriate for young children. If a child eats two of these, they have blown past the AHA/AAP daily sugar limit recommendations for the day. These bars do not feed the microbiome or the brain, and the sugar content is shocking and damaging to the metabolism. I would not recommend these products for any child, especially as a regular staple in their diet. Even the healthier-appearing popular granola bars contain 6 grams of added sugar per bar (12 grams per serving) from four different sugar sources, with only 1 gram of fiber. And what about the ever-popular toaster pastries for a quick breakfast? A staggering 30 grams of added sugar *plus* 40 grams of refined high glycemic index flour per two pastries with only 1 gram of fiber and 3 grams of protein. We are well over the AHA sugar limit and not even past breakfast yet.

*Healthier alternative*

There are some healthier bars on the market, although there are better breakfast choices. Save these bars as a backup option for when life gets especially busy. First off, look for a bar with minimal to *no added sugar.* That means the sugar is from a natural source such as fruit. Fruit juice concentrate is just another added sugar, so don't be fooled by this ingredient. Second, I would choose a bar with no artificial flavors, sweeteners, dyes, or fillers and featuring *simple natural ingredients* like nuts, fruit, and/or whole grains. Look for products that are relatively high in fiber (3-5 grams or more) and also have moderate fat and protein content to give them better balance. One brand of higher protein bar boasts only 2 grams of added sugar from honey, 10 grams of fiber, and 15 grams of protein with no artificial sweeteners or preservatives. Consider making homemade breakfast/snack bars using basic (healthy) ingredients that are rolled flat and baked in the oven, then cut into single serve bars for kids to grab and go. (see recipes on the book website) Better yet, choose a healthier breakfast that feeds a child's brain and microbiome and avoids the programming for chronic disease that comes with high sugar foods.

### Fruit snacks/strips/rolls

Don't even get me started. None of these highly processed "fruit snacks" can be called healthy. Yes, there is *some* vague form of fruit in a few of these sugar bombs disguised as food, but they are no substitute for the real thing. These food imposters contain multiple types of sugar, and not much else in terms of nutritional value. The primary ingredient in most of these "fruit snacks" is corn syrup, but also may contain any number of other added forms of sugar including fruit juice concentrate. Some of them actually contain a fruit puree containing fruit, but does this make them healthy? Any high-sugar, low-fiber food like this has the potential to put children on the "blood sugar roller coaster" (the "amusement" park ride that no parents want their children to take!). We will discuss this more in Chapter 17. Some also have the added "bonus" of containing multiple artificial colors and flavors. One pack of these snacks provides about 8 to 10 grams of added sugar per serving (do children really eat just one serving at a sitting?). These sugar-laden products almost guarantee that children will exceed the recommended daily maximum of 25 grams of added sugar set forth by the American Heart Association and *are not recommended for toddlers*. There are better snack options.

*Healthier alternatives*
How about actual fruit for a good alternative? A sliced apple, some raisins, an orange (especially the little "cuties") are easily transportable, and kids love them. Plus, there is the added benefit of fiber and other nutrients. Or consider a healthy trail mix with nuts and some dried fruit for an older child. However, recall that nuts are not appropriate for young toddlers and represent a choking risk. Once we eliminate the super-concentrated sources of sugar from our diet, it is amazing how sweet real natural fruit tastes. Apple slices or a banana with 100% almond or peanut butter is a healthy snack that will keep them going with a balance of simple and complex carbohydrates, fiber, fat, and protein.

### Breakfast cereals

From my perspective, even the "healthiest" cereals are not the best break-fast choice for any child. Most cereals are sorry excuses for breakfast and are simply sugar delivery devices for kids. These highly processed foods are pumped full of multiple forms of sugar and often artificial coloring to make them more appealing. They are relentlessly marketed to kids. Under the best of circumstances, cereal is not the optimal breakfast for children because of the excessive amounts of added sugar and the highly-processed carbohydrates that quickly metabolize as sugar. The United Nations classifies most breakfast cereal as an "ultra-processed food".[67] The road to diabetes, obesity, and fatty liver disease can start with excessive sugar and ultra-processed foods. One of the most popular cereal brands that is marketed heavily towards children delivers 12 grams of added sugar per cup, plus 20 grams of processed carbohydrates, no fiber, only 1 gram of protein, and multiple types of artificial flavors and colors. According to research, children's portion sizes of the high-sugar cereals tend to be higher compared to high fiber, low sugar cereals. Children tend to over-eat on the highly sweetened varieties because of the excessive sweetness (hyperpalatability) and appetite stimulation. It would be relatively easy for a child to get well over 20 grams of added sugar from their breakfast cereal alone, soon leaving the AHA guidelines in the rearview mirror. Based on the AAP guidelines of no added sugar under 2 years of age, these products would not be appropriate for a young toddler.

Don't be fooled by some of the "whole grain" options that have just as much added sugar, but a bit more fiber. One serving of typical instant oatmeal still contains 12 grams of added sugar even though it has 4 grams fiber and 4 grams of protein. There are a few cereals (such as regular Cheerios and low-sugar/no-sugar muesli) that have minimal to no added sugar plus 4 to 5 grams fiber and 5 grams of protein. While not perfect, they are considerably healthier than the high sugar varieties.

*Healthier alternatives*
Start reading labels. If you choose to eat cereal for breakfast, avoid the ones with artificial coloring and look for options with the *lowest added sugar*. Again, reference the list of other names for added sugar to look out for. Consider steel cut or rolled oats as an alternative breakfast rather than instant oatmeal. Some folks put oats in a slow cooker or InstaPot the night before so they can be ready first thing in the morning. To add flavor or sweetness, try cinnamon, real fruit, or a small drizzle of honey (1 teaspoon is 5 grams of sugar). This way a child can get the flavor and fiber with a small fraction of the added sugar.

## The PB & J
How can I question this "gold standard" of kids' foods? The old standard PB+J sandwich was made with ingredients that were less than healthy. Highly processed white bread, commercial peanut butter with partially hydrogenated oil (trans fat) as well as added sugar, and jelly that was largely high fructose corn syrup. That leaves a lot of room for

improvement. One PB+J with standard white bread, regular peanut butter and standard jelly totaled around *19 grams of added sugar per sandwich*, approaching the AAP/AHA 25 gram added sugar limit with one sandwich, and not considered appropriate for young toddlers. Not to mention that some commercial white breads have an ingredient list that reads like a chemistry set. Remember that the FDA finally banned trans fat from partially hydrogenated oils in the food supply after increasing evidence of the dangers for over a decade. This was a big improvement in peanut butter. Trans fats were implicated in damaging cells leading to heart disease, cancer, and potentially contributing to brain disorders like Alzheimer's. Partially hydrogenated has now been replaced with "fully-hydrogenated oils" by some companies which reportedly carry no trans fats anymore. Getting rid of the trans fat was a good step forward. The research on fully hydrogenated oils is still limited, but they appear to be better than partially hydrogenated oils. However, if one is not paying attention to the quality of the ingredients that make up their PB+J, it can still become a low-fiber sugar bomb that can have questionable health quality.

*Healthier alternatives*

With a little scrutiny, it is possible to make a healthier PB&J option if one takes several steps. First, choose a better bread such as 100% whole grain bread with higher fiber. Read labels to find a bread with higher fiber. Be aware that most popular brands of 100% whole wheat and the real whole grain breads, while containing 8 to 10 grams of fiber, are also going to carry 6 to 10 grams added sugar per two slices. There were a few breads I found with only 2 grams added sugar per two slices so look for one with higher fiber and lower sugar if possible.

Second, use natural peanut butter with no added sugar or consider using almond butter instead. Keep in mind that almond butter contains more fiber, monounsaturated fat, vitamin E, and calcium than peanut butter, but both can be a good source of fat and calories for children. Standard brands of peanut butter may contain one or more types of added sugar. Read labels and choose a "no sugar added" variety if possible. There are "natural" peanut butters with no added oils, or sugars, made with just peanuts and salt. There are also some with some non-hydrogenated oils like palm oil added. Often local health food stores will grind their own peanut and almond butters, which can be light and fluffy and easily spreadable with absolutely no additives, just the ground nuts.

And lastly, choose a jam, preserve, or fruit spread with the least amount of added sugar. There are low or no sugar added sugar fruit spreads with half as much added sugar as standard jelly. Read labels to compare sugar content and think about choosing a fruit preserve or fruit spread with low added sugar content and avoid the high fructose corn syrup. Making better choices of bread, peanut butter, and lower sugar fruit spread, the grams of added sugar can be reduced to around 8 grams of added sugar per sandwich. One could argue this is far better than the standard PB +J, and the moderate amount of sugar is offset by the much higher fiber content that one gets from making better choices.

## Ramen noodles

This staple consumed by many children could be cause for concern. With the flavor packet, a package of noodles has more than 1500 mg of sodium (salt). This is the entire day's allotment for a younger child. It contains 50 grams of highly processed carbohydrate (starch) that turn quickly to sugar in the intestines, with almost no fiber (2 grams) to slow it down. It doesn't offer much nutrition save for a few B vitamins and minerals added during the enrichment of the flour and is typically composed of empty starch-based calories along with a host of additives and preservatives.

*Healthier alternatives*

Look for whole grain ramen or other whole grain noodles that have 3 to 5 grams of fiber per serving and the fewest number of additives. At the very least, skip the flavor packet and add some diced or shredded vegetables to the noodles to improve the nutritional value. Consider a lower-salt vegetable broth seasoning that has nothing artificial and about a quarter of the salt. Offer kids other healthier noodle options such as chickpea/lentil pasta, or zucchini noodles which can be purchased frozen or made with a cool device called a spiralizer.

## Prepackaged lunch packs with crackers, cheese, and lunch meat

I know that these are the ultimate in parent convenience foods, but I would encourage looking for alternatives, since these are about the most highly processed of all lunches. What could be a relatively simple fare of crackers, cheese, and meat, ends up being a less than optimal meal for a young child. These lunch packs generally contain multiple food additives and preservatives, and significant amounts of added sugar if you opt for the packs with a dessert and/or juice. Adding the dessert and juice skyrockets the sugar content from a reasonable 5 grams to an eyebrow-raising 37 grams. This is combined with a complete lack of fiber (essentially zero grams), and wrapped in environmentally unfriendly plastic packaging. If going this route, I recommend skipping the juice and dessert options. However, with a tiny bit of effort parents can create their own fun, healthier meal for their child.

*Healthier alternatives*

Break down the ingredients and make healthier lunch packs that are quick, convenient, and inexpensive. We purchased durable and environmentally-friendly metal reusable trays and made our kids "lunch packs" that provide all the benefits and convenience of a fun transportable finger food meal. PlanetBox makes a modern version of this compartmentalized "bento box." Fill these environmentally-friendly containers with healthy antibiotic/hormone/nitrate free lunchmeat (as is, or cut into cool shapes with a cookie cutter), whole grain crackers (with 2 to 3 grams of fiber per serving and lower in salt and preservatives), real cheese (cut into slices, strips or cubes), sliced veggies (carrots/peppers/cucumbers) and fruit, and a homemade dipping sauce. The child gets to choose what and how they eat out of this fun and nutritious pack without the plastic and endocrine disrupting chemicals. It is well worth the effort and the results to take ten minutes of prep time to cut up the ingredients and load the box with a healthy lunch.

There is considerable quality difference when it comes to choosing lunchmeat. Meat from the deli may (or may not) have fewer chemicals and preservatives than prepackaged lunchmeat so this may be a better bet. Another option is to purchase a precooked chicken or turkey breast and cut it into slices, cubes or strips at home. Options for healthier lunchmeat should include a short list of simple ingredients such as turkey (or chicken), broth, rice or potato starch and salt and/or lemon juice, possibly rosemary extract with no other additives or preservatives.

## BEVERAGES: JUICE AND JUICE BOXES

Depending on the type and brand, a juice box may be 100% juice or a blend of juice and high fructose corn syrup. Even if it says 100% real juice, it doesn't make it a healthy food, especially for young children. *Some 100% grape juice has 50% more sugar per ounce than soda.* There may be some vitamin C, antioxidants, and phytonutrients in juice, but it is far better for children to get these nutrients from eating whole fruit that has less sugar and all the fiber for their microbiome. It is way too easy for a child to guzzle a number of these boxes daily when they are thirsty, leading to a dangerous level of sugar intake. One box of grape juice can have up to 25 grams of sugar (the entire days allotment), which is high for a toddler. The American Academy of Pediatrics (AAP) recommends *no juice for children under a year of age and a maximum of 4 ounces daily* for toddlers.

*Healthier alternatives*
Juice should be a minimal part of children's diets. Encourage children to drink plain water as much as possible to quench their thirst. Alternatively, make kid-friendly "spa-water" with twists of lemon or lime, splashes of juice, or some fresh fruit or mint.

## BASIC TIPS FOR INCREASING FRUIT AND VEGETABLE INTAKE

Fruits and vegetables are an important part of a growing child's diet. However, it may not always be easy to convince them of this. So how can we help children consume more fruits and vegetables? There are a few strategies that can be used to not only increase fruit and vegetable consumption, but also improve their overall diet.

### 1. Role model the behavior

Kids will be much more likely to try different varieties of foods if they see the rest of the family trying them as well, especially parents. To encourage children to eat fruit and vegetables on a daily basis, parents must do the same. Avoid negative talk and really "sell" them on how good vegetables are. This goes for the siblings as well as the parents. Many kids will respond if it is explained that vegetables are good for their "belly bugs" (the friendly bacteria in their tummies) and will make their bodies stronger and help them poop.

### 2. Encourage kids to help buy and prepare food

Getting kids involved in the growing, shopping and cooking process helps them become more invested in food, which will make them more likely to try whole food options. Let them pick out one new fruit and vegetable at the grocery store and cut them up together. Let them help stir ingredients together or sprinkle seasoning or sometimes cheese on top of vegetables before they go in the oven. Cooking skills are associated with healthy eating throughout life (less reliance on processed foods), so be patient and encouraging.

### 3. Don't give up

Encourage kids to keep trying new foods even if they don't love them the first time. It can take up to 20 or more exposures to a new food before kids will accept and enjoy that food, so even trying one bite several times (the "no thank you bite") can help the child acquire a taste for it. Don't make it stressful or punishing; rather keep gently encouraging them. Pair a new food like a vegetable with an old familiar food to improve acceptance. It is a bad idea to reward vegetable eating with candy or sweets, as this sets a bad precedent and will become a trap for rewarding good behavior.

### 4. Eat together

Keep a routine where children are served meals at approximately the same time each day can improve appetite and allows them to be exposed to a variety of different foods. The family meal also creates a healthy and positive atmosphere around eating, which is likely to promote healthy food choices.

### 5. Make it fun

Allow children to experiment with their food, such as creating edible fruit and vegetable artwork as this can help them make a positive association with these foods. Cut them into cool shapes and designs and give them exciting names like "power-vision carrots" or "brontosaurus broccoli." Dip it! Serve their fruit and veggies with healthy dips such as natural peanut butter, yogurt, hummus, or guacamole to make them more flavorful and exciting. Make a healthy ranch dip using unsweetened yogurt, spices, mustard, and lemon.

### 6. Sneak it in

Add greens or avocado to smoothies; mix crumbled or riced cauliflower into rice, chili or scrambled eggs; grate, shred or dice zucchini, mushrooms, cabbage, spinach or carrots into hamburger patties or meatloaf; bake grated veggies (zucchini or carrots) into bread; finely chop vegetables into pasta sauces; or turn veggies into fries (sweet potatoes, zucchini, or green beans, with oil and seasoning, baked or air-fried until slightly crispy).

### 7. Eat vegetables first

Start with just the vegetable on the child's plate at lunch and dinner (or as a pre-dinner snack) to encourage them to eat the healthiest item first, while they are the hungriest. When parents get the "I'm hungry, when are we gonna eat… can I have a snack?" pre-dinner request from an older child, reach for some carrot sticks with a healthy dip or quick cut up a cucumber or bell pepper to quell the hunger in a healthy way. Food always tastes better the hungrier we are!

### 8. Roast with flavor

Roast vegetables in the oven with healthy olive or avocado oil, a flavorful seasoning or even some diced bacon for an easy and flavorful side dish. The more flavor the vegetables have, the more likely they are to be accepted. (Everything tastes better with bacon–it works with Brussel sprouts, cauliflower, broccoli, and most any vegetable; while I don't endorse eating bacon daily, if it is used once in a while to get a child eating more vegetables, that is a good thing.)

### 9. Make it convenient

Always keep fruits and vegetables washed and in plain sight for quick snacks or to add to lunches. Apples, pears, bananas, carrots, and celery sticks are all easy "grab-and-go" options.

### 10. Frozen is still good!

While fresh veggies are the best nutritionally, frozen vegetables still retain most of their nutrients and benefits for the child. In fact, frozen organic vegetables from Costco or Sam's club as well as Walmart are really helping to make eating organic more affordable. Our family uses the organic frozen Normandy vegetables all the time, and these can be roasted or steamed relatively quickly. Frozen stir fry vegetables can also be a lifesaver for quick healthy meals. Keep the freezer stocked at all times.

# NUTRITION R$_X$

**1** If a child is not primarily eating regular table food and they are over 12 months of age, talk to the child's PCP and have them evaluated.

**2** Lead by example. Kids should eat what the adults eat, and the adults should be eating healthy, real food.

**3** Eating vegetables and healthy food should be a family affair. Consistently, repetitively offer healthy food in a positive supportive environment.

**4** Don't fall into the trap of the "kids' menu" of unhealthy food items. There are much healthier alternatives that will appeal to children.

**5** Try to choose foods with the least amount of added sugar and the lowest amounts of potentially harmful food additives.

# CHAPTER TWELVE

# COMMON NUTRIENT DEFICIENCIES IN CHILDREN

One in four kids are eating a diet that leaves them deficient in multiple nutrients. These nutritional shortcomings can affect our children's ability to fight off infections and damage their school performance.

While it is relatively uncommon in the Western world to see a child suffering from classic nutritional deficiencies such as scurvy (vitamin C deficiency), beriberi (thiamine deficiency), or kwashiorkor (severe protein deficiency), more subtle or **subclinical deficiencies** are much more common and can have insidious effects on our children. The Western diet full of processed food may lack several important nutrients that we will explore in this chapter. Increasingly, research shows that children with brain conditions like ADHD or autism may be especially at risk for nutrient deficiencies. We will highlight some specific associations between nutrients and the child's brain in each of the upcoming sections. Becoming aware of possible subtle nutritional deficiencies in the **Standard American Diet (SAD)** can help us better sculpt a diet for our children that is nutritionally complete and promotes optimal health and brain functioning.

## THE CURRENT STATE OF NUTRITION IN US CHILDREN

Overall, it has been reported by the Children's Defense Fund that only 2% of US children are meeting all the food guide pyramid recommendations (which are less than optimal to say the least), 16% meet *none* of the recommendations and only 22% of children eat five or more servings of fruits and vegetables daily (this is in a country that considers ketchup a vegetable).[1]

According to a recent study looking at the most up to date National Health and Nutrition Examination Survey (NHANES) nutritional intake data on US citizens over 9 years of age, our diets left 31% of US citizens at risk of at least one vitamin deficiency or anemia, with *23% at risk of deficiency in at least 2 vitamins and/or anemia*. A significantly higher deficiency risk was seen in women (37%) and was most common in pregnant or breastfeeding women (47%), non-Hispanic blacks (55%), individuals from low income households (40%), and underweight (42%) or obese individuals (39%).[2]

> Although researchers do their best to minimize inaccuracies, nutritional studies based on self-reporting of food intakes are notoriously inaccurate, as they are prone to "recall bias" where participants "remember" what they ate more selectively than reality. Some of the NHANES study data uses blood tests to check levels of certain vitamins and minerals to back up the survey data, which does increase the validity of some estimates of nutrient adequacy. This data is valuable for understanding who is at risk for which deficiencies. However, for an individual child or adult, keeping a 3-day food diary and meeting with a qualified dietician may be more revealing for that person's individual risk of nutritional deficiency based on current eating habits.

## COMMON DEFICIENCIES IN US CHILDREN

Based on research looking at food intake data and past deficiency studies, the following list of important nutrients are commonly lacking in a surprising number of today's kids. These should be considered "nutrients of interest" for today's parents. We will briefly go over each of these and describe why low levels of these nutrients can have adverse effects on the growth, development, and brain function of our children.

### Iron

Iron is vitally important for red blood cell formation, immune function and muscle **metabolism**. Iron is also an essential nutrient for brain structure and function. It is vital for the production of **neurotransmitters** such as dopamine, serotonin, and norepinephrine, and helps to keep neurotransmitter levels balanced in the brain. In addition, iron is needed to make the brain insulation known as **myelin** and is necessary to create new **synapses**.[3] We have previously discussed the serious ramifications of prenatal and neonatal iron deficiency on brain development. The need for iron in proper brain function and development is ongoing in toddler and school-aged children.

Deficiency is common worldwide with 25% of children not getting enough iron. In developed countries like the US, deficiency rates are closer to 10% in younger children. Unrecognized iron deficiency may result in brain dysfunction, learning disabilities, and fatigue leading to potentially poor academic performance and reduced quality of life for the child.[3,4] Low iron levels have been associated with ADHD in multiple studies and **meta-analyses**.[5-7] Iron deficiency also impairs the immune system, leaving a child more vulnerable to infections.[8-10]

Food sources of iron include meat, poultry and seafood, green leafy vegetables, legumes and fortified grains and cereals. As explored in detail in chapter 10, while the iron *content* of plant-based foods may appear adequate, the amount that gets absorbed may be insufficient to support optimal health and iron status in a growing child. It is important to remember that dietary iron can be blocked by certain **anti-nutrients** in the diet and that non-animal (**non-heme**) sources of iron are not well absorbed. An **omnivorous** child who eats meat, poultry, and fish regularly is at lower risk for deficiency. However, if children do not consume adequate amounts of more highly absorbed iron, this increases the risk of iron deficiency that could negatively impact their brain and immune function.[16]

The Institute of Medicine states that the iron requirements of vegetarians are 1.8 times higher than non-vegetarians. There are *recommendations for the estimated average requirement (EAR) for iron be increased by 80% for vegetarian children* due to the decreased absorption from plant-based sources.[11] A child who is vegetarian or eats very little meat may be at risk of iron deficiency unless they are eating iron fortified foods and taking the proper steps to boost intake and absorption.[12] High milk intake (more than 16 oz per day) in young children also blocks the absorption of iron, which may further increase the risk of anemia and iron deficiency. If a child is a big milk drinker, they are at risk for iron deficiency.

Vegetarian and vegan kids, children with obesity, children who are not growing well, children with feeding disorders or a poor diet, children who were born prematurely or born to mothers with anemia or iron deficiency, and kids from lower income families are also at higher risk of iron deficiency and should be screened with the appropriate lab tests.

It is vital to conduct proper early screening for the at-risk child. Iron deficiency develops in phases, and anemia (low blood counts as measured by reduced **hemoglobin** or hematocrit) appears as a late-stage presentation. By the time anemia happens, the child's brain is already iron deficient. Hemoglobin or hematocrit tests which are currently used to screen for low iron will miss a great many cases of earlier stage iron deficiency that still impacts a child's brain development. *Studies show that a child can have insufficient iron levels for proper brain and biological functioning without being anemic.*

If there is suspicion for iron deficiency based on a child's medical condition or diet, it should be discussed with their medical provider. Some experts feel that *all* young toddlers should be screened specifically for iron deficiency at their 12 or 15 month well child visit to ensure adequate iron for brain development during the **first thousand days**.[138] Proper testing with the correct iron studies includes a **complete blood count (CBC)** in addition to a **ferritin** level. *Ferritin levels below 12 ug/L in a younger toddler or below 15 ug/L in a school aged child are consistent with iron deficiency.* These are the minimum acceptable levels for children rather than the goal.[137-140] However optimal ferritin levels for brain development are likely higher, with past studies showing the average level in healthy young toddlers around 30 ug/L.[137,138] Ferritin levels can increase when there is infection or inflammation, skewing the iron results. To account for this, it has been recommended to also check a marker of inflammation called a CRP in a child where there is suspicion for increased inflammation or infection. Since too much iron can be detrimental and even toxic, it is recommended to get the child's levels monitored with a medical provider when supplementing and ask their guidance on a safe dose of iron that is not excessive.

The subject of iron deficiency and ADHD is somewhat controversial. A fair number of studies show an association with low iron levels measured by serum ferritin in children with ADHD, but others do not. Proper testing is crucial to determining the actual rate of iron deficiency in this population.[13-15] In one study, 60% of kids with ADHD consumed less than two servings of meat or meat alternatives per day, leaving them at risk for low iron and zinc.[17]

## TABLE 12.1 RECOMMENDED DAILY INTAKE FOR IRON

| Age | Recommended Daily Allowance (RDA) (mg/day) | Estimated requirement for vegetarian children (mg/day) [133, 134, 136] |
|---|---|---|
| 7-12 months | 11 | unclear |
| 1-3 years | 7 | 12.5 |
| 4-8 years | 10 | 18 |
| 9-13 years | 8 | 14.5 |
| Teen, male | 11 | 20 |
| Teen, female | 15 | 27 |

IOM suggestion that iron requirements are increased 80% in vegetarians. May require supplementation. Consider testing. Data from 133,134,136

## TABLE 12. 2 IRON AND ZINC CONTENT OF FOODS

| Food (per 2.5 oz serving) | Iron (mg) | Zinc (mg) |
|---|---|---|
| Ground beef | 1.85 | 4.4 |
| Liver, beef | 4.8 | 4.0 |
| Chicken thigh | 1.0 | 2.0 |
| Chicken breast | 0.8 | 0.75 |
| Turkey dark meat | 1.1 | 2.6 |
| Turkey white meat | 0.5-1.0 | 1.3 |
| Salmon | 0.6 | 0.6 |
| Trout | 1.4 | 0.6 |
| Sardines | 2.0 | 1.0 |
| Black beans* | 1.6 | 0.85 |
| Lentils* | 2.3 | 0.9 |
| Spinach (cooked)* | 2.0 | 0.6 |
| Egg (1)* | 0.8 | 0.6 |

*non-heme iron sources, less efficiently absorbed.

Data from National Institutes of Health (www.NIH.gov), USDA Nutrient Database (https://fdc.nal.usda.gov/), Health Link British Columbia (www.healthlinkBC.ca), Linus Pauling Institute (https://lpi.oregonstate.edu/mic/minerals/iron)[141-144]

## Zinc

Vital for a host of enzyme functions (in the neighborhood of 200+) including digestive enzymes, zinc also is involved with maintenance of the lining of the intestines and lungs, growth and tissue repair, and immune system function. Zinc is required for brain development and function and is especially important in the first thousand days during rapid brain development.[18] Zinc interacts with numerous enzymes involved with neurotransmitter production in the brain, notably dopamine, norepineph-rine, serotonin, and GABA.

Food sources of zinc include seafood, meat, green leafy vegetables, seeds and nuts, and *fortified* grains. The main sources of zinc in the US diet are meat (50%), beans and cereals (30%) and dairy products (20%).[19] The latter fact is somewhat ironic as dairy products are not a good source of zinc and may actually inhibit zinc absorption; however, dairy products provide a disproportionate percentage of calories in many children's diet.[20,21]

Worldwide zinc deficiency is a major issue. **Phytates** that occur naturally in grains, nuts and legumes can bind to zinc in the GI tract and render it less absorbable, potentially more so when combined with calcium from dairy products. The Institute of Medicine has reported that vegetarians may require up to 50% more zinc because so much of the zinc gets bound up by phytates, and other experts have reported that zinc requirements may more than double on a high-phytate vegetarian diet.[23] It is esti-mated that 6 to 7% of kids in the US are not meeting the basic zinc intake requirements, without consideration of source or how much of that zinc is actually being absorbed. Even a modest amount of meat or poultry in the diet enhances zinc absorption.[22] Without proper planning or access to the correct foods, plant-based diets with little or no meat or seafood are at increased risk of being zinc deficient or insufficient.[11]

Deficiency of zinc can result in poor immune function and healing, fre-quent illnesses and infections, impaired growth, chronic diarrhea, and is now known to be associated with ADHD, depression and anxiety. Even in developed nations like the US, it is possible that zinc insufficiency could be impairing our children's immune systems and increasing their risk of infections. Could insufficient zinc also be contributing to the epidemic of ADHD and other brain disorders?

Multiple studies show low zinc intake and low zinc levels in children and adults with ADHD. A study in British Columbia on children with ADHD reported that 28% of children 6 to 8 years old and 61% of 9 to 12 years old with ADHD were not meeting dietary requirements for zinc.[5] In addi-tion, a **meta-analysis** of studies looking at zinc levels in kids with ADHD found significantly lower levels measured in their blood, hair, and urine.[19] Several of these studies showed improvement in symptoms and response to medications when zinc was supplemented in these individuals.[26-32] Whether deficiency in zinc and other nutrients directly contribute to symptoms (or is merely an association) remains a matter of investigation, but the improvements seen with supplementation in some studies could suggest a direct link.

The decision for supplementing to correct zinc deficiency can be based on diet history and clinical suspicion by a qualified healthcare provider.[24] If a child does not eat meat or seafood and eats a lot of grains and beans they are at increased risk of zinc deficiency. If a child drinks a lot of milk (more than 16 oz per day), they are at increased risk. Children with chronic diarrhea, celiac disease, or poor growth should be suspected to be zinc deficient. Testing for zinc levels in the blood is notoriously inaccurate and there is not yet a great test available to tell if someone is deficient, especially if the deficiency is minor.[24]

My recommendation is that children first try to improve the zinc content of their diet by including zinc-rich foods. If a child has poor growth, chronic diarrhea, frequent infections or has a diet low in meat or seafood, then supplementation with a safe dose of zinc may be warranted. Consider zinc supplementation in the child with ADHD as well. As discussed previously, avoid supplementing with zinc oxide or carbonate, as these forms may not absorb well. I prefer zinc glycinate, citrate, gluconate or amino acid chelates as they may have superior absorption, but zinc sulfate may be an acceptable form as well. Avoid excessive supplementation in children. I do not recommend more than 5 to 10 mg daily in a younger child, 10 to 20 mg in a teenager. Many good multivitamins will contain this level of zinc, so we must take care to avoid "double dipping" and accidentally giving children an excessive dose of zinc.

### TABLE 12.3 RECOMMENDED DAILY INTAKE OF ZINC

| Age | RDA (mg/day) | Estimated requirements for Vegetarians (mg/day) | Recommended supplemental zinc (at-risk children) mg/day[25] |
|---|---|---|---|
| 6-11 months | 3 | 4.5 | 5 |
| 12-36 months | 3 | 4.5 | 5 |
| 4-8 years | 5 | 7.5 | 10 |
| 9-13 years | 8 | 12 | 10 |
| 14-18 years (f/m) | 9/11 | 13.5/16.5 | 10 |

IOM suggestion that zinc requirements increase 50% for vegetarians. (2006 Dietary Reference Intakes) Data from Brown KH, et al. *Food Nutr Bull*. 2004.[25]

## Magnesium

Magnesium is another vitally important mineral involved in hundreds of enzyme reactions in the human body. Involved in glucose and fat metabolism, magnesium is also anti-inflammatory, and vitally important for cardiovascular health. Magnesium has also been shown to enhance insulin sensitivity and adequate intakes are potentially protective against **type 2 diabetes**; the higher the magnesium intake (from food), the lower the risk for type 2 diabetes.[33-36]

Magnesium is another essential brain nutrient involved in many enzyme reactions, including the rate-limiting step in dopamine synthesis (the "pleasure neurotransmitter") and helping dopamine and serotonin (the "happy neurotransmitter") work more effectively in the brain. Magnesium is also known to "calm" the nervous system by controlling the release of some of the excitatory neurotransmitters and increasing the release of the calming ones.[44,45]

Interestingly, recent research shows that we need adequate magnesium intakes in order to metabolize and properly use Vitamin D, which is also commonly deficient in children. Supplementing magnesium may help normalize Vitamin D levels in those who are resistant to supplementation. Magnesium deficiency, especially in childhood, may contribute to weak bones and osteoporosis. Current thinking suggests we should focus more on optimizing magnesium and vitamin D levels in our children, as well as increasing their exercise, and not focus so much on excessive calcium intake to build and maintain strong bones.[35,36,46]

Food sources of magnesium include green leafy vegetables, whole grains like quinoa, brown rice and oats, legumes, seeds and nuts. Magnesium in the body may be depleted by not only caffeine and alcohol (hopefully not a concern for most children) but also by excessive *dietary salt and sugar,* which are unfortunately the cornerstones of the Standard American Diet (SAD). Almost *half (48%) of the US population* and 36% of children consumed less than the required amount of magnesium from food in 2005 and 2006, and this does not account for the reported significant drop in the magnesium content of foods over the last thirty years caused by extensive processing and the amount getting leached from our bodies due to the high salt and sugar content of the Western diet.[33,37] With the rates of magnesium deficiency in the US approaching more than half of the general population, this is a nutrient every parent should be working toward increasing in their child's diet.[34]

Low magnesium is associated with ADHD and anxiety; correcting its deficiency may help improve symptoms of these disorders. Several studies have found up to 70% or more of children with ADHD are subclinically deficient in magnesium, significantly higher than the general population.[26,41,38] While previous magnesium intervention trials for ADHD were not large, double-blind placebo-controlled studies, they do suggest that magnesium supplementation in certain populations may be worth further investigation.[26,40,42] Magnesium can have potential positive effects on the brain and mood, and act as an anti-anxiety and calming agent, and may have effectiveness in treating depression.[43-45] Early promising studies need more extensive follow up to verify their findings.

### TABLE 12.4 RECOMMENDED DAILY INTAKE FOR MAGNESIUM

| Age | mg |
|---|---|
| 1-3 years | 80 |
| 4-8 years | 130 |
| 9-13 years | 240 |
| Teens | 360-410 |

**Low magnesium intakes and blood levels have been associated with the following:**

+ Type 2 diabetes and insulin resistance
+ Metabolic syndrome
+ Elevated inflammation
+ Hypertension
+ Atherosclerosis
+ Sudden cardiac death
+ Osteoporosis
+ Migraine headache
+ Anxiety
+ ADHD
+ Asthma
+ Colon cancer

### TABLE 12.5 MAGNESIUM CONTENT OF FOODS

| Food | mg/serving |
|---|---|
| Cashews (1 oz) | 83 |
| Brown rice (½ cup) | 43 |
| Almonds (1oz) | 80 |
| Peanuts (1oz) | 48 |
| Pumpkin seeds (1oz) | 156 |
| Spinach/chard (½ cup) | 78 |
| Black beans (½ cup) | 60 |
| Pinto/refried beans (½ cup) | 43 |
| Lentils (½ cup) | 36 |
| Baked potato w/ skin (1 med) | 48 |
| Oatmeal (½ cup) | 32 |
| White rice (½ cup) | 25 |
| Peanut butter (2 tbsp) | 50 |
| Raisins (1 cup) | 46 |
| Yogurt (1 cup) | 43 |
| Banana (1) | 32 |
| Avocado (1) | 58 |
| Lima beans (½ cup) | 63 |
| Squash (½ cup) | 22 |

Data from National Institutes of Health (www.NIH.gov), USDA Nutrient Database (https://fdc.nal.usda.gov/), Health Link British Columbia (www.healthlinkBC.ca), Linus Pauling Institute (https://lpi.oregonstate.edu/mic/minerals/iron)[141-144]

Standard blood testing for magnesium is inaccurate for picking up deficiency. Research into testing intracellular magnesium (the amount of magnesium *inside* the cells) holds some promise but is not commonly available. We may have to assume a child is deficient in magnesium if their diet is inadequate. If a child is not consuming regular amounts of these magnesium rich foods, and/or has a diet that contains high amounts of processed foods and sugar, they are likely sub-clinically magnesium deficient. The first step is always to increase magnesium rich foods in the diet, but children who may be symptomatic (i.e., asthma, ADHD, anxiety) may benefit from a supplement of 100 to 300 mg magnesium daily.

The Food and Nutrition Board (FNB) of the US Institute of Medicine (IOM) set the tolerable upper intake level for magnesium *supplementation* at 110 mg/day for younger children, 350 mg/day for kids 9 and above. This is thought to be the highest level of daily supplemental magnesium unlikely to cause diarrhea or gastrointestinal issues in almost all individuals. Overall supplementing with magnesium at these levels is safe, and at worst causes some looser stools. Remember, we are not megadosing (using potentially harmful high dose supplementation), we are correcting deficiencies and supplementing the amounts lacking in the diet and leached out of our bodies by increased salt and sugar intake. I do not recommend using magnesium oxide which is relatively poorly absorbed. Magnesium citrate, glycinate or other amino acid chelates such as threonate are preferred forms for better absorption. Check with the child's primary or specialty physician to make sure they do not have issues with their kidneys or take medications that would make supplementation unsafe. Given the importance of this mineral to the human body, more attention needs to be paid to getting adequate magnesium intakes through diet or supplementation.

## Calcium

Calcium is a major component of bone health, density, and strength. Calcium also plays a role in muscle contractions, cellular and neurotransmitter signaling, and blood clotting.

A reported 47% of American children are not meeting the US recommended daily intake levels of calcium. However, other nations and the **World Health Organization** (WHO) recommend a calcium intake that is significantly less than what is recommended in the United States.

### TABLE 12. 6 RECOMMENDED INTAKE OF CALCIUM (MILLIGRAMS PER DAY)

| Ages (years) | USA | WHO | United Kingdom | Japan |
|---|---|---|---|---|
| 1-3 | 700 | 500 | 350 | 400-450 |
| 4-8 | 1000 | 600-700 | 450-550 | 550-600 |
| 9-18 | 1300 | 1300 | 800-1000 | 650-800 |

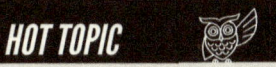

**HOT TOPIC**

In fact, the US is the only country in the world with calcium recommendations set this high. Why such a big difference? The Harvard School of Public Health states that we could do just as well with the European recommended calcium levels versus the current US levels that some scientists feel may be set too high. In general, children are not eating enough vegetables, which are a good source of calcium, but many of them do consume plenty of milk and cheese (perhaps too much in place of other nutrient rich foods like vegetables). This is demonstrated by the leading twenty sources of calories consumed by US children, of which dairy products occupy three of the top twelve foods consumed.

Clearly osteoporosis (weak bones) continues to be a problem for American women, and it is known that bone density (or lack of) is established in childhood and teenage years. There is a bit of a disconnect going on. Are the US recommended calcium intake levels justified or are they set too high? How much calcium do our bodies actually need?

Surprisingly, increased calcium intake beyond a certain baseline is *not* associated with increased bone density in several large epidemiological studies. In some studies, increasing dairy consumption either had no effect or actually *increased* fracture risk long term. The nations with the highest milk intake have the highest osteoporosis rates. Women with the highest intakes of low-fat dairy products had the highest risk of osteoporosis. How can this be? This has been referred to as *the milk paradox*. Scientists who research calcium metabolism have identified *increased calcium excretion* and *inadequate calcium utilization* as risk factors for low bone density, indicating that we are not absorbing or retaining it or using it for its intended purpose in the body.[50-53]

Rather than elevating calcium requirements, we need to look at other key nutrients like vitamin D and magnesium which are crucial for calcium metabolism and may be deficient in the diet. Milk is notoriously low in magnesium. There is also evidence that the Western diet makes the body slightly acidic, with lots of grains and salt, processed meat, and too few of the foods that buffer this acidity, namely fruits and vegetables. Meat, dairy and animal protein is acid forming in the body unless balanced with vegetables and fruits. This excessive acid formation (called the net renal acid load) will cause the body to pull calcium, magnesium and phosphorus out of the bones in order to buffer the acid. This is potentially a driver of both osteoporosis and kidney stones in adults.[54-57]

Another thing to consider is the possible effect of acid blockers (proton pump inhibitors or PPI) for reflux and abdominal pain that are overprescribed in kids. By reducing the levels of stomach acid in children, we may be decreasing their absorption of key nutrients like calcium, magnesium, and vitamin $B_{12}$. This has been grossly understudied in children, but in adults there is evidence linking PPI use to increased fractures in early adulthood and later life.[58-60]

And lastly, the number one factor in determining bone density is exercise. Examination of bones of our hunter-gatherer ancestors and of indigenous peoples eating a traditional diet with plenty of meat and plants and no dairy products reveals incredibly strong bones. It is highly unlikely that they were getting 1300 mg of calcium in their daily diet. However, it is likely that they were getting plenty of exercise and sun exposure for vitamin D.[61,62] If children are inactive during the critical bone forming years, their bones will suffer the consequences.

Children need adequate calcium in order to grow and maintain strong bones, and dairy products (especially yogurt) can be a significant source of that calcium. However, there is little evidence that a high milk or high calcium intake is associated with stronger bones. Should the US consider following the international recommendations of 500 to 700 mg daily for most pre-teen kids? It is an ongoing debate. It is important for their bones that children get sufficient calcium and vitamin D (exposure to sunlight or supplement) and magnesium in addition to acid-buffering fruits and vegetables. Finally, plenty of daily exercise is important to assure healthy metabolism and to maintain calcium in the bones.

## TABLE 12.7 CALCIUM CONTENT OF FOODS

| Food | mg/serving |
|---|---|
| Yogurt (8oz) | 415 |
| Cheddar cheese 1.5 oz | 300 |
| Milk (8oz) | 275 |
| Almond milk (8oz) | 300 |
| Tofu (½ cup) | 430 |
| Canned salmon (3oz) | 180 |
| Sardines (3oz) | 325 |
| Turnip greens (½ cup) | 100 |
| Collard greens (½ cup) | 180 |
| Bok Choy (½ cup) | 80 |
| Kale (½ cup) | 90 |
| Broccoli (½ cup) | 30 |
| Orange (1) | 55 |

Data from National Institutes of Health (www.NIH.gov), USDA Nutrient Database (https://fdc.nal.usda.gov/), Health Link British Columbia (www.healthlinkBC.ca), Linus Pauling Institute (https://lpi.oregonstate.edu/mic/minerals/iron)[141-144]

## Omega-3 fatty acids

As discussed in the prenatal and infant nutrition sections, long-chain **omega-3** fatty acids (EPA/DHA) are crucial for brain and eye development. They are concentrated in the synapses of brain cells, make the brain cell membranes more fluid and robust, and omega-3 control inflammation at the cellular level. There is also growing evidence that EPA/DHA are **epigenetic modifiers** helping to shut off the genes for inflammation and chronic disease and stimulate a brain boosting nerve growth factor called **brain derived neurotrphic factor (BDNF)**. Failure to get adequate omega-3 in the diet may lead to suboptimal growth and functioning of the brain and increases the potential for a subtle "short-circuiting" effect and increased susceptibility to inflammation. Deficiency of omega-3 may result in suboptimal brain function, contribute to ADHD, mood disorders such as depression and anxiety, and promote inflammation that is a precursor of cancer, heart disease, diabetes and autoimmune disease.

Individuals with brain disorders such as ADHD may need much higher omega-3 intakes to correct an undiscovered deficiency. Studies show an unhealthy imbalance of **omega-6** and omega-3 fats in children with ADHD.[63-68] Diets rich in seafood are being shown to be protective against ADHD.[64,69] Multiple extensive review studies have shown overall favorable symptom improvement in ADHD using fish oil supplements, but results from individual studies have been variable.[70-74]

Food sources of omega-3 EPA/DHA include fish, and eggs from pasture-raised chickens and chickens fed additional omega-3. There are smaller amounts in beef and game meat. The plant source short chain omega-3 (**ALA**) found in soybean, canola, and flaxseed oil, hemp and chia seeds, walnuts, and a few other plant oils is not the biologically active form and requires conversion in the body to get the necessary EPA and DHA.

The majority of children in the US are not getting remotely close to adequate intakes of the short or long chain omega-3 fatty acids in their diet, and many children actually have close to zero intake of EPA/DHA daily. Unless children regularly eat fish like salmon, trout, sardines, herring, or cod or eat omega-3 enhanced eggs regularly, they are most likely suboptimal in their brain levels of DHA. As illustrated previously, plant source omega-3 does not get converted by the majority of people at a level to support optimal brain function, especially in a rapidly developing child. The efficiency of this conversion likely varies between individual children based on their genetics and nutritional status so some children may need more omega-3 than others. Many children are low in zinc, magnesium, and B6 required to convert ALA to EPA/DHA.

Omega-3 fats get crowded out in our children's bodies and brains by high amounts of omega-6 refined vegetable oils and trans fats from diets high in processed foods, further increasing the need for long chain omega-3s. Recent estimates of child omega-3 intake showed at least a 10:1 omega-6 to omega-3 ratio and possibly up to 20:1, leaving children at considerable risk of having insufficient levels of omega-3.[75,76]

Although not commonly performed, one can test for omega-3 and omega-6 fatty acid levels in the body. *Red blood cell membrane (erythrocyte) fatty acid* levels are more accurate than serum fatty acid levels, and there are validated studies using this test, typically for research purposes.[82,83] However, if a child's diet lacks fish and contains lots of processed foods, we can assume they are likely suboptimal in omega-3 unless they take a supplement containing EPA/DHA.

I believe that during the vitally important early years of rapid brain development, we need to emphasize adequate long-chain omega-3 (EPA/DHA) intake in our children, in addition to incorporating ALA rich foods such as leafy greens, nuts, and flaxseed in their diet. Optimally children should eat a minimum of 200 mg combined EPA/DHA daily. Make low mercury, high omega-3 fish part of their regular diet. Use high omega-3 eggs. Care should be taken to limit excessive omega-6 oils in the diet as well. Cook with olive or avocado oil that do not have excessive omega-6. Minimize deep fried foods and highly processed foods that contain the damaged oils that displace the vital omega-3.

If a child will not eat fish, I feel a fish oil supplement is warranted. 200-500 mg of EPA/DHA daily for the younger child is a safe adequate dose. Their brain will be thankful. Alternately, 1 tbsp of cold pressed flaxseed oil contains 7,600 mg of ALA, the short chain omega-3. Under *optimal* circumstances, this may yield up to 400 to 600 mg of EPA in the child's body, helping to control inflammation, but will likely not yield much in the way of DHA for their brain.[84,85] An additional algae source 200 mg DHA could be considered for vegetarian/vegan children.

If an omega-3 supplement smells off or excessively fishy, it may be rancid, and needs to be returned. Quality matters, more so with omega-3 than any other nutritional supplement and several companies have a higher quality standard for their omega-3 products. Nordic Naturals, Carlson's, and Barleans are a few of the omega-3 products that I often recommend for their quality and taste.

### B6, B12, Choline, and Folate: The Methyl Donors

Known as methyl donor vitamins, all of these nutrients are needed for neurotransmitter formation in the brain, for detoxification processes, and all have been found to be low in some studies of children especially those with ADHD.[63,86] Methyl donor vitamins are involved with the process of epigenetic modification described earlier and can effect a child's **gene expression**, significantly affecting their health. A preliminary study looking at genes involved in nutrient metabolism showed a possible association with several genes affecting folate and B6 metabolism in patients with ADHD.[87] There is also a link between low folate and vitamin $B_{12}$ and depression. Folate works with Vitamin $B_6$, $B_{12}$ and choline to reduce a potentially damaging amino acid called **homocysteine**. High homocysteine levels in adults are linked to heart disease, stroke, cancer, and homocysteine may be related to a number of brain disorders including autism, ADHD and Alzheimer's. Homocysteine levels are associated with increased risk of all-cause mortality (dying from any cause), which means the higher the homocysteine levels in the body, the higher the chance of dying from a number of diseases.[95,96] We will briefly explore each of these important methyl donor vitamins in turn.

*Vitamin $B_6$*

Also known as pyridoxine or its active form P-5-P, $B_6$ may work synergistically with magnesium and zinc to produce neurotransmitters in the brain. $B_6$ is widespread in foods and found in meat, fish, poultry, beans, grains, vegetables. However, the more bioavailable form P-5-P is found in animal products. Being more widely available in the food supply makes overt deficiency unlikely except for really picky eaters consuming only highly processed food. However, some researchers feel that there may be a disordered metabolism of $B_6$ in some children with ADHD that could be amenable to supplementation.[91] There has also been research using a high dose form of $B_6$ called metadoxine in small studies on adults with ADHD, with reported positive results on inattention, but this needs more research and is not appropriate for children at present.[92-94] While I do not think there is any evidence supporting isolated $B_6$ supplementation in children, a multivitamin containing $B_6$ or the pyridoxine-5-phosphate (P-5-P) form of $B_6$ in safe doses could have the potential to help improve ADHD symptoms in a deficient child, and may be warranted for children with a very poor diet. The **RDA** for vitamin $B_6$ is 0.5 to 1 mg per day, and safe upper limit of supplementation is listed at 30 mg per day for younger children.

*Vitamin $B_{12}$ (cobalamin)*

Vitamin $B_{12}$ is involved in multiple bodily processes including DNA synthesis, blood cell formation, neurotransmitter synthesis and nerve myelination (**myelin** is a layer of insulation made up of protein and fatty substances that protect nerves in the brain and spinal cord). This vital sheath ensures that electrical impulses in the nerve cells function efficiently.

Estimates range from 2.5 to 5% of the US population over 9 years old are deficient in $B_{12}$, but rates as high as 22% of children in Israel have been reported.[98,99] Inadequate levels of $B_{12}$ are associated with increases in homocysteine with potential effects on the brain during growth and development including possible impairments in learning. $B_{12}$ deficiency may cause **macrocytic anemia** (a condition in which the body has overly large red blood cells and not enough normal red blood cells). Research shows that vitamin $B_{12}$ deficiency and elevated homocysteine levels may contribute to the development of depression.[100]

### TABLE 12.8 RECOMMENDED DAILY INTAKE OF $B_{12}$

| Age (years) | mcg |
|---|---|
| 1-3 | 0.9 |
| 4-8 | 1.2 |
| 9-13 | 1.8 |
| 14-18 | 2.4 |

Vitamin $B_{12}$ is found in fish, meat, poultry, eggs, milk, and milk products. $B_{12}$ is not found in adequate levels in a typical vegetarian or vegan diet, so steps need to be taken to monitor and prevent deficiency with supplementation in that population. Nori seaweed and shitake mushrooms are two of the only plant-based foods that may have *some* $B_{12}$ activity, and are not commonly eaten by younger children.

Other at-risk groups for $B_{12}$ deficiency are those taking long-term acid blockers for GERD, those with celiac or Crohn's disease, those with *H. pylori* infection of the stomach or **small intestinal bacterial overgrowth** (SIBO). The most accurate way to screen for deficiency is with a serum $B_{12}$ level and methylmalonic acid level, which is a sensitive marker that is increased during $B_{12}$ deficiency.

*Choline*
This B vitamin plays triple duty in the brain. It is a key structural component of a building block called phosphatidylcholine, a part of the nerve cell membrane. It is also a crucial part of the neurotransmitter **acetylcholine** and part of the methyl donor group of vitamins involved in detoxification and neurotransmitter synthesis. It is essential for developing babies before and after birth but likely continues to have developmental importance in the older child. The effects of low choline intake on children are not well studied at this point. Given its importance

in several aspects of brain metabolism, it is reasonable that subclinical deficiency could have adverse effects on the child's brain function.

Recommended choline intake is 250 mg for younger children, 375 mg for older children 9 to 13 years and 550 mg for teens.[103,104]

Eggs (yolks) are probably the best source for kids, as well as meat, poultry, pork, liver, and fish (especially salmon). Sources of choline are listed in Chapter 6. A child with a poor diet or one that is strictly vegetarian could be insufficient in choline. If a child is not eating any choline-rich foods, make an effort to start including some of these foods into their diet. If this is not possible, it is reasonable to consider a supplement like choline bitartrate or choline chloride, lecithin, or phosphatidylcholine at a safe level to support their brain function and to reach the recommended daily choline intake.

*Folate*
Folate is involved in DNA synthesis during growth, red blood cell formation, and **methylation**/detoxification reactions. It is also involved with production of brain neurotransmitters (serotonin, dopamine, norepinephrine). Low levels of folate in the body are associated with depression, autism, increased risk of heart disease and certain cancers including cervical cancer in adults, and macrocytic (as opposed to iron deficiency) anemia.

Food sources of folate include green leafy vegetables, liver, and beans. Because of increased fortification of processed grain products with folic acid (the synthetic version of folate), frank folate deficiency in children in industrialized countries is relatively rare. However, many children are not getting adequate amounts for optimal health.

### TABLE 12.9 RECOMMENDED DAILY INTAKE FOR FOLATE

| Age | mcg |
| --- | --- |
| 1-3 years | 150 |
| 4-8 years | 200 |
| 9-13 years | 300 |
| Teens and adults | 400 |

## HOT TOPIC

Individuals with a genetic variant called an *MTHFR mutation* have reduced activity of the enzyme that acts to convert folic acid (the synthetic form used in fortification) or dietary folate into the active form of folate used in the body (L-methylfolate). This potentially leaves that person at risk for *functional* folate deficiency despite seemingly adequate intakes, putting them at increased risk for adverse effects associated with dietary deficiencies of folate and elevated homocysteine. People with these genetic variants may have a higher requirement for dietary folate in order to get optimum levels of the active form L-methylfolate in their bodies. More severe forms of these variants are present in 25% of Hispanics and 10 to 15% of Caucasians. Research increasingly is investigating the role that folate and MTHFR variants play in development of cardiovascular disease and stroke in adults. A study done in 2005 showed *20 times increased risk of stroke* in those adults with the more severe MTHFR variant.[97] There is also interest in how MTHFR and homocysteine may impact ADHD, autism, and other neurological disorders including refractory depression and Alzheimer's.[100,86,87]

I'm a little concerned about the current percentage of children who may be sub-clinically deficient or insufficient in folate resulting from marginal folate intake and their decreased ability to use the folic acid found in fortified products if they carry abnormal copies of the MTHFR genes. I am not suggesting everyone get their MTHFR genes tested, but I think there needs to be more research in this area.

As discussed in the pregnancy chapter, there are supplements containing the L-methylfolate forms of this vitamin that bypass the rate-limiting step that is less efficient in people with MTHFR mutations. Supplementing with this form of the vitamin can result in significant reductions in potentially damaging homocysteine in these folks, lowering their risk for related disorders. Higher quality prenatal and children's multivitamins are starting to incorporate the L-methylfolate form of folate at a safe dose (150 to 250 mcg for children, 400 to 800 mcg for pregnant women). Increasingly, L-methylfolate supplementation is being used in adult and adolescent cases of treatment-resistant depression.[106,107]

## Vitamin D

Vitamin D is necessary for calcium absorption and bone metabolism, but also has receptors on almost every cell in the body and is considered as much a hormone as a vitamin. It has receptors in the nucleus, the control center of our cells, and impacts gene expression and therefore can be considered an epigenetic modifier. It has essential roles in supporting the immune system, controlling inflammation, and supporting the brain.

Vitamin D may have a significant impact on brain health. There are vitamin D receptors throughout the brain and growing evidence that adequate Vitamin D levels help support the ongoing health of the **neurons** by releasing growth factors. Vitamin D also supports the production of the neurotransmitters dopamine and serotonin, which are known to be altered in depression and ADHD.[109] Vitamin D deficiency is common in ADHD, and several early studies on Vitamin D supplementation in kids with ADHD have improved their cognitive performance.[110-112] Vitamin D deficiency is also known to be associated with depression and development of Alzheimer's in older adults. Adequate vitamin D levels in the pregnant mother and in the infant and young child may help protect against autism.[116-118]

Deficiency of vitamin D has the potential to result in poor bone density and rickets, which had been epidemic in the US in the earlier 1900's, especially among African Americans. Rickets is a condition of low body calcium due to an inability to absorb the calcium because of vitamin D deficiency, or from inadequate calcium intake in the diet. It results in bowing of the legs and leg pain in toddlers and young children from inadequately calcified bones. Studies are showing that rickets is again on the rise in the United States, likely because of inadequate vitamin D intake and inadequate time spent outdoors in the sun. We have become a sun-fearing culture because of concern about skin cancer, but the reality is that too little sun exposure is also bad for us and our children and can have serious health ramifications.

Probably the larger concern for vitamin D deficiency or insufficiency is immune system dysregulation including the development of **autoimmune disease.** Vitamin D is involved with both **innate immunity** (the body's front-line defense against all invaders) as well as **adaptive immunity** (the part of the immune system that learns how to defend against specific invaders). A dysregulated immune system is thought to potentially result in autoimmune disease, where the body's immune system turns and attacks its own tissue. The fact that vitamin D has effects on decreasing pro-inflammatory gene expression and increasing anti-inflammatory gene expression also suggests its importance in preventing the major diseases of Western civilization, all of which are inflammatory in nature. There is speculation that the rampant insufficiency of vitamin D could be playing a role in the rising rates of autoimmune diseases like **type 1 diabetes,** thyroid disease, multiple sclerosis, celiac disease, **inflammatory bowel**

**disease**, as well as increased susceptibility to respiratory infections like influenza and the worst effects of COVID-19.[113-115]

Vitamin D comes mainly from sunlight exposure on our skin, but also from fortified dairy products, fatty fish and fish oil, liver, and mushrooms. The human body makes vitamin D from cholesterol with a key reaction requiring UV sunlight exposure to the skin. For most of human evolution, vitamin D was not an issue as we were outdoors 90% of the time, getting plenty of sun exposure. Contrary to human evolution, our modern lives indoors make inadequate vitamin D an epidemic, especially among darker skinned individuals and those living in northern climates. The rise of the "screen culture" with kids spending most of their time indoors, inactive in front of a computer or TV screen, also raises the risk of vitamin D deficiency and insufficiency. Estimates are that 10% of US kids are deficient in vitamin D (with blood levels less than 20 ng/ml), but up to 60% may have suboptimal levels (<30 ng/ml). This may have significant health implications.

The AAP recommends all breastfed children up to one year of age receive a supplement of 400 IU of vitamin D daily. Recommend daily vitamin D intake is 600 IU for older children and teens. Supplements are recommended if those children are not meeting these dietary intake recommendations (which few kids are). This means many children should be receiving daily vitamin D supplements and we should probably be screening a lot more children for vitamin D deficiency as well.

Given the evidence, vitamin D screening should be considered for kids with ADHD, with chronic GI or autoimmune diseases like Crohn's or celiac disease, as well as darker skinned children or children living in northern climates. There is an interesting relationship between low vitamin D and overweight and obese children, so this may be a population that should be screened as well. At risk children may be screened by their primary healthcare provider for deficiency.

The screening test of choice is a 25-OH vitamin D level in the blood. With the explosion of research into the epigenetic roles, the immune regulatory and anti-inflammatory roles, as well as the roles in the brain, we should target optimal vitamin D levels in our children. Levels should be above 30 ng/ml, and the Endocrine Society (a group of doctors that study hormones) would say 40 to 60 ng/ml is the "sweet spot," but optimal levels remain somewhat controversial. Blood levels above 100 ng/ml are not recommended and above 150 ng/ml could be considered toxic. In the northern climate where I practice, the majority of kids I test are below 30, lots are below 20, and a significant number have been below 10!

Supplement dosing varies on age and the degree of vitamin D deficiency. Younger children can receive 400 to 600 IU. For the school age child, I usually start with 1000 IU Vitamin D3 (cholecalciferol) supplement daily. Vitamin D supplementation at these levels is very safe. If blood levels are very low, I endorse a physician monitored vitamin D loading protocol. For teens and adults this is a dose of 50,000 IU of vitamin D3 (the more bioavailable form) given weekly with a fat containing meal for a total of six weeks; for younger children 25,000 IU is the dose. The child is then returned to a lower maintenance dose and levels rechecked in four to six months. *Vitamin D megadosing should only be done under the supervision of a qualified healthcare provider.*

### Fiber

Both soluble and insoluble fiber are needed to maintain proper colon function. Soluble fiber supports a healthy **microbiome** and production of important **short chain fatty acids** by feeding bacteria in the colon. Soluble fiber also helps to create a protective coating or gel on the intestinal walls, preventing leaky gut and slowing absorption of nutrients to improve metabolism. Insoluble fiber acts like a broom to "sweep" waste out of the intestines, and it also carries beneficial bacteria to the lower intestines. The best fiber is "intact fiber" from real food that hasn't been overly processed to the point that diminishes or negates the benefits – many food manufacturing techniques destroy the fiber in foods with ultra-processing, then add fiber back in as an additive. This is a questionable approach.

The Institute of Medicine (IOM) recommends 19 to 25 grams of fiber daily for children. Average fiber *intake* is estimated at 11 to 14 grams daily for children, falling short of recommendations. Food sources of fiber include vegetables, fruits, and whole grains.

The vast majority of Americans are significantly deficient in fiber of both types, but especially soluble fiber from fruits and vegetables. NHANES data from 2010 showed *only 5% of Americans* were meeting their fiber requirements. Fiber is more than just "roughage" that keeps us "regular" – it is now listed as a *"nutrient of concern"* by the Dietary Guidelines Advisory Committee (DGAC). If the average adult is only getting 16 grams of fiber daily, how little is the average child getting?[124,125] If a child is not eating five servings of fruits and vegetables daily and is not eating the whole grain versions of their carbohydrates (bread, pasta, rice, etc.) they are likely not getting enough fiber and are not supporting their gut microbiome as much as they should.

Is your child a daily pooper? A diet with sufficient fiber should result in soft daily bowel movements, not two to three difficult stools a week. Deficiency of fiber can lead to constipation, **dysbiosis**, and an unhealthy microbiome. We as a nation are starving our good gut bacteria and feeding the bad ones with all the processed foods lacking in fiber. There is increasing evidence that an imbalance of gut bacteria may contribute to everything from constipation to ADHD and autism via the **brain-gut-microbiome axis**. (See ramifications of an altered microbiome and the "Five Things Needed for a Good Number Two" in Chapter 15.) Children need adequate fiber in their diet. Increase their vegetable intake, give them whole fruit instead of juice and choose 100% whole grain products to boost their fiber intake.

### Phytonutrients

Mind the phytonutrient gap! The modern Western diet with all its processed foods is likely leaving many children and adults with a lack of **phytonutrients** referred to as the "phytonutrient gap." This class of compounds incorporates hundreds if not thousands of nutrients not officially classified as vitamins yet playing important roles in maintaining health.[126-132] If a child is on a "white food" diet, eating mostly bread, pasta, crackers, macaroni, cereal, and milk, then they are likely deficient in phytonutrients. Phytonutrients are the compounds that give fruits and vegetables their wonderful color and are one of the main reasons why all of us need to "eat the rainbow" of red, orange, yellow, green, blue and purple colored fruits and vegetables in order to protect our health. *We cannot get these nutrients from taking a vitamin.* "Eating the rainbow" ensures that we are getting a spectrum of compounds including polyphenols, flavonoids, carotenoids, limonoids, thiocyanates and indoles that act to protect our bodies in multiple ways.

## TABLE 12.10 FOOD SOURCES AND ACTIVITY OF PHYTONUTRIENTS

| Phytonutrient | Food Sources | Activity in the Body |
|---|---|---|
| Carotenoids | Red, orange and yellow vegetables | vitamin A precursor, eyes, anti-cancer, antioxidant |
| Lycopene | Tomato, pink grapefruit | antioxidant, anti-cancer, cardioprotective |
| Limonoids | Citrus fruit | anti-cancer, anti-viral |
| GLS | Broccoli, cauliflower, cabbage, brussels sprouts | antioxidant, anti-cancer |
| **Polyphenols** | | |
| Flavonoids | Fruits, vegetables, tea, chocolate | anti-inflammatory, antioxidant, anti-cancer |
| Anthocyanins | Grapes, berries, cherries | antioxidant, neuroprotective |
| Flavonols | Onion, kale, tea, broccoli | anti-cancer, anti-diabetes |
| Flavones | EVOO, oranges, whole wheat | cardioprotective, anti-diabetes |
| Isoflavones | Legumes and lentils | anti-cancer, anti-diabetes |
| Resveratrol (stilbenes) | Red grapes, blueberry, peanuts | antioxidant, anti-cancer |
| Curcumin (phenolics) | Turmeric | anti-cancer, anti-inflammatory |
| Lignans | EVOO, flaxseed, whole grains | anti-cancer, anti-inflammatory |

Evidence shows these compounds enhance detoxification and epigenetic signals that activate the body's anti-inflammatory and anti-cancer pathways. Phytonutrient variety also helps to support a healthy diverse gut microbiome which has many downstream health benefits. The blue and purple fruits and vegetables like grapes, blueberries, plums, and cabbage are shown to be protective of the brain and may help delay cognitive decline later in life. Red and orange fruits and vegetables have powerful **antioxidant** and anti-inflammatory activity. Yellows and greens contain antioxidants and heart protective compounds. Phytonutrients are one of the reasons it is felt the Mediterranean diet is so healthy. This diet is heavy in many of the richest sources of these protective nutrients, while the Western diet is not.

Low intake of fresh fruits and vegetables among American children (and adults) means fewer phytonutrients are available to their body. In fact, the top ten foods eaten by American kids are devoid of phytonutrients and 8 out of 10 adults are not meeting the minimum levels of fruit and vegetable consumption, thereby cutting out the main source of phytonutrients in the diet. There is no Recommended Daily Allowance (RDA) set for these nutrients, but that does not mean they are not vital to human health. Having a low intake of phytonutrients may not result directly in a "deficiency" like scurvy, but it could increase risk of cancer, heart disease, diabetes, autoimmune disease as well as other inflammatory and neuro-degenerative diseases. Most modern diseases are inflammatory in nature, and brain conditions like ADHD are being linked to markers of increased inflammation and **oxidative stress** (insufficient **antioxidant** activity in the body to prevent cellular damage). Closing the phytonutrient gap therefore makes sense from a prevention and treatment perspective for all kids, especially ones with these conditions. As a caveat, we discussed previously how some otherwise beneficial fruits and vegetables, if conventionally grown, may have significant amounts of pesticide residues that can be potentially neurotoxic and have been linked with increased risk of ADHD and other brain disorders. Organically grown fruits and vegetables have been shown to be higher in phytonutrients as well as significantly lower in pesticide residues. I recommend choosing organic or locally grown whenever possible, especially for the "Dirty Dozen" fruits and vegetables that are known to have the highest levels of agrochemical exposure and pesticide residues. We do not have to worry as much about the "Clean Fifteen" least pesticide exposed fruits and vegetables.

## Plant-based diets

While it has been stated that a well-planned vegan diet can be suitable and nutritionally complete for any age group, there are large caveats for children.[133-136] Children are not little adults. Their bodies and nutrient requirements are different and still developing. Children on vegetarian and vegan diets are at particular risk of deficiency in certain crucial nutrients including $B_{12}$, iron, zinc, choline, and omega-3 fats (EPA/DHA).

If choosing to raise a child vegetarian or vegan, the correct steps *must* be taken to fill in nutrient gaps as there are developmental windows that may close, leaving children with deficits that may not be recoverable. If making this choice for children, then do it as safely as possible and make sure they are getting adequate nutrition. I am not trying to raise the dander of folks who follow a vegetarian or vegan diet for moral, ethical or religious reasons, but this does not change the fact that this type of diet could potentially put a child at nutritional risk if one is not paying careful attention to the foods being provided.

The biggest risk for vegetarian/vegan children is vitamin $B_{12}$ deficiency. $B_{12}$ cannot be found in adequate amounts in plant-based foods. Therefore, all children raised on a vegan/vegetarian diet need vitamin $B_{12}$ supplementation and testing. The RDA is 0.9-2.4 mcg per day depending on age, and many children's multivitamins contain the RDA for $B_{12}$. One European academic group recommends supplementation of 5 mcg per day for younger vegan children up to 3 years, and 25 mcg per day for older children. It was also recommended by these authors to monitor blood levels of $B_{12}$, homocysteine, and methylmalonic acid to ensure adequate intakes.[135]

Making sure a young child has adequate iron and zinc intake is a bit trickier as described earlier in the chapter on first foods. Iron and zinc *content* of a plant-based diet can be adequate on paper if the right foods are selected. Iron and zinc *absorption* on a plant-based diet may be questionable. Soaking and rinsing beans and grains prior to cooking, slow cooking, and including a source of vitamin C with each meal to enhance mineral absorption can help but may not be enough.

I cannot endorse feeding the plant-based child a diet high in processed foods and low in fiber to enhance the absorption of iron and zinc as recommended by some plant-based nutrition groups. As illustrated earlier in this book, fiber is vital to the health of the child and their microbiome and should be encouraged early in childhood. However, I do recognize that iron and zinc fortified foods and supplements can help fill in these nutrient gaps in the plant-based diet and can be an important source of iron and zinc. These deficiencies may be less of a concern in older children and adults following a plant-based diet, but during the critical developmental windows of younger children (and during pregnancy) a nutritionally complete diet requires even greater attention.

As reviewed earlier, there is no adequate testing for low zinc, but a supplement of 5 to 10 mg daily for the vegetarian or vegan child may be warranted. Vegetarian and vegan children need a complete iron profile checked at least annually to catch iron deficiency early. Complete blood count (CBC) with a serum ferritin are both needed to detect deficiency; merely checking a hemoglobin is not sufficient. Markers of low iron in a child should prompt supplementation and repeat monitoring by a qualified health professional.

Children on a purely plant-based diet should strongly consider an omega-3 DHA supplement. As discussed earlier, the conversion of plant-based **ALA** (flaxseed oil, walnuts) to the biologically active EPA is inefficient (5-8% at best), and conversion to the brain friendly DHA is even lower (often less than 1%). The child's brain needs DHA. Vegetarians can get DHA through DHA-enhanced eggs but vegans should consider 200 mg of algae-derived DHA daily for the growing child's brain. Choline may also be low in a plant-based diet, and is important for the growing brain. Consider a supplement of 200 to 500 mg daily if intakes are low.

Let's take a quick look at three fairly realistic diets for a younger school-aged child.

## ANALYZING THE CHILD'S DIET

### Child #1-

- Breakfast- 2 toaster pastries and 1 cup orange juice
- Lunch- PB+J on white bread and 1 cup chocolate milk
- Snack- 2 fruit snack packs and a juice box
- Dinner- macaroni and cheese and 8 oz orange flavored drink

This diet is very unhealthy and imbalanced with lots of sugar (almost 150 grams of added sugar!), almost no fiber (4 grams which is less than a quarter of the requirement) with limited quality protein and few phyto-nutrients other than those in the juice, and possibly the jelly. This diet is close to meeting the RDA for iron on paper, but much of this iron is from fortification and will not be well absorbed or bioavailable to the child's body because of other factors in the diet. This diet is inadequate in zinc, folate, choline, $B_{12}$, magnesium and omega-3 fats, and what little zinc is in this diet is being blocked by other dietary factors. Long-term, this type of diet puts a child at risk for constipation and dysbiosis, iron deficiency, immune system and brain dysfunction, and the future development of diabetes and heart disease.

## Child #2-

- Breakfast- 2 fruit and grain breakfast bars, 1 cup 2% milk
- Lunch- Pre-packaged lunchpack with ham, cheese, crackers, and cookie. 1 cup 2% milk
- Snack- 1 container "kids'" yogurt
- Dinner- 2 oz spaghetti with ½ cup canned sauce, ½ cup frozen peas and carrots, 1 cup water

This diet is marginally better than the first diet, but has lots of room for improvement. This diet still contains 72 grams of added sugar, far too much for a child. It contains 45 grams of protein but still only 8 grams of fiber (half the recommended daily total for a younger child) and is short on servings of fruits and vegetables. This diet is also low in magnesium, folate, and choline. On paper this child meets the RDA for both iron (9 mg) and zinc (4.4 mg), but when accounting for the limited absorption of these minerals this child could still be at risk for nutritional deficiency and insufficiency. There are almost no omega-3 fats in this diet as well.

## Child #3-

- Breakfast- 2 scrambled eggs with diced spinach, 1 slice whole grain toast, 1 cup 2% milk
- Lunch- Turkey and cheese on 100% whole grain bread, baby carrots, 1 cup water
- Snack- Trail mix with nuts and dried fruit (1 serving), flavored seltzer water
- Dinner- Chickpea pasta with marinara meat sauce, ½ cup steamed broccoli, water with lemon

By reading labels and making a few better choices on breakfast, snacks and drinks, it was possible to significantly improve the quality of the diet. We reduced the added sugar of this diet to only 14 grams. The fiber content of this diet is much better at 25 grams for the day, supporting both the microbiome and better bowel movements. This diet is more in balance and it has multiple servings of fruits and vegetables for the important phytonutrients. Folate, choline, and B12 intakes are adequate. The iron (14 mg) and zinc (8 mg) are both higher and more bioavailable in this diet, lowering the risk for deficiency. With the eggs and the nuts, there is at least some omega-3 in this diet. There is also nothing in this diet that is considered a highly-processed food, significantly cutting down on the number of food additives and preservatives the child is exposed to.

By paying a little more attention to food labels and making better food choices, we can reduce the risk of chronic disease in our children.

## NUTRITION R$_X$

**1** Common nutrient deficiencies in children, especially those with ADHD may include iron, zinc, magnesium, omega-3 fats, vitamin D, phytonutrients and fiber. Efforts should be made to sculpt a diet that includes all the important nutrients for a growing child.

**2** Omega-3 insufficiency in our children is rampant. Two to three servings per week of high omega-3 fish can really boost their brain levels. Check the website for kid friendly fish meals and snacks.

**3** If a child won't eat fish, or is being raised vegetarian, consider an omega-3 EPA/DHA supplement for their brain in the range of 500 mg combined EPA/DHA daily; alternately consider 200 mg of algae derived DHA plus 1 tablespoon of cold-pressed, high quality flaxseed oil for vegans.

**4** Vegetarian and vegan children need to be monitored closely for B$_{12}$, iron, zinc and omega-3 deficiency and likely need supplements for all these nutrients. A visit with a pediatric trained dietician is recommended.

**5** Many children are at risk for vitamin D deficiency. If they are in a high-risk group, consider getting their levels tested and start a vitamin D$_3$ supplement of 600 IU per day.

# CHAPTER THIRTEEN

# FOOD ALLERGIES AND INTOLERANCES

Are you concerned that something in your child's diet could be causing rashes, constipation, diarrhea or other tummy troubles? If so, you are not alone.

Many parents have concerns about possible food reactions during solid food introduction or early childhood. Young children might develop eczema, hives or other rashes, difficulty gaining weight, frequent vomiting, reflux, abdominal pain, diarrhea, or other bowel concerns. Common foods like bread, crackers, milk, cheese, eggs, and peanut butter are all staples of the American child's diet but may be causing health issues in millions of children.

Food allergies and intolerances are increasingly common in today's children. Because of differences in the presentation and severity of food allergies and intolerances, confusion exists surrounding what constitutes a food allergy, an intolerance, or a sensitivity so hopefully, this chapter can offer clarification and guidance.

Adverse food reactions are divided into **immune-mediated** food allergies (food reactions which are known to involve the immune system) and **non-immune mediated food intolerances** (food reactions which do not directly involve the immune system). Food "sensitivities" (a term which is not universally defined, and therefore usually better avoided with some exceptions) often encompass more general food reactions such as infant reflux and colic, chronic constipation, **non-celiac wheat/gluten sensitiv-ity** (NCGS) and **irritable bowel syndrome.**

About 6-10% of US kids have a food allergy; these numbers keep increasing.[1-7]

Up to 15% of infants have adverse reactions to cow's milk proteins found in standard infant formulas.

2-5% of infants have diagnosed cow's milk allergies that are lasting well into childhood.

Up to 3% of children have an egg allergy.

One in 100 US children have *Celiac disease*, a specific adverse reaction to gluten in wheat, barley, and rye.

About one in 200 children have a *wheat allergy*.

Food intolerances and other adverse food reactions, apart from food allergies, also seem to be increasing.

Accurate estimates of the actual prevalence of "sensitivities" and intolerances (as opposed to true allergies) are often difficult due to lack of accurate testing. These conditions commonly go undiagnosed.

**HOT TOPIC**

The reason adverse food reactions are increasing in kids is hotly debated but in my opinion is likely caused by a breakdown of **immune tolerance** from a combination of environmental factors during the critical **first thousand days**.[8] Immune tolerance refers to the natural state of balance wherein the immune system does not get activated by foods that are being eaten, and does not react. When there is a breakdown in tolerance, exposure to specific foods causes the immune system to recognize proteins in food as an enemy.

Breakdown in tolerance may occur in susceptible individuals from multiple factors: damage to the gut **microbiome** (the master immune regulator), increased intestinal permeability (leaky gut), breakdown in the skin barrier (as seen in eczema), and altered regulation of the immune system itself.

Increasingly, many factors conspire to foster the development of allergic reactions.[2,8,9] A high rate of C-section births and formula feeding may increase the risk of allergies in children, as do use of acid blockers for infant reflux, the widespread use of antibiotics in medicine and the food supply, and food additives and chemicals that disrupt gut bacteria and immune cells. Deficient diets in mothers and children that lack important nutrients like zinc, vitamin D, fiber, and **omega-3** fatty acids contribute to inflammation and dysfunction of the immune system. By following the recommendations in this book for pregnant mothers and young children, perhaps we can reverse this trend of adverse food reactions.

What are the differences between an allergy and an intolerance? How common are they? What are the symptoms to look for in children and how do we work to prevent these conditions? Let's explore the answers to these crucial questions.

## TYPES OF FOOD ALLERGIES

The topic of food allergies can be confusing. Physical responses commonly referred to as an "allergy" could represent any number of adverse reactions to foods. The term *food allergy* should be used to describe an unpleasant reaction to a food that is caused by the immune system. Below we will clarify the different immune reactions to get more specific.

**Classic food allergies (IgE-mediated food allergies and anaphylaxis)**
"Classic" allergies are caused by a specific type of reaction of the immune system, referred to as an **IgE-mediated** reaction. These classic food allergies now affect up to 10% of children although prevalence can vary by geography and ethnicity.[1] Of those affected, about 3% of children are estimated to have severe allergic reactions to foods. The most common IgE-mediated food allergies are to milk, egg, peanut, tree nut, sesame, soy, wheat, and fish/shellfish.

IgE (immunoglobulin E) is an antibody (immune protein) produced in our immune systems by specific white blood cells called B cells. With classic allergic reactions to foods, there is a breakdown in immune tolerance that

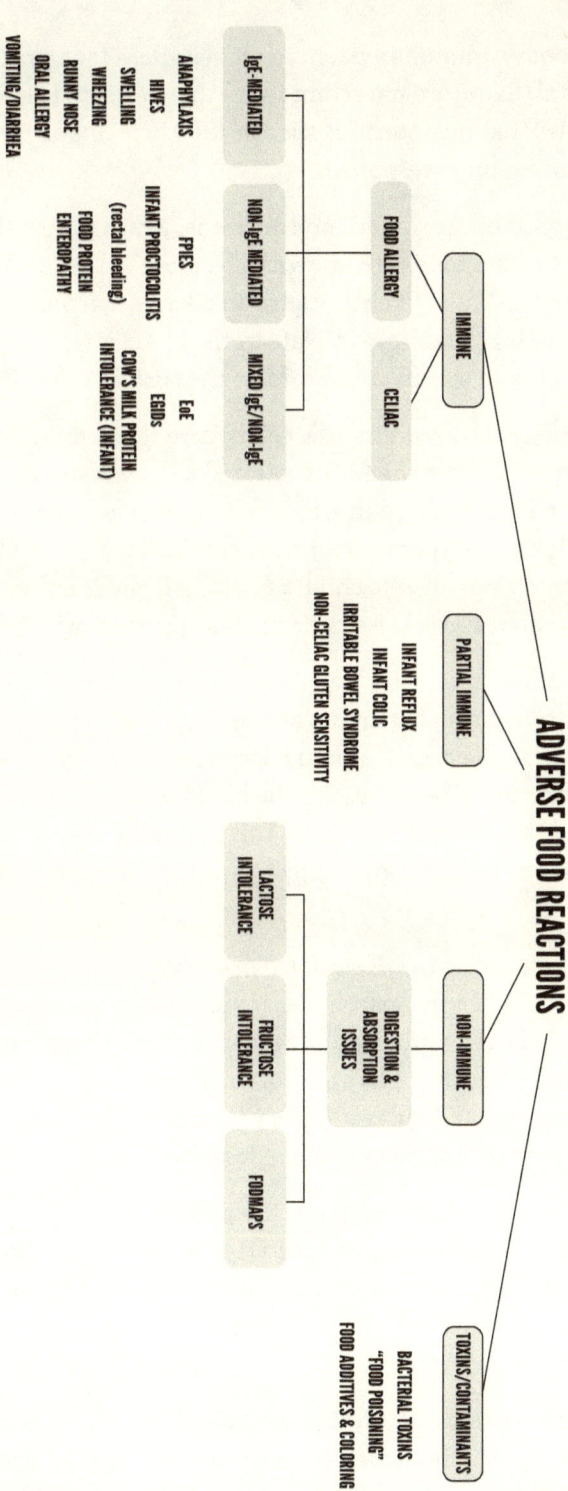

causes the body's immune system to see harmless food proteins as potentially harmful. Exposure to certain foods then leads to the production of IgE molecules that misinterpret specific food proteins as threats leading to significant immune responses.

These food proteins are called food antigens, which means they generate antibodies. Certain foods are known to be more antigenic than others, meaning they are more likely to cause an allergic reaction. Once IgE-antibodies are formed, they circulate in the blood stream and in the body where they bind to specific receptors on the surface of **mast cells**.

Mast cells are specialized immune cells where the body stores **histamine** (and a number of other chemicals referred to as *mediators*). They are found throughout the body, often in sites where the body comes into close contact with the environment, like the skin and gut. When IgE binds to a food allergen in an allergic child, a classic allergic reaction begins. Mast cells are activated and release their mediators into the bloodstream.

The release of histamine is a "call to arms" for the immune system, and when produced in small amounts at a local site of injury, it aids healing. However, in the case of a food allergy, histamine may be secreted in massive quantities all at once into the bloodstream, which can result in **anaphylaxis** or anaphylactic shock. This potentially severe, even fatal reaction can be caused by an allergy to any food, medication, insect stings, or latex.

*Up to half of the kids with IgE mediated food allergies have had an anaphylactic reaction.*[9] During anaphylaxis, hives, itching, facial and airway swelling, runny nose, nausea, vomiting and wheezing can all occur within minutes. Anaphylaxis, left untreated, can result in a rapid drop in blood pressure (also known as shock) and respiratory failure as the airway closes off. Immediate proper treatment can be lifesaving.

Treatment for anaphylaxis requires the prompt use of an auto-injectable epinephrine device (Epi-Pen or Auvi-Q) that injects an emergency dose of epinephrine (adrenaline) into the muscle of the thigh. The epinephrine is absorbed rapidly into the bloodstream, thereby reversing the effects of histamine and other mediators.

Antihistamines (Benadryl, Zyrtec, etc.) also block the effects of histamine and should be given immediately on the way to the closest emergency room or while waiting for the paramedics. However, it is the epinephrine that is the life-saving treatment and needs to be given promptly during an anaphylactic reaction. The child with a severe anaphylactic reaction will be treated and closely monitored in the hospital until all symptoms of the anaphylactic reaction have subsided.

Up to 5% of the US population has suffered an anaphylactic reaction at some point in their lives, and rates continue to increase.[10] Medications are the most common cause of anaphylaxis, but food and insect sting reactions are also common causes. Failure to recognize and treat anaphylaxis early in an episode results in several hundred deaths annually in the US and worldwide in both children and adults.

Not all IgE-mediated reactions cause anaphylaxis, the most extreme form of this allergic reaction. Milder IgE-mediated reactions can cause less severe wheezing, rashes, itching, hives, or vomiting.

IgE-mediated reactions are rapid onset, occurring within minutes to hours after the food is eaten. Typical IgE mediated allergic reactions include[11,12]

+ Anaphylaxis
+ Hives and facial swelling (angioedema) with or without anaphylaxis
+ Asthma and allergic rhinitis (nasal allergies)
+ Eczema flares (although eczema may be a predisposing factor for allergies as well as a symptom)
+ Vomiting and diarrhea (typically in conjunction with other skin findings or swelling)
+ Oral allergy syndrome: itchy mouth after eating certain fruits and vegetables. This is now called Pollen Food Allergy Syndrome
+ Food and exercise-induced anaphylaxis: food only causes the reaction if eating the food is followed by exercise

Foods that cause IgE-mediated allergies can be identified using blood tests and skin prick testing (SPT) performed by a certified allergist (a healthcare provider specializing in allergy and immunology). IgE levels to specific foods can be detected in the blood by obtaining a food allergen-specific IgE level in the blood (immunoCAP test). SPT can be used to verify if there is a visible reaction consisting of a bump surrounded by an area of redness within minutes of introducing a tiny amount of food allergen into the skin, indicating an IgE-mediated sensitivity to the food. Frequently, a child can have a mildly elevated IgE level to a specific food in the blood but not physically react to the food, making the situation somewhat confusing. The same can happen with skin testing where a child has a mild reaction on SPT but can eat the food without a reaction.

These "false positives" are a main reason why testing should be done by a qualified allergist who knows how to interpret the results and avoid unnecessary food restriction.[1,12] Thus, a food allergy is diagnosed by a history that strongly suggests a food reaction along with a positive skin or blood test. The gold standard for diagnosing these and any allergies is still the initial elimination of the food from the diet followed by a medically supervised oral food challenge of the suspected food in the allergist's office or medical center (the proof is in the pudding).

If a child has severe allergies or suspicion for severe allergies, testing must be done in a medical office equipped to react if there is an anaphylactic reaction. (Parents, don't try this at home.) If there is suspicion for food-related allergic reactions, discuss their symptoms promptly with their primary provider, who may want to refer to a certified allergist for appropriate testing. It is important to remember that food allergies are not generally diagnosed with a single test.

One of the other common misunderstandings with IgE blood tests and SPT is that people often believe it rules out any type of allergic or adverse reactions to foods. Parents or primary care providers can be lulled into thinking a particular food is safe when it may very well still be causing an adverse reaction in their child. For example, IgE blood tests and SPT do not test for other relatively common adverse food reactions like delayed food **hypersensitivity**, food protein-induced enterocolitis syndrome (FPIES), celiac disease, non-celiac gluten sensitivity, or lactose/fructose intolerance. We will dive into these other food reactions shortly.

It is common for an infant with milk or egg allergy to go on to develop other food allergies. These children are more likely to develop the "atopic triad" consisting of food allergies, eczema, and asthma. It is also well established that the baby with eczema is more likely to develop other allergies and asthma in what is known as the "atopic march." While a significant portion of the children with milk and egg allergy outgrow these IgE reactions by the time they are in kindergarten, other allergies to peanut, tree nuts, fish and shellfish may be lifelong.

Percentage of children who outgrow food allergies during childhood[1]

| | | |
|---|---|---|
| Milk – over 50%<br>by ages 5-10 years | Egg – 50%<br>by ages 2-9 years | Wheat – 50%<br>by age 7 |
| Soy – 45%<br>by age 6 | Peanut – 20%<br>by age 4 | Tree nut –10%<br>during childhood |

Fish, Shellfish, & Seeds – low percentage outgrow these allergies. More research is needed.

In short, food allergies need to be taken seriously and evaluated by a certified allergist. Food allergies are increasingly common; they are lasting longer and potentially have more serious ramifications. Early recognition is crucial to avoid severe reactions. At the end of the chapter, we will list a few thoughts about preventing allergies, starting in pregnancy and early infancy.

## Mixed and Non-IgE Mediated Food Reactions

There are many adverse reactions to foods that are not classic IgE-driven allergic responses but can still cause significant gastrointestinal distress and other symptoms. These **non-IgE mediated reactions** generally do not have available tests to identify them accurately and dietary elimination must be used to confirm the reaction. (Celiac disease is an exception, see Chapter 14.) As the symptoms of non-IgE food reactions often overlap with many other GI disorders including diarrhea, abdominal pain, vomiting, and reflux, there is often a significant delay in diagnosing these food-related disorders. These disorders can generally be categorized as:

+ mixed IgE/non-IgE mediated allergic conditions like eczema or Eosinophilic GI Disorders (EGIDs)
+ delayed food allergies (non-IgE mediated allergies) like FPIES
+ non-immune mediated food reactions like lactose or fructose intolerance

*Eczema (a.k.a. Atopic Dermatitis)*

Atopic dermatitis (eczema) is a common rash in infants and children believed to represent a mixed IgE/non-IgE mediated disorder. Like other allergic diseases, the incidence of eczema in the US and other industrialized countries has risen sharply in the past twenty years.[13] As described earlier, loss of immune tolerance contributes to both development of eczema and food allergies in the first thousand days of a child's life.

The relationship between allergies and eczema is well known. For example, data from the medical literature show that 35 to 40% of young children with eczema also have diagnosable food allergies, and that 80% of children with egg allergy have eczema.[7,11,12,14] Sensitized children have an eczema flare when exposed to certain trigger foods, and dietary elimination can improve some cases of eczema. Eczema may *contribute* to the development of food allergies or may *co-evolve* at the same time with food allergies. One of the known pathways linking the development of eczema and food allergies is the breakdown of the skin barrier, allowing allergic sensitization through the skin and subsequent immune system activation and inflammation. It is interesting to note that breakdown in both skin and intestinal barriers predispose to development of allergies. Maintaining skin and gut barrier integrity should then be a primary focus of allergy prevention and treatment.[1,2]

Still, not all eczema is directly related to a food allergy. New lines of thinking suggest that there could be two types of eczema: intrinsic (not caused by allergens or antigens) and extrinsic (caused by environmental triggers) or that perhaps eczema could exist on a spectrum with components of both.[15] While the exact role of food in eczema is still being evaluated and likely varies by individual, an expert panel of allergists recommends food allergy testing for children under five years with moderate to severe eczema.[16]

---

### HOT TOPIC

Food elimination in order to treat eczema is recommended by some allergy groups, but not others.[13] It has become a controversial topic, with some providers focusing only on healing the skin barrier without addressing the role of foods. As a gastroenterologist, I question this approach. In my opinion, to deny the potential involvement of foods in causing or exacerbating eczema may be doing a disservice to a significant number of children who could benefit from

dietary restriction. I would think that the ongoing ingestion of a food that is causing inflammation and further damaging the skin and intestinal barrier would be counterproductive. I feel
eliminating problematic foods makes sense for these children. The flip side is the concern by
some allergists that overly restricting foods could lead to delayed development of immune
tolerance and increased risk for anaphylactic reaction. It is a conundrum with no easy answer.

While eczema therapy may or may not involve food allergy testing and
avoidance in younger children, treatment is primarily focused on healing
the skin barrier. Frequent skin hydration and use of emollient creams
is a mainstay of therapy. It is advised to avoid soaps and cleansers with
harsh detergents as well avoiding moisturizers containing chemicals
like phthalates, preservatives, and perfumes.[13] Several new medications
targeting specific inflammatory pathways involved in eczema are now
starting to be used.[15]

But can we also support the skin barrier through diet? There may be a role
for nutrients like vitamin D, omega-3 fatty acids, as well as **probiotics** in
the prevention and treatment of eczema. Vitamin A and zinc are also vital
nutrients for maintaining skin and gut barrier integrity, so it is important
to ensure that the mom's diet while pregnant and breastfeeding, and the
child's diet after weaning are adequate (but not excessive) in these nutrients. Recall that while vitamin A deficiency is uncommon in the Western
world, **subclinical** zinc, vitamin D, and relative omega-3 fatty acid deficiencies are common. Could these deficiencies be playing a role? The diet
and environment of the child in the first thousand days significantly
impacts the risk for developing eczema and food allergies. We will discuss
potential ways to prevent allergies later in the chapter.

*Eosinophilic Gastrointestinal Disorders*
Aside from IgE-mediated food allergies, everyday foods may be the trigger
of Eosinophilic Gastrointestinal Disorders (EGIDs), which are interesting food-related immune reactions.[17-20] We will discuss Eosinophilic
Esophagitis (EoE) primarily, as it is the most common of these disorders.
EoE was relatively unheard of until the 1990s (go figure that one out) but
has become fairly common in the US and other Westernized countries,
likely due to immune system dysregulation from multiple environmental
influences.

While EoE is more common in kids and families with a history of food
allergies, asthma, eczema (atopic disease), it can also present with no

prior allergy history. EoE is thought to be a combination of IgE and non-IgE mediated immune reactions. This disorder is an example of a food reaction that could be missed if we rely on the allergy blood tests and skin tests to define an "allergy." In many cases, allergy testing is negative, even in kids with obvious instances of EoE. Eosinophils (sometimes abbreviated as "Eos") are part of the immune system that are typically enlisted to fight parasites and increase in response to an allergic exposure. In EoE, the Eos migrate and congregate in the esophagus (the tube that connects our mouth with our stomach). In significant numbers, Eos cause inflammation, pain, and impaired swallowing. Although less common, it is possible to see congregations of Eos in the stomach (eosinophilic gastritis), small intestine (eosinophilic duodenitis or enteritis), or colon (eosinophilic colitis). These are conditions that come with a unique set of symptoms but may have the same root cause. Together these disorders make up the EGIDs.

The top four foods that trigger EoE are dairy, wheat, soy, and eggs (essentially, the American diet). Nuts and fish can also be triggers and added to the top four foods become the "Big six." An elimination diet excluding some or all of these six foods is often the treatment for EoE.

EoE can present in the older infant or toddler with solid food refusal, choking, or gagging with more solid foods, recurrent vomiting, and severely picky eating (refusing meats and chewier foods), as well as holding food in the cheeks after chewing rather than swallowing them. In the older child or teen, EoE often presents with a chunk of food getting stuck halfway down the esophagus (food impaction) or frequent transient self-resolving food sticking episodes. A list of concerning symptoms for EoE are listed below.

In my practice, I have found EoE to be more common in children who had a history of feeding issues or excessive reflux as a baby and who needed **hypoallergenic** formula but were told they "grew out of it." It is also more common in families and children with a history of atopy–allergies, eczema, and asthma. Just like food allergies and eczema, there is a breakdown in the *esophageal* barrier that in part leads to the sensitization and loss of tolerance seen in EoE. EoE can present at any time in childhood and into adulthood as well.

A fairly common scenario for the pediatric gastroenterologist is to get called into the emergency room to endoscopically remove a piece of meat that has gotten stuck in the esophagus of a child or teenager who turns out to have EoE. These children often report that they had been having meat or other foods getting stuck for months or years but weren't telling anyone or thought it was normal.

I was fortunate to train in one of the top EoE research centers at Children's Hospital Colorado, with Dr. Glenn Furuta, a pediatric gastro-enterologist, and Dr. Dan Atkins, an allergy and immunology specialist. These dedicated researchers have developed a comprehensive multi-disciplinary clinic for EoE and EGIDs (Eosinophilic Gastrointestinal Disorders–don't worry, I have a hard time saying it too). Treating more complicated EoE and EGIDs often "takes a village," and having pediatric gastroenterologists, allergy and immunology specialists, pediatric dieti-cians, and speech/feeding therapists involved can help get these kids back on track more quickly; however, most well-trained pediatric gastroenter-ologists should be able to diagnose and treat cases of EoE.

Warning Signs of Possible EoE

+ Inability of a young child to wean onto solid foods—choosing mostly liquids and purees
+ Frequent choking and gagging with feedings or meals
+ Frequent vomiting, especially with feeding
+ Excessively picky eater—avoiding meat, bread, and other foods with dense texture
+ "Cheeking" or pocketing food in the cheeks, spitting out food rather than swallowing
+ Feeling of "food getting stuck" when swallowing
+ Washing foods down by drinking large amounts of liquids during meals
+ "Dipping" all foods in a sauce like ranch dressing or ketchup (to prevent sticking)
+ Persistent heartburn or chest discomfort that doesn't resolve with acid-blocking medication
+ Excessively slow eating—chewing foods to a liquid consistency, taking tiny bites; last one at the table

If your child has these symptoms, talk to a primary health provider who may want to refer them to a pediatric gastroenterologist or certified aller-gist well versed in diagnosing and treating EoE.

## Non-IgE mediated allergic reactions

Several food reactions (referred to as cell-mediated reactions) are not IgE-mediated but involve different parts of the immune system, including T-cells.[21-23] These reactions do not cause anaphylaxis and are much sneakier than immediate IgE reactions. They sometimes take hours to days to manifest, so they are easier to miss or misdiagnose. Note that *allergy testing by blood or skin is mostly negative in all these cases*, but the food-induced damage can still occur nonetheless. It is hard to estimate how many kids suffer from non-IgE allergic reactions because these reactions are less severe than an IgE-mediated anaphylaxis or not as obvious as hives. This situation is compounded by lack of accurate blood or skin testing for these reactions. As a result, these reactions are grossly underreported and often unrecognized. Delayed non-IgE allergic reactions to foods are more common than we think. Western medicine does not like when things do not fit into a nice, neat box, and food reactions are not always as well defined as we would prefer. Medicine is often not black and white. *It is incorrect to think that anaphylactic reactions or IgE confirmed food allergies are the only adverse food reactions that exist.* This false assumption is the reason why a great deal of non-IgE mediated reactions, including celiac disease, are missed for *years*. I would like this mindset to change so that more of these cases are caught early to prevent needless suffering among children. Let's look into a few of these non-classic food reactions. As with any adverse food reaction, infants and children with these symptoms should be followed closely by their PCP and a pediatric gastroenterologist or allergist. The following are the main types of pediatric non-IgE reactions to foods.

*Infant food protein-induced allergic proctocolitis (FPIAP)*
This is a common infant condition where food proteins in the baby's formula or, less frequently, present in mom's breast milk, cause inflammation in the large intestine leading to stools with blood and mucous that resolve upon elimination of that food from mom's diet or by switching to a hypoallergenic formula. Often the child otherwise appears healthy. At times, this reaction can be more severe with grossly bloody stools, which increases risk for iron deficiency.

Typical maternal foods causing this reaction are cow's milk protein from milk, cheese, or yogurt; or from soy, eggs, and occasionally wheat. Breastfeeding mothers may need to eliminate these foods from their diet for several months to allow the baby's immune system to calm down before reintroducing them. Formula-fed infants may need hypoallergenic formula without intact cow's milk or soy protein to stop the reaction. Blood in the stool generally stops within one to two weeks after removing the offending foods.

I sometimes recommend that breastfeeding mothers of one of my patients having this reaction take 500 to 1,000 mg of EPA/DHA fish oil (if they are not big fish eaters) and consider a high-quality, multi-species pro-biotic supplement or probiotic foods. All infants are recommended to take 400 IU of Vitamin D3 drops daily to support their immune system. While not a treatment or a cure, these items all help support immune tolerance in a child. Breastfeeding mothers should wait until 6 to 9 months of age before reintroducing these foods with close monitoring for return of any GI symptoms, and I recommend formula-feeding parents keep their infants on hypoallergenic formula until the time of weaning.

*Food protein enteropathy*
Food protein enteropathy is a non-IgE food reaction (typically to milk or soy) in infants and toddlers, which damages the small intestine causing chronic diarrhea and/or intermittent vomiting, but typically without blood in the stool. Symptoms resolve upon removal of the offending food or going to a hypoallergenic formula. These children often are not grow-ing well, so it is vital to recognize these symptoms, which closely mimic celiac disease—but often without any gluten in the diet and at an earlier age than celiac is diagnosed. Other triggers in older infants may include wheat and eggs. Children may outgrow this by about two years of age, but more research is needed in this area.

*Other non-IgE mediated food reactions*
These reactions include **celiac disease** and **gluten sensitivity** (see the chapter on celiac and gluten sensitivity for more detail). Many cases of **infant and child reflux, colic,** and **constipation** may result from delayed allergies and non-IgE mediated reactions that are under-recognized as food related. I always keep non-IgE mediated food reactions in mind when I see a super fussy or refluxing infant or child in my clinic with significant constipation. In my opinion, an elimination diet should be tried before resigning the child to years of acid-blocking medication or laxatives.

*Food Protein-Induced Enterocolitis Syndrome*
Food Protein-Induced Enterocolitis Syndrome (FPIES) is a frightening but not typically life-threatening reaction to foods that can occur in the infant

or toddler or occasionally older children.[24-27] FPIES presents after the triggering food is introduced into the diet, usually for the second or third time once the immune system has been "primed" to react. It can occur in an infant who has been switched to a milk or soy-based formula or an older infant just starting solid foods like rice or oats. The presentation is scary. It begins with repetitive projectile vomiting and is often followed hours later by diarrhea. The child turns pale and limp. They are often rushed to the ER by parents who think they are going into shock. Unlike the IgE mediated allergies, there are no skin reactions or breathing issues. About 15% of these children can develop real shock with dangerously low blood pressure.

Typically, they look awful, and this is terrifying for the parent and often the healthcare provider. However, when these children are examined and tested, there is no evidence of infection, no signs of trauma, and a few hours after rehydration, they snap out of it like nothing ever happened. Occasionally they have a little blood in their poop the next day and some transient diarrhea, but otherwise, they are fine until the next time they consume the trigger food; then the reaction repeats itself. While the exact immune reaction is still under investigation, FPIES is thought to involve reactions by T cells toward certain foods, referred to as a cell-mediated reaction, as well as mast cells, which produce histamine. It does not involve antibodies like an anaphylactic IgE-mediated reaction.

The FPIES reaction typically takes place two to four hours after the trigger food is eaten. Once the reaction starts, few medications are effective but ondansetron (Zofran) can slow or halt the worst of the reaction in some cases. An untreated FPIES reaction has to run its course and can result in dehydration and low blood pressure. For this reason, severe reactions should be managed in the emergency room with intravenous fluids, ondansetron, and close monitoring.

FPIES reactions are typically acute but a variant of *chronic FPIES* can develop in an infant repeatedly exposed to the trigger, which is usually a protein in formula. Chronic FPIES in an infant can result in inadequate weight gain, anemia, and low blood protein levels. These infants need to be followed closely by their PCP and a pediatric allergist or gastroenterologist. They typically need to be on a hypoallergenic formula. An infant doesn't usually have an FPIES reaction to breast milk proteins, but there are case reports of FPIES reactions to food proteins from mom's diet coming through the breast milk. An elimination diet by mom usually resolves this. Once the causative food is identified and removed from the diet, the child recovers within a few days, often dramatically, with weight gain, improved mood, and gains in developmental milestones. "Chronic FPIES" in an older child is often some other type of food reaction that has been mislabeled.

FPIES trigger foods are relatively common: dairy, soy, oats, rice, barley, sweet potato, squash, banana, avocado, chicken, and turkey are all on the list, but trigger foods may vary by geography. An estimated 65 to 80% of children with FPIES react to a single food, with milk, oats and rice being top of the list. Still, a significant minority of infants react to multiple foods, but rarely more than three.[26] Due to the estimated prevalence of FPIES, it should be one of the disorders suspected if children have severe reactions when introducing new foods. There is no test for FPIES; skin or blood tests are not accurate or diagnostic. The clinical diagnosis is based on a history of recurrent reactions with the symptoms described in the previous paragraph, occurring two to four hours after an exposure to the same food or foods. Generally underdiagnosed, delays may occur in diagnosis of FPIES unless the healthcare provider is already familiar with the condition.

I first learned about FPIES from Dr. Dan Atkins at Children's Hospital Colorado during residency while presenting the case of a toddler with projectile vomiting and lethargic episodes that I now know are classic FPIES. These cases are hard to forget! Because it is commonly unrecognized or misdiagnosed, it is challenging to say accurately how common this reaction is in children. Luckily, most, but not all kids outgrow the reaction once they are out of the toddler phase, but a medically supervised food challenge is the only way to tell if they have outgrown the reaction. It is advisable to wait 12 to 18 months after the last reaction to challenge the offending food again. For kids reacting to several foods, meeting with a qualified dietician may help make sure they are getting a nutritionally complete diet. For more information, check out one of the websites listed in the recommended reading section.

# ISSUES WITH COW'S MILK: ALLERGIES, INTOLERANCES, AND CONSTIPATION

When babies are weaned from breastmilk or formula, they are commonly given whole milk. This is such an established practice and is pushed so hard by the medical establishment and pediatricians, that most of the time it is never even questioned. But what does the evidence say? Do children really need to go on milk as soon as they are done with breast milk or formula? Is this safe for all kids?

While some children do just fine with milk and dairy products, others clearly do not. There is actually no biological need for cow's milk in the human diet, and a child raised without dairy *on a well-balanced diet with lots of vegetables and other sources of calories and calcium* will generally not be deficient in key nutrients. As we already established, cow's milk is not the same as mothers' milk.

Here are some interesting facts:

+ Cow's milk is the most common allergen in the human diet. There are classic IgE-mediated allergic reactions, delayed reactions, mixed IgE/non-IgE reactions like eczema and EoE, and non-immune mediated adverse reactions to cow's milk. Reactions can run the full spectrum of severity and presentation with skin and gastrointestinal symptoms. Adverse reactions to cow's milk in the diet are grossly underdiagnosed in children.

+ Adverse cow's milk protein reactions are estimated to affect up to 15% of infants; 2 to 7% of these classify as a classic (IgE mediated) milk allergy.[3-5,28] In the infant, adverse milk protein reactions can present as reflux or vomiting, colic, diarrhea, constipation, bloody stools, rash, poor growth, or feeding issues. Milk allergy or intolerance in the infant often requires hypoallergenic formula or maternal avoidance of dairy products if breastfeeding.

+ Evidence suggests that the likelihood that a child will outgrow an infant milk protein allergy is 30 to 50% at one year, 50 to 77% at two years, and up to 70 to 87% at three years.[3,7,29,30] That means that many children who were milk protein intolerant as babies (needing special formula) *will continue to have some degree of sensitivity until they are well into toddler years* and closer to school age. The more severe the reaction, the lower the chances that the child will outgrow it very quickly. This should give pause to those who automatically want to wean a child onto cow's milk when they have shown signs of intolerance in the past. Caution and awareness of ongoing reactions may be warranted.

+ Common toddler milk reactions include rash or eczema, vomiting or "reflux," diarrhea or mucus in the stool, or significant constipation. Even though the common mindset is that babies who need to be on a special formula for cow's milk intolerance will outgrow it by the age of one, in my practice, this is often not the case. I see kids all the time who get incredibly constipated, have significant reflux, or vomiting when dairy products are reintroduced into the diet.[3-5,31-37] I am curious about the number of milk sensitive infants that go on to develop EoE in later childhood.

+ Cow's milk is the most common food trigger of EoE, which often presents in the young child with recurrent vomiting or feeding issues.

+ Cow's milk is the most common trigger food in FPIES.

+ The AAP recommends that no child under the age of one year be offered cow's milk because of the risk of gastrointestinal bleeding. Does this risk somehow magically disappear the second the child turns one year old? Milk intake also directly interferes with iron absorption, so heavy milk drinkers and infants given cow's milk are at increased risk of iron and zinc deficiency, which can be associated with anemia and neurodevelopmental issues.[38,39]

+ Milk intake over 200 ml (6.5 oz) per day has long been associated with constipation. Multiple studies on children with persistent constipation showed improvement upon milk elimination. Several studies in the medical literature have shown constipation is more common than diarrhea as a symptom of milk protein intolerance and resolves with elimination of milk in the diet.[40-48]

To be clear, a child can wean from mothers' milk (or formula) onto many items, including just water (if they are a good eater). They do not invariably need milk added to their diet by default, and the necessity of milk for bone health has been called into question.[49-55] There is no question that dairy products are a good source of calcium and good fat for kids brains and can be a healthy part of some children's diets, but not for everyone. Can they get calcium and fat from other sources? Yes, and many people and cultures do just that. Non-dairy calcium sources include broccoli, green leafy vegetables, beans, tofu, almonds, and almond milk.

## Lactose intolerance vs. milk protein allergy

**Lactose intolerance** is not a milk *allergy* and does not involve the immune system. It is the inability to digest and absorb the milk *sugar* lactose, leading to gastrointestinal issues.[56-59] We previously discussed that true lactose intolerance is rare in infants and very young children, as most are born with the ability to digest lactose from mother's milk. However, between *70 to 80% of older children and adults worldwide are lactose intolerant.* Only northern European cultures generally hold on to the ability to digest lactose into adulthood. Based on studies, 30% or fewer adults of Hispanic, Native American, African, or Indian descent tend to tolerate lactose later in life. Those from southeast Asia only have a 10% chance or less of maintaining lactose tolerance. The age of onset and severity of lactose intolerance varies by individual and ethnic groups. Lactose intolerance can start after age five in Caucasians and at two years in children of African descent.

Secondary lactose intolerance, when the intestines are inflamed and the child temporarily loses the ability to digest lactose, is not uncommon in young children and can piggyback on other disorders like celiac disease or food protein enteropathy. However, when the gut is healed, the lactase enzyme and the ability to digest lactose usually (but not always) comes back.

Interestingly, there is evidence that probiotics may improve lactose intolerance in some people, so probiotic supplementation is being evaluated as a possible therapeutic measure.

A lactose-free diet does not equal a dairy-free diet.

There is a common misconception with parents and healthcare providers that a lactose-free diet is the same thing as a dairy-free diet. Almost always, when we are putting a child on a restricted diet for a food related immune-mediated condition the goal is to remove most of the cow's milk *protein* (the part that the immune system reacts to), which means eliminating milk, ice cream, yogurt, cheese, and foods with cheese and cream in them. *Substituting lactose-free milk does not eliminate the problematic milk protein* for these kids and does little to help them clinically unless they also suffer from secondary lactose intolerance. If the child's medical provider recommends a *dairy-free diet*, this might involve substitutes such as almond milk, rice milk, coconut milk, etc., that do not contain any *milk protein*.

Additionally, it is necessary to look at food labels for ingredients containing milk for those on a dairy free (but not lactose free) diet. Many milk-based food items will contain low to no lactose, but plenty of milk protein. Small quantities of milk baked into food are less likely to cause a reaction in some children with either a milk allergy or intolerance, but it is best to discuss this with a healthcare provider. Other names for milk ingredients in food products include **casein** or caseinate, milk protein isolate or hydrolysate, milk solids, dairy solids, **whey**, butter or cheese flavoring, cream, and curds.

Many kids tolerate dairy just fine, with no GI symptoms, and should be free to enjoy full-fat (not skim) dairy products without added sugar. Toddlers need fat in their diet, so there is no place for skim milk products. Replace the skim milk, chocolate milk, processed dairy foods, and sugar-laden "kid's yogurt" that are flooding children's diets with healthier versions like cheese made from whole milk, and full-fat unsweetened yogurt. Berries or fresh/frozen fruit can be added to make unsweetened yogurt more appetizing to kids. I don't believe schools should be serving chocolate milk or highly sweetened yogurts because of the unnecessary added sugar (more on this later).

However, based on the data just presented, many children don't tolerate milk or are having adverse reactions and are essentially being pressured to drink milk by their healthcare provider, school, or daycare under false assumptions.

> As the US becomes more culturally diverse and food allergy rates continue to rise, the ethics of pushing milk on a growing population of children who may have an adverse reaction is questionable.

It also doesn't make sense that mother nature would design a system wherein a food that is viewed as essential to health, in actuality, causes significant gastrointestinal symptoms in the majority of older children and adults who consume it. My take-home point on milk is this: milk does not do *every*-body good, so watch for signs of intolerance or allergy. If a child has persistent eczema, chronic constipation or diarrhea, frequent abdominal pain, reflux or vomiting, they could be showing signs of milk intolerance. A healthcare provider should be consulted to determine whether food allergy testing or a four to six-week trial of a dairy-free diet is warranted. If a toddler becomes seriously constipated after introducing milk, a cow's milk elimination trial can be implemented, removing almost all dairy products while keeping a record of their poops (the poop calendar). Then milk can be challenged back in the diet. If the constipation returns within 3 to 5 days of reintroducing dairy, then the source of the issue is evident.

Consider the possibility of lactose intolerance in school aged children with ongoing bloating and diarrhea after consuming milk or ice cream. Discuss allergy testing if the reactions are more severe. While allergy testing for more severe reactions is advisable with a certified allergist, allergy testing is *only* suitable for classic IgE-mediated allergies and can be misleading as a great many adverse reactions to milk and other foods are delayed intolerances (T-cell not IgE-mediated).

Some medical providers order IgG-based allergy blood tests, but these tests are not recognized as being very accurate. IgG is another antibody produced by the immune system that lasts longer in the body and is controversially thought to be related to delayed-type food reactions. My issue with this test is that it is expensive, almost always paid out of pocket, and it is relatively unvalidated by rigorous scientific methods. Almost everyone tests positive for dairy and wheat and gluten sensitivity, which are the items I would start with for someone doing an elimination diet for **food sensitivities and intolerances** anyway, thus saving them hundreds of dollars. That being said, I look forward to more studies on new modes of allergy testing and would welcome a more accurate testing method to evaluate food allergies and intolerances. I am just not convinced that the IgG test is it.

Bottom line: remember, it is your *choice* to wean a child onto milk and dairy products, but contrary to common convention, it is not a nutritional *necessity*. Be aware of possible reactions.

**A quick word on goat and sheep milk products.** There is a high risk of "cross-reaction" in children who have more severe IgE-mediated milk protein allergy and anaphylaxis when given goat milk or sheep milk products, so these products should be avoided in these kids. However, growing evidence indicates that for some children (and adults) with a cow's milk intolerance (non-IgE mediated), goat and sheep products may be better tolerated. This is due to different forms of casein, the main allergenic protein in milk products. Goat and sheep milk have a form of casein called alpha-2 beta casein, whereas cow's milk has both alpha-1 and alpha-2 beta casein. The alpha-1 form of casein is now suspected to cause the adverse reactions in significant numbers of sensitive people and may even mimic lactose intolerance. Blinded studies comparing the gastrointestinal effects of alpha-1 versus alpha-2 casein show improvements in GI issues in a significant number of people who are given the alpha-2 form found in goats, sheep and some specialized breeds of cows.[60-65] More studies are needed on the role of dairy products that do not contain the more allergenic alpha-1 casein in allergic disorders in children.

## Other non-immune related food reactions

In addition to lactose intolerance, several other adverse food reactions can occur in a child that do not involve the immune system per se and are rather issues with digestion and absorption. These reactions include toddler's diarrhea, fructose intolerance, and reactions to **FODMAPs.**

### Toddler's Diarrhea—a.k.a. "The Diaper from Hell"

Toddler's diarrhea is not necessarily an allergic issue, but a common parental concern when the young child (most likely still in diapers) starts to produce really interesting poops. In toddler's diarrhea, there may be three to ten loose stools per day without other concerning symptoms. Sometimes there can be undigested food in the stool that looks identical to the way it looked going in. This is typically not concerning if the child is growing and gaining weight, not having abdominal pain, and not having excessively high-volume loose stools. Toddler's diarrhea is a common cause of blowout stools during this phase and can represent a relative intolerance to fructose and other sugars, but it is not an allergy.

Often cutting out the juice and cutting back significantly on the sugar and fruit intake will minimize the number and severity of diaper blowouts. On other occasions, symptoms may result from the toddler's gastrointestinal motility getting turned up a few notches for unclear reasons, causing food to pass quickly through their system. Increasing fat in the diet of a child who has a very carbohydrate heavy diet may improve symptoms, as this will slow down the intestinal transit. Most of the time, this condition is no cause for concern and resolves on its own. However, if there is increased mucus or any blood in the stool, the child is not growing well, or the issue is not resolved by reducing or eliminating sugar, juice, and fruit, then the child should be evaluated by a medical provider for concerns, such as celiac disease, infection, IgE and non-IgE food allergies.

*Fructose Intolerance*

Fructose intolerance, like lactose intolerance discussed previously, is the inability or decreased ability to digest and absorb fruit sugar. This condition is a relatively common and underrecognized source of pediatric tummy issues. Fructose is found in fruit juice, table sugar (sucrose), and high fructose corn syrup, agave nectar, honey, and most sweetened foods and drinks. Our fructose intake has gone up exponentially in the past fifty years, mostly thanks to high-fructose corn syrup sweeteners. Fructose intolerance is not an allergic reaction; it is an absorption issue. Poor absorption of fructose can cause belly pain, gas, bloating, diarrhea, or nausea when that unabsorbed fructose pulls water into the digestive tract and starts to get metabolized by the gut bacteria. A large number of people with "irritable bowel" (up to 30% in one study) may have some degree of fructose intolerance.[66] In another recent study, kids presenting to a pediatric GI clinic for unexplained abdominal pain, bloating, or diarrhea, were given a breath test to identify fructose intolerance. Among those tested, 54% were positive, and when placed on a low fructose diet, 77% of these kids reported that their symptoms disappeared.[67] Given this information, a low fructose diet is certainly something to try if the child has otherwise unexplained GI issues like pain, bloating, gas, diarrhea, and nausea.

Food sources high in fructose:

+ apples
+ pears
+ mangoes
+ cherries

+ figs
+ pears
+ watermelon
+ dried fruit

+ honey
+ agave
+ high fructose corn syrup

Putting a child on a low fructose diet means cutting back or eliminating the fruit juice, these listed fruits, soda, sweetened drinks, dried fruit, candy, and sweets to see if symptoms improve. Since foods containing higher amounts of concentrated sugar are not suitable for children in general (see the section on sugar), there is no worry about this affecting them nutritionally. Even if juice is not tolerated, eating whole fruits may often be tolerated as there is ample fiber and much lower concentrations of fructose involved.

*FODMAPS and the low FODMAP diet*

In addition to fructose specifically, another group of foods that have been associated with gastrointestinal symptoms and "irritable bowel" is the **FODMAPs**. FODMAP stands for *fermentable oligo and disaccharides,* *monosaccharides, and polyols.*[68-71] When people with these intolerances eat foods high in FODMAPs, they may become gassy, bloated, or experience abdominal pain and diarrhea. This is because if certain food items aren't digested, the gut bacteria will ferment. When there is excessive fermentation, the bacteria make by-products from the food that cause GI distress, including severe stomach aches. Remove the trigger food or foods, and symptoms improve. FODMAP triggers include lactose, fructose, "alternate" sugars like sorbitol, and some carbohydrates found in vegetables like broccoli, cauliflower, and beans (the gassy vegetables). Wheat is high in FODMAPs and can trigger reactions irrespective of gluten sensitivity. Not everybody is sensitive, and some of the FODMAP foods are quite healthy (fruits and vegetables) and should not be removed long term. There may be a crossover between FODMAP sensitivity and gut **dysbiosis** or **small intestinal bacterial overgrowth (SIBO)** and for some individuals if their dysbiosis is corrected, their FODMAP intolerance improves. FODMAPs fall under the heading of non-immune mediated food intolerance, not an allergy, and there are no tests other than elimination and reintroduction to tell if someone is sensitive. For more information on FODMAPs and a more comprehensive list of FODMAP containing foods, refer to the recommended reading section at the end of the chapter. Note that it is important for a child to be tested for celiac disease prior to trying any elimination diets for gastrointestinal issues.

### Prevention of food allergies and introduction of foods

Past recommendations for introducing potentially allergenic foods have been confusing. Growing evidence indicates that if potentially allergic foods like eggs and peanuts are introduced during breastfeeding around six months of age, the food is less likely to cause a reaction because of the process of immune tolerance mentioned earlier. Previously, experts believed that if wheat gluten was introduced while the baby was breast-feeding, the chances of developing celiac disease would be reduced. Unfortunately, recent data is refuting that claim.

The most recent consensus statements from the AAP and associations of allergists are recommending the introduction of potentially allergenic foods from 4 to 6 months of age, and not waiting until after weaning at 12 months. However, it is a good idea to wait until at least 4 months of age to introduce solid foods (preferably starting between 5 and 6 months) and whole cow's milk at 12 months. Allergy prevention data is most robust for eggs and peanuts with earlier introduction lowering the chances of developing an allergy.[72-76]

Breastfeeding provides a vital role alongside these foods to prevent allergy, as the immune regulating effects of breastmilk helps prevent overactivity of the immune system leading to food allergies. The microbiome also plays a huge role. A child with healthy intestinal bacteria has a much better regulated immune system and lower intestinal permeability (less leaky gut), making the chances of developing a food allergy lower. If the child has eczema or a strong family history of food anaphylaxis, discuss food introduction with a qualified allergist before introducing peanut and egg, but otherwise I would recommend offering some scrambled eggs as an early food and a little peanut butter sometime after 6 months; however, watch for any adverse reactions and discuss them with a medical provider.

### What other ways can I try to prevent allergic food responses in my child?

A great deal of epigenetic programming in the first thousand days of the child's life likely leads to the development of allergies in children. As discussed earlier, two main epigenetic influences are nutrition and the microbiome. Several early mechanisms for preventing the development of food allergies and sensitivities involve these two factors. Abundant evidence exists that the microbiome of the infant influences risk for allergies and eczema.[77,78] One means of prevention then is for the mother to maintain a healthy maternal microbiome while pregnant and pass this on to her child during natural childbirth. Choices such as avoiding antibiotics when possible, eating a fiber-rich whole-food-based diet with lots of vegetables, and emphasizing nutrient-rich foods for immune regulation (discussed in the pregnancy chapter) may all help swing the pendulum for the newborn infant.[8,79]

Several recent meta-analyses showed some evidence that taking probiotics during later pregnancy and lactation may reduce the risk of eczema and food allergies in the child. Additionally, supplementation of fish oil during this time reduced the incidence of egg and peanut allergy in children.[80-82] The World Allergy Organization (WAO) recommends probiotics for pregnant and lactating women with a child at increased risk of allergies and probiotic supplementation of the at-risk child.[6,83] To be clear, I do not think all mothers need to be on probiotic supplements, but some studies are suggesting probiotics may be useful for at-risk children of allergic families, milk-allergic children, or those with eczema.[84–86] I would add to this list children born by C-section, or those who had early exposure to antibiotics. Again, studies suggest that a multi-species probiotic with strains of both *Lactobacillus* and *Bifidobacteria* may be more effective than single strain varieties.

Regardless of allergy risk, I believe that all pregnant mothers need to be good stewards of the microbiome of both mother and child to improve health outcomes. Rates of allergies are lower in children born vaginally and breastfed; while circumstances may make vaginal birth and breastfeeding impossible, being mindful of our children's microbiomes may help in any case. Minimizing a child's exposure to pesticides, antibiotics, unnecessary acid reducing medications, and harmful food additives may also help. It is worth noting that having a family dog when a child is born and family farming or gardening both positively impact microbiome health and reduce the risk of allergies in children. Refer to Chapters 2 and 3 on **epigenetics** and the microbiome for more information.

Omega-3 fish oil supplements may hold promise for those suffering from eczema.[87,88] A high intake of **omega-6** oils may contribute to an increased risk of allergy development and should be avoided.[89] Balance is the key. Adequate intake of the key immune nutrients during pregnancy, lactation, and early diet is essential. Sufficient intake of zinc, vitamin A/beta-carotene, vitamin D, omega-3 EPA/DHA, and iron as well as the **phytonutrients** and fiber from fruits and vegetables gives the immune system the nutrients needed to function correctly and control excessive inflammation and immune dysregulation that contribute to the development of allergies.

Lastly, we need to be mindful of the link between eczema and food allergies. As discussed earlier, a disrupted skin barrier is one route by which food allergies develop. Maintaining a healthy skin barrier in the baby may prevent development of food allergies by blocking skin sensitization. Avoid bathing infants with harsh soaps that could harm their skin barrier. Essential nutrients for skin health include the essential fatty acids (balanced omega-6 and omega-3), zinc, and vitamin A; adequate intake of these nutrients will help support a healthy skin barrier. Daily use of an emollient moisturizer on the baby's skin was hoped to be protective, but several recent large studies found no effect in preventing infant eczema in the general population or a high risk group.[90–92] Studies are ongoing to determine if other creams or topical moisturizers may prevent eczema.

# NUTRITION R$_X$

**1** Children may experience many different allergic and non-allergic reactions to foods. If they have frequent diarrhea, vomiting, reflux, feeding difficulties, poor weight gain, blood in their stool, hives, or eczema, they may be having a food reaction. They should be evaluated by their primary provider and potentially a pediatric gastroenterologist or allergist.

**2** A child may still be having a food reaction even when blood or skin tests for allergies are negative.

**3** Offer potentially allergenic foods (egg and peanut) starting at 6 months but consult the child's healthcare provider if they have a history of severe eczema or a strong family history of anaphylactic reactions to foods. They may want to refer the child to a pediatric allergist first.

**4** Always watch for adverse reactions when introducing new foods. These reactions include vomiting, rash, wheezing, mucus, or blood in the stool. Promptly bring these issues up with the appropriate healthcare provider.

**5** Remember that weaning to cow's milk is a choice, not a necessity. Milk is the most common food allergy and intolerance, and at least 70% of the people on the planet are lactose intolerant. Schools and daycare providers should be required to offer a non-soy milk alternative for children.

## RECOMMENDED READING

1.   For more information on eosinophilic esophagitis:
     https://www.childrenscolorado.org/doctors-and-departments/departments/diges-
     tive-health/programs/eosinophilic-gastrointestinal-diseases/
     www.GIkids.org
     www.apfed.org.

2.   Asthma and Allergy Foundation of America:
     https://www.kidswithfoodallergies.org/

3.   For more information on FPIES:
     https://www.fpies.org/
     https://fpiesfoundation.org/

4.   For more information on the low FODMAP diet:
     https://www.monashfodmap.com/.

# CHAPTER FOURTEEN

# CELIAC DISEASE AND GLUTEN SENSITIVITY

Could your child be among the millions of people getting sick from eating wheat? Based on the science, it is increasingly possible.

Thirty years ago, if someone said they were gluten-free, they mostly got blank stares. These days, almost everyone has heard the term, and it gets a variety of reactions, from eye-rolling ("one of THOSE people") to acknowledgment ("oh, me too!").

First off, what is **gluten**? Contrary to what Seth Rogan says in the 2013 movie *This is the End*, a "gluten" is not everything bad.

> *Seth Rogan: "If you stopped eating gluten, you'd feel way better."*
>
> *Jay Baruchel: "You don't even know what gluten is."*
>
> *Seth Rogan: "Sure, I do. Gluten is a vague term—it's used to categorize everything that is bad. Calories, that's a gluten, fat, that's a gluten."*
>
> —Seth Rogen and Evan Goldberg, *This is the End* (Colombia Pictures, 2013), Film

The term "gluten-free" has become a fashionable buzzword. A 2013 study found that 65% of American adults believed gluten-free foods were healthier and 27% chose gluten-free products to aid in weight loss.[1] Is this trend founded in science? There are many misconceptions about gluten issues.

In reality, gluten refers to a specific protein found in wheat, barley, and rye, but not in other grains like corn, rice, or quinoa. A cousin of gluten is found in oats (called avenin) but only causes trouble for a few susceptible celiac patients. Wheat and gluten are everywhere in the Western diet, so they are hard to avoid unless we pay attention and actually know which ingredients contain gluten and read ingredient labels. Bread, crackers, pasta, cookies, cakes, bagels, muffins, pretzels—anything made from wheat flour—is a high gluten food.

The gluten in wheat, barley, and rye is composed of two main proteins, glutenin and gliadin. Because these proteins have a remarkable elastic property, bread made with gluten has a chewy springy texture (gluten-free bread generally does not). These proteins are uniquely tough to digest because their shape makes it hard for digestive enzymes in our intestines to break them down. Why can this be bad? Our bodies like to have proteins broken down to the smallest possible units (amino acids) in our intestine before absorbing them. Larger chunks of incompletely digested protein are harder to absorb. Any bigger pieces that happen to slip past the intestinal barrier into the bloodstream can trigger immune reactions and are said to be more *antigenic and allergenic*.

The other interesting fact discovered by the pediatric gastroenterologist Dr. Alessio Fasano is that eating gluten appears to increase the production of a unique protein called **zonulin**.[2,3] Zonulin increases the permeability (leakiness) of the gut. In addition to gluten, it has also been discovered that **dysbiosis** (a state of bacterial/**microbiome** imbalance in the gut) can also increase this protein. So, if eating gluten appears to increase the gut's leakiness and the protein itself is hard to digest, it is more likely that higher amounts of gluten can activate the immune system, making it a potential troublemaker in a susceptible person.

### Reactions to Wheat

Wheat products and bread have become a seemingly irreplaceable part of our diet. Understandably, a lot of doubt, denial, and disinformation surround nutritional scenarios that remove this staple food. However, far from being rare, an estimated one in every fifteen to twenty people has an adverse reaction to wheat whether they know it (and admit it) or not. How can this be? There exists a spectrum of wheat and gluten-related disorders, including but not limited to celiac disease.

### Classic wheat allergy

First, there is a **wheat allergy,** which is a classic (**IgE-mediated**) food allergy. Wheat allergy can present with hives, wheezing, facial swelling, eczema, and **anaphylaxis**: the life-threatening allergic reaction that can be fatal. Wheat allergy is more common than most people believe, with 1 in 100 to 1 in 200 children being overtly allergic to wheat.[4] This allergy is defined by an elevated wheat IgE level in the blood, and usually confirmed with a positive skin prick test (scratch test). There is an interesting phenomenon known as wheat-dependent exercise-induced asthma (WDEIA), where patients only get symptomatic asthma when they eat wheat and exercise afterward. Wheat allergy is commonly outgrown as a child gets older.

### Eosinophilic esophagitis

Wheat also triggers some cases of **EoE** (eosinophilic esophagitis). EoE is a newer allergic disease that doesn't play by conventional rules. Instead, this allergy causes choking, chronic vomiting, or chronic GERD (reflux) symptoms. Dairy, wheat, soy, and eggs are the top four triggers of this immune-mediated disease of the esophagus, which often improves when the trigger foods are eliminated. EoE is both IgE and **non-IgE mediated,** which means that the eosinophils (the allergic cells causing inflammation and all the problems) take their marching orders from several different parts of the immune system. Therefore, it is possible to have a rip-roaring case of EoE and a completely negative allergy test. Wheat, but not necessarily gluten, may be one of the food triggers for this disease. Review Chapter 13 for more detail about allergies.

### Celiac disease

Celiac disease is an **autoimmune disease,** where the body's immune system attacks itself. This unique reaction depends on the presence of gluten in the diet. Take out the gluten, and the reaction stops. Celiac is far more common than people think, affecting more than 1% of the population and a total of three million Americans or more.[5] A common misconception is that it only affects children, but celiac disease is diagnosed in adults into their seventies and eighties with increasing frequency. As many as 80% of adult celiac patients have been undiagnosed or misdiagnosed (often with **irritable bowel syndrome**), sometimes for decades. Another misconception is that celiac only happens to people of Irish and Scottish ancestry. While it is undoubtedly more common in northern Europe and Caucasian people of northern European descent, it is also relatively common in the Middle East, Italy, Northern Africa, India, Central and South America, and other parts of the globe. It is less common in Asia or people of Asian descent.[5,6] Studies in China have demonstrated that the celiac genes are tenfold less common in the Chinese than Caucasians, but also that celiac in China is likely underdiagnosed.[7,8] A recent study confirmed that 10% of the people with celiac living in the United States were non-Caucasian.[9]

Certain groups are at higher risk of getting celiac disease and should be screened.

### TABLE 14.1 CONDITIONS ASSOCIATED WITH INCREASED RISK FOR CELIAC DISEASE IN CHILDREN AND ADULTS[10-14]

| Condition | Percent with celiac disease |
|---|---|
| Type 1 diabetes | 8%–16% |
| Down syndrome | 3%–15% |
| Turner syndrome | 4%–8% |
| Williams syndrome | 8%–10% |
| IgA deficiency | 2%–8% |
| Autoimmune thyroiditis | 4%–8% |
| First degree relatives with celiac | 5%–18% |
| Second degree relatives with celiac | 3% |
| Dermatitis herpetiformis | 80%–100% |
| General population | 1% |

Like all autoimmune diseases, the incidence of celiac disease is increasing faster than population growth. More people are getting celiac disease, likely because of environmental factors that damage our immune systems. However, not everyone is susceptible to celiac disease; having celiac disease requires carrying at least one of the two celiac genes, DQ2 and DQ8. These genes are quite common in the Caucasian population, with an estimated 30% to 40% of Caucasians carrying at least one of these genes. However, not everyone with these genes gets celiac disease. Something has to activate the gene and cause a breakdown of **immune tolerance,** like an infection that stimulates the immune system. Dysbiosis or an altered microbiome may also predispose a susceptible child to get celiac disease.[15]

There may be higher celiac disease rates in children born by C-section and lower rates in breastfed children. The mother and child's environment and diet in the **first thousand days** influence a child's risk for developing celiac and other autoimmune diseases.

The DQ2 and DQ8 genes code for the ability of immune cells to recognize and attack gluten fragments when they are present. With ongoing exposure to gluten in the diet, the immune system goes into "war" mode and keeps trying to "kill" the gluten every time it is consumed. In the average American diet, gluten is consumed three or more times a day. Unfortunately, this battle takes place in our intestines, at the site of the intestinal villi. The villi are small, finger-like projections from inside the small intestine that are the site of nutrient absorption into our bodies. The villi are the "collateral damage." Over time, they get damaged in the fray, leading to villous blunting, where they get stubby and inflamed, which reduces their ability to absorb nutrients, vitamins, and minerals. This reduced absorption can lead to anemia, vitamin and mineral deficiencies (including iron), weight loss, poor growth, and delayed puberty in children.

Celiac disease is not a classic IgE-mediated allergy. It will *not* show up on routine allergy testing. It is considered a T-cell mediated reaction, which is run by a different part of the immune system. It needs to have a separate (but accurate) screening test called a TTG (tissue transglutaminase), EMA (anti-endomysial antibody), or DGP (deamidated gliadin peptides). Testing for the celiac genes does not tell us if someone *has* celiac disease; it only tells us if someone *could get* celiac. If someone doesn't have the DQ2 or DQ8 genes, they can't develop celiac disease but may still have other reactions to wheat.

*Symptoms of Celiac*
Celiac disease has been called "The Great Imitator" or the "The Great Masquerader" because it features nonspecific symptoms that gets confused with other diseases. It can even be "silent" and asymptomatic despite lab abnormalities and positive biopsies. However, even in silent celiac disease, the intestinal damage is ongoing, and the long-term health risks continue as long as gluten remains in the diet.

The most common chronic complaints are diarrhea, abdominal pain, nausea, vomiting, or constipation. The younger the patient, the more commonly they will have these obvious gastrointestinal symptoms.

However, in some children, adults, and many individuals with type-1 diabetes, celiac disease does not present with GI symptoms and can be asymptomatic. Some may also present with unexplained anemia and fatigue, elevated liver tests, headaches, and other vague symptoms. Celiac rarely affects the colon, so blood isn't usually found in the stool with this condition. Children and adults will often get diagnosed with "irritable bowel" without first properly being screened for celiac or other GI diseases. This oversight is a mistake.

### TABLE 14.2 MANIFESTATIONS OF CELIAC DISEASE

| Classic Celiac Symptoms* | Non-intestinal Symptoms* | Neurologic/Psychiatric Symptoms |
|---|---|---|
| Poor growth | Dermatitis herpetiformis | Ataxia (increased dizziness) |
| Chronic diarrhea | Dental enamel defects | Epilepsy +/- cerebral calcifications |
| Abdominal distension | Anemia (unexplained) | Migraines |
| Recurrent vomiting | Aphthous stomatitis (mouth sores) | Depression |
| Chronic abdominal pain | Arthritis/arthralgias | Fatigue/malaise |
| Chronic constipation | Abnormal liver function tests | Anxiety |
| Fatty stools | Pubertal delay/short stature | Peripheral neuropathy (tingles) |
| | Osteoporosis/weakened bones | |

*Strong evidence for symptom association (non-neurologic symptoms)–consider screening tests for celiac disease

Older children and adults with celiac disease sometimes develop an itchy rash called dermatitis herpetiformis, which often shows up on the back, elbows, and knees and can be confused with eczema. A family member of mine with celiac lovingly refers to it as "the itchy butt rash" if he gets gluten in his diet. Dermatitis herpetiformis is classified as its own disease, but at least 75% of folks with this form of dermatitis also have the classic intestinal damage of celiac disease. The rash goes away on a gluten-free diet. This rash is rare in younger children.

Gluten can affect far more than just the gut (or an itchy butt). Some of the most interesting celiac and gluten sensitivity complaints are neurologic manifestations of headaches, brain fog, peripheral neuropathy ("tingles" in the hands and feet), and dizziness (ataxia) as well as psychiatric complaints of depression and anxiety.[16] There may be a link between schizophrenia and gluten. The term "bread madness" was used in a historical context to describe schizophrenia and other mental conditions, and some so-called "mental patients" have recovered spontaneously when they ceased consuming bread products and other gluten-containing foods. Indeed, not everyone with headaches or depression has celiac disease or gluten sensitivity, but most patients or their medical providers aren't aware of this connection and therefore it goes undetected.

Why does it matter? Aside from suffering from the ongoing gastrointestinal symptoms of celiac disease, long-term ramifications of undiagnosed or untreated celiac disease in a child can include *growth stunting, short stature, iron deficiency and anemia, delayed puberty, weakening of the bones, chronic fatigue, and increased risk of other autoimmune disorders.* Undiagnosed or untreated celiac disease in the adult increases the risk of gastrointestinal cancer.

Children need to be tested for celiac if they are not growing adequately, regardless of whether they have GI symptoms (see how to screen for celiac below). Celiac never happens in infants prior to the addition of gluten-containing cereals, so babies should not be tested unless they are closer to a year old, symptomatic, and have been eating gluten for several months.

### NCGS (non-celiac gluten sensitivity) /NCWS (non-celiac wheat sensitivity):

What is the real story with gluten intolerance and gluten sensitivity? Is this a real thing or all media driven hype? Although denied for years, NCGS is now well accepted in the medical literature as a valid medical condition. For our purposes we will use NCGS interchangeably for NCWS, although wheat sensitivity may be a more accurate term. Because specific diagnostic testing is lacking, accurately estimating the numbers of people who suffer from NCGS is challenging. Still, up to 5 to 7% of the population may be affected, which makes it 5 to 7 times more common than celiac disease.

NCGS is a different immune reaction than celiac disease or wheat allergy because it is not IgE or T-cell mediated. There is another part of the immune system called the *innate immune system* that is likely to be involved. *NCGS does not cause damage to the intestines like celiac* but can cause a lot of the same symptoms of diarrhea, bloating, constipation, and abdominal pain (the same as irritable bowel syndrome symptoms). Research indicates that a host of non-GI symptoms can also manifest in relation to gluten sensitivity, including chronic fatigue, headache, brain fog, and joint pains.[14,17-20]

## TABLE 14.3 SYMPTOMS ASSOCIATED WITH NCGS

| Gastrointestinal Symptoms | Non-Intestinal Symptoms |
|---|---|
| Bloating | Brain Fog |
| Diarrhea | Fatigue |
| Constipation | Anxiety |
| Abdominal pain | Headache |
| Heartburn/reflux | Joint Pain |
| Nausea | Muscle pain/fibromyalgia |

Unfortunately, there are no definitive diagnostic blood or skin tests for NCGS, but the current proposed diagnostic criteria for this disorder are as follows:[21]

+ Irritable bowel-like symptoms (diarrhea, bloating, constipation, abdominal discomfort)
+ Negative celiac blood tests (TTG IgA/EMA)
+ Negative intestinal biopsies (normal villi or very mild inflammation on endoscopy not consistent with celiac)
+ Negative wheat allergy IgE testing (either blood or skin prick)
+ Symptoms must resolve on a gluten-free diet (GFD) after four to six weeks and return on a dietary gluten challenge

Studies report one in ten people living in the US, Canada, and Europe have *irritable bowel syndrome* (IBS). That means 30 million people in the US are currently suffering from IBS, a staggering number. A few studies have published data showing that *up to 30% of people with IBS may suffer from gluten/wheat sensitivity.*[22] If this were true, upwards of 10 million people could therefore be enduring gastrointestinal symptoms caused by NCGS. Based on these numbers, if a person has IBS, a trial of a gluten-free diet may be warranted *after* celiac disease and other disorders have been effectively ruled out by a qualified health professional. The professional recommendation is that *any adult or child with irritable bowel symptoms needs to be screened for celiac disease before labeling them as having IBS.*

Typically, people with NCGS do not need to be as strict with gluten avoidance as those with celiac disease. With celiac, even tiny amounts of gluten such as crumbs can cause a potentially severe reaction. Individuals with NCGS can often "get away with" small exposures. Unfortunately, this leads many restaurants and restaurant workers to be very lax with the "gluten-free menu," which is often *not* actually gluten-free or suitable for the person with celiac disease. Restaurants need to be educated on proper food handling. Items cross-contaminated by being cooked in a fryer, toaster, or grill with gluten-containing items should not be falsely advertised as gluten-free.

Food allergies and celiac disease need to be taken seriously. Imagine telling a mother, "I'm sorry ma'am, these peanut-free cookies do actually contain some peanut, so we apologize in advance for your child's anaphylactic reaction." One would be hard-pressed to find humor in this situation if you were this parent. It is the same when restaurants say, "Please accept gluten-free fries that do actually contain some gluten for your child with celiac disease." The only difference is that gluten exposure is not immediately life-threatening.

*All that glitters is not gluten*

There are ongoing debates if gluten is even the culprit in many cases of "gluten sensitivity." Several other compounds in wheat are under scrutiny. A protein in wheat called *amylase trypsin inhibitor* protects the wheat from pests; this protein has been bred into new, heartier wheat strains and may irritate the intestines in susceptible people, leading to GI complaints.[23,24] Wheat is also high in FODMAPs (fermentable oligo and disaccharides monosaccharides and polyols). FODMAPS are compounds in foods that some find difficult to digest, causing IBS symptoms independent of gluten. Numerous studies show improvement in IBS symptoms in large numbers of patients placed on a low FODMAP diet, irrespective of gluten content.[25,26]

*How to screen for celiac disease*
The proper screening for celiac disease is a *tissue transglutaminase immunoglobulin A level (tTG IgA)*. This is sent along with a *total IgA level* to ensure the person is not deficient in the IgA protein, which would invalidate the test. Up to 5 % of the population has some degree of IgA deficiency and is more common in patients with celiac disease. For younger children with a high index of suspicion for celiac disease, or with patients who are at increased risk, I also test for DGP IgA and IgG (deamidated gliadin peptides). These celiac blood tests are reasonably accurate, in the range of 90% when performed correctly, which is about as good as screening tests get. The EMA (endomysial antibody) is also a good screening test, but generally more costly. It can be sent in conjunction with TTG, but I generally

send the TTG and DGP along with a total IgA level to screen for celiac disease in my patients.[27]

Any child with a positive celiac screening should be referred to a pediatric gastroenterologist for possible endoscopy assessment. This flexible camera allows the gastroenterologist to sample the intestinal villi to look for damage and rule out other GI diseases. Damaged and inflamed villi that have a characteristic pattern of disease confirms the diagnosis. With children, the endoscopy is performed under anesthesia; it is a ten-minute procedure that is both safe and well-tolerated. Both the blood tests and endoscopy need to be done *while eating gluten* to prevent a false negative result (thinking a child doesn't have celiac when, in fact, they do). *Before removing wheat and gluten from a child's diet, be sure to get the proper testing performed.* A correct diagnosis is essential for long-term monitoring and diet compliance from friends, family, and the schools.

*The treatment for celiac disease*
The only treatment for celiac disease is a strict lifelong adherence to a gluten free diet. Despite attempts with other therapies like gluten digesting enzymes, medications for a leaky gut, and immune-based treatments, none have been effective or appropriate for celiac patients.[15] Some of these remedies may help people with gluten sensitivity tolerate some gluten in their diet, but for now avoidance is the only true therapy for celiac disease. The role of **probiotics** in helping alleviate NCGS is being looked at, and some folks with gluten sensitivity say they tolerate sourdough breads without issue. Sourdough products are the result of a fermentation process by bacteria and yeast that may help break down gluten and other items in wheat that may cause sensitivity. I would caution against use of sourdough products for children with celiac disease, as the safety of this is unproven and the risk to their health and development is too great. *Prevention* of celiac disease has been investigated and is an area of interest likely involving epigenetics and the microbiome, as well as intestinal permeability.[15,28–31]

*Common gluten related questions:*
**Is it challenging to go gluten-free?** It can be, especially at first. Having resources and support are crucial. It gets much more comfortable with time. There are more gluten-free products available than ever before.

**Is going out to eat frustrating at times?** Absolutely. Especially when the restaurant staff does not take it seriously or offer any gluten-free options. Thankfully, with raised awareness, this is getting better.

**Would I ever go back to eating gluten?** Not on your life. However, this decision is based upon my personal experience and the impact on my health and not a mindless desire to join the gluten-free lifestyle movement.

**Does everyone need to be on a gluten-free diet?** Clearly, no. Many people tolerate wheat and gluten without any issues.

**Is a gluten-free diet healthier?** Not necessarily. Going gluten-free *can* be healthier if the right foods are chosen, but plenty of "gluten-free" foods are highly-processed garbage based on other forms of starches, such as rice, corn or potato. "Gluten-free" does not equal "healthy." Many people gain weight unintentionally on a gluten free diet.

**Should more people be on a gluten-free diet?** Looking at the numbers, I say yes. Combining celiac disease, wheat allergy, non-celiac gluten sensitivity and its role in IBS, and the FODMAP factor, an estimated of 5 to 10% of the population, totaling millions of people, could be experiencing adverse reactions to gluten or wheat-containing food. That being said, there are many people following a gluten-free diet that don't necessarily need to be, but that is their choice.

Celiac and NCGS are underdiagnosed, and many people are needlessly suffering the consequences. I find it ironic that many people openly criticize gluten-free folks, all the while suffering themselves from gut-wrenching pain or explosive diarrhea after every meal. How's that working out for you? Why cast judgement on a dietary change without properly investigating the rationales and benefits behind it? There is a pervasive mindset that there is no life without gluten. But for tens of millions of people, there is no life WITH gluten. I have lost track of how many families I have treated where I have had to remove wheat from a child's diet, prompting the whole house to go gluten-free with improvement in multiple other family members' gastrointestinal, neurologic, or behavioral symptoms. This is not "all in their heads," and I find this attitude counter-productive, closed-minded, and potentially dangerous.

**Are there other reasons to consider a gluten-free trial for my child?** As we will discuss in the section on diet and the brain, studies show a significant number of children with ADHD and other brain disorders such as autism improve when certain foods are removed from their diet. We are slowly waking up to the fact that some dietary staples like wheat and dairy may be causing or exacerbating a number of health issues, including brain disorders in certain people. This inconvenient truth inexplicably offends many healthcare providers and some members of the general public despite the fact that dietary connections with these issues are evidence based. Most would not question a diagnosis of a peanut allergy, so why the skepticism with gluten?

## RECOMMENDED READING

1. Gluten Intolerance Group: www.gluten.org

2. Celiac Disease Foundation: www.celiac.org

3. North American Society for Pediatric Gastroenterology, Hepatology and Nutrition: www.gikids.org

# NUTRITION R$_X$

**1** Adverse reactions to wheat are common in the Western diet.

**2** Anyone with unexplained GI symptoms, especially "irritable bowel," needs to be screened for celiac with a TTG IgA and total IgA. Younger children should also have DGP IgA and DGP IgG screening.

**3** If a child is not growing as expected or has unexplained delayed puberty, anemia, or an autoimmune disease like **type 1 diabetes** or thyroid disease, get them screened for celiac disease.

**4** If there is suspicion for a child reacting to wheat-containing products, *get them tested by a qualified healthcare provider for celiac disease and wheat allergy.* If those tests are negative, consider a four to six week gluten-free diet, with a gluten challenge at the end to see if the symptoms return (which may indicate a non-celiac gluten or FODMAPs sensitivity).

**5** Contrary to common concern, going on a gluten-free diet is safe with *zero* risks for nutrient deficiencies if the diet is balanced with vegetables, meat, fish, poultry, fruits, nuts, healthy fats, and alternate grains.

**6** If a gluten-free diet has been recommended, don't go it alone. Going gluten-free can be uncomfortable and challenging at first. Work with a celiac-trained dietician. Many websites, support groups, cookbooks, podcasts, and other resources are also available to help people on this journey.

# CHAPTER FIFTEEN

# CONSTIPATION
# —THE STRAIGHT POOP

Does your child sometimes go three to five days or more between bowel movements? Is passing a BM a traumatic event for you and them? If so, this chapter may offer some help.

Since this is such a common and frustrating problem that many parents face, I devote this chapter to some of the causes and remedies for constipation. Why include constipation in a book about nutrition? Because a child's constipation may have everything to do with their nutrition!

The scope of the problem? We are a constipated nation.[1,2]

| | |
|---|---|
| 1 in 20 visits to the pediatrician is for constipation | 1 in 4 visits to the pediatric gastroenterologist is for constipation |
| 30% of US children experience constipation each year | Kids with autism and developmental delays are 5 times more likely to be constipated |
| 30% of children with constipation have pooping issues as adults | |

Constipation has been defined by something referred to as the Rome criteria.[3,4] This was created by a group of top gastroenterologists who met up in Rome to discuss gastrointestinal disorders now known as Disorders of Gut-Brain Interaction (DGBI), with pooping issues being a major topic. During this conference they reviewed current research and developed some standardized criteria to help define and promote better recognition of these gastrointestinal issues.

Constipation in an otherwise healthy child is now defined by the Rome criteria as having two or more of the following symptoms for more than one month:[5]

+ Two or fewer bowel movements per week
+ One or more episodes of incontinence (stool leaking or accidents) per week
+ History of stool withholding behavior (e.g., the "I gotta poop" dance)
+ History of painful defecation (the child who cries when they poop)
+ Presence of large stools in the rectum or palpable on abdominal exam
+ Large diameter stools that clog the toilet (*how did THAT come out of my child*?!)

Defining constipation in an infant is a little more difficult, as stool output, especially in breastfed infants, is highly variable. Breastfed infants can go several days without pooping, and as long as they are not straining to stool, having explosive "blowout" stools frequently, having hard pebble poops, or having blood in their stool, they are usually OK. Formula-fed infants should be pooping daily to every other day, but the other rules apply to them as well. We discussed the constipating effect of standard palm oil used in many infant formulas in Chapter 9. The cow's milk protein used in many formulas can also constipate a sensitive infant. The addition of **prebiotics** and **human milk oligosaccharides (HMO)** to infant formula can help to prevent infant constipation. Any onset of constipation in the first year of life should be a red flag and prompt discussion with the primary care provider, who may refer the child to a pediatric gastroenterologist.

The most common times of onset for constipation to occur are

+ During weaning from formula or breast milk to cow's milk and a regular diet (40% of cases)
+ During potty training (the peak time that pooping issues start)
+ When starting school. (Who likes to do their business in a school bathroom? Fear of public restrooms can cause anyone to "hold it" for a few hours, or a few days...or longer. The longer a child holds it, the harder it is to pass the BM.)

Constipation is not "normal" or "natural." It is an indicator that the system is not working correctly and that something needs to be fixed—behaviorally or physiologically. No child ever suffered from a Miralax deficiency. Throwing laxatives at the problem without looking for underlying causes is not good medicine.

Ignoring constipation or pretending it will go away can lead to long-term difficulties. Short-term use of age-approved laxative products can be safe and beneficial but are not an optimal long-term solution. Although much constipation is described as "functional constipation," assumed to be behavioral and often disregarded by many medical practitioners, something isn't working correctly in the intestines in many people suffering from constipation. Recent research shows altered intestinal motility and colon dysfunction in close to 50% of constipated patients.[6-9] What could be possible underlying causes of a child's pooping issues? Let's start by ensuring they meet the five basic requirements to have a good poop before looking into other causes.

## THE FIVE THINGS WE NEED FOR A GOOD NUMBER TWO

Assuming that a child has an intact and functioning nervous system and anatomy, five essential factors ensure they have healthy daily poops. Let's take a look at the basics.

### 1. Fiber

Fiber is an indigestible carbohydrate that plays a vital role in our health.[10-13] Dietary fiber comes in two forms, soluble and insoluble. Soluble fiber comes mostly from fruits and vegetables; this kind of fiber dissolves in water and forms a gel (think of the psyllium fiber supplements like Metamucil). Insoluble fiber is found in whole grains and in the "roughage" part of vegetables. Both types are essential, but the soluble part is especially critical because it softens up the stool and is the primary prebiotic food for our good bacteria. *Soluble fiber feeds the microbiome!*

Without adequate fiber, good poops don't happen. Fiber can make the difference between a child passing rock-hard poop pebbles or boulders, or soft, easy-to-pass BMs that do not cause pain. As it stands, the modern diet is shockingly low in fiber, with serious health ramifications.

**The Institute of Medicine (IOM) currently recommends 19 to 25 grams of fiber daily for children.** The average estimated intake in US children falls short at only 11 to 14 grams of fiber daily, with many getting less than 10 grams daily. The vast majority of Americans are significantly deficient in fiber of both types, but especially soluble fiber from fruits and vegetables. Data from 2010 showed *only 5% of Americans* were meeting their fiber requirements. Fiber is listed as a "nutrient of concern" by the Dietary Guidelines Advisory Committee (DGAC).[10]

This lack of fiber impacts health. Highly processed foods, with all their fiber removed, starve kids' healthy bacteria, feed harmful bacteria, and cause many bathroom woes. The lack of fiber in our modern diet also causes some of the starving intestinal bacteria to break down the protective layer of the intestines, promoting **leaky gut** and inflammation.[14,15] Fiber adds bulk and softness to the stool and protects the healthy intestinal bacteria and the protective mucus lining of the intestines, which are all important for good poops. We need to do our best to select high fiber foods as a regular part of our children's diet.

*Do whatever possible to increase a child's fruit and vegetable intake.* Give them whole fruits for fiber, not fruit juice! Juice may temporarily help soften their stool but is far too high in sugar. Choose whole-grain products like rolled or steel-cut oats that still contain intact fiber, as well as 100% whole-grain bread, pasta, and crackers. Incorporate some peas, beans, or lentils for the fiber—they are now making these foods into high fiber pasta that kids enjoy. Almonds and almond butter are a good source as well.

Consider adding a fiber supplement for kids not eating much in the way of vegetables. I often recommend psyllium fiber because of its bulking effect on the stool and prebiotic effect, but other options are listed below. I don't find the fiber gummies containing inulin as effective, but they will add some prebiotic fiber for the **microbiome** and have been shown to be helpful for some individuals.[16] Inulin does not have the same bulking and softening effect as psyllium.[17] Many of the fiber gummies contain large amounts of added sugar, so be wary. Psyllium has been shown in research studies to be an effective fiber supplement for constipation and often superior to other forms of supplemental fiber.[18-20] Psyllium can be taken as a capsule or powder mixed with applesauce, oatmeal, or a smoothie to give a child a fiber boost. Metamucil now makes an orange flavored fiber drink sweetened with stevia with no artificial colors or flavors. Start low with one to two teaspoons per day and increase slowly to avoid bloating and cramping. Push water with the fiber to increase effectiveness. Ground flaxseed can also be effective for constipation and, like psyllium, can also be added to foods like oatmeal, smoothies and baked goods to boost fiber intake.[21,22]

*A note of caution: In a child who is extremely impacted with stool, the impaction must be resolved prior to increasing the fiber through diet or supplements to avoid worsening the impaction. Discuss this with the child's medical provider.

## TABLE 15.1 HIGH FIBER FOODS

| Food Source | Grams of Fiber |
| --- | --- |
| Oats (½ cup) | 4.1 |
| Quinoa (½ cup) | 2.6 |
| Brown rice (½ cup) | 1.6 |
| Frozen corn (½ cup) | 2.0 |
| Whole wheat spaghetti (½ cup) | 3.0 |
| Whole wheat bread (1 slice) | 2.0 |
| Quinoa pasta (½ cup) | 4.0 |
| Chickpea pasta (1 oz) | 4.0 |
| Red lentil pasta (1 oz) | 3.0 |
| Split pea/Lentils (½ cup) | 8.0 |
| Refried beans (½ cup) | 5.7 |
| Almond flour crackers (1 oz) | 2.0 |
| Wheat Thins whole grain crackers (1 oz) | 3.0 |
| Multigrain crackers (1 oz) | 2.0 |
| Almonds (1 oz) | 3.5 |
| Pear (1 small) | 4.6 |
| Raspberries (½ cup) | 4.0 |
| Apple (1 small) | 4.0 |
| Squash (½ cup) | 3.3 |

| Food Source | Grams of Fiber |
|---|---|
| Brussel sprouts (½ cup) | 3.2 |
| Spinach (½ cup) | 3.5 |
| Cauliflower (½ cup) | 2.5 |
| Broccoli (½ cup) | 2.0 |
| Carrots, cooked (½ cup) | 2.2 |
| Green peas (½ cup) | 3.6 |
| Avocado (half) | 4.6 |
| Psyllium husk (1 tbsp) | 3.5 |
| Flaxseed, ground (1 tbsp) | 1.9 |

## 2. Probiotic bacteria and a healthy microbiome

Unless you are an expert in poop-ology, you probably don't know that 30 to 50% of the weight of our poop is dead bacteria and that a healthy intestinal microbiome drives the stooling process. So if we don't have a good number of beneficial bacteria in our intestines, how could we possibly have a good poop?

**Probiotic** bacteria in a healthy microbiome help proper bowel movements in a number of ways:

+ They provide a large proportion of the weight of the stool.
+ They eat the soluble fiber and make short-chain fatty acids (SCFA), which are the fuel for our intestines.
+ They interact with the gut's nervous system and immune system to promote proper motility—the squeezing motion of our colon that pushes the poop out.
+ They utilize prebiotic fiber to help maintain the protective mucus layer on the inside of the intestines.

As discussed previously, our children's intestinal probiotic bacteria may be altered from too many antibiotics, inadequate fiber in the diet, things like C-section birth and formula feeding, pesticides, and food additives. While all the probiotics are essential for health, *Bifidobacteria* species are especially important for pooping (think *Bifido* for the BM). Before repeatedly offering laxatives or resigning children to a lifetime of Miralax, healthcare providers should consider recommending increased dietary fiber and a trial of multispecies probiotic with several strains of *Bifidobacteria* as well as *Lactobacillus*. (Probiotics with only *Lactobacillus* species have not been shown in studies to be very effective for constipation, whereas *Bifidobacteria* has shown its effectiveness for both constipation and intestinal motility.[23–31]) Make sure to feed those probiotic bacteria in the intestines with good dietary and/or supplemental soluble fiber to maximize effectiveness, as taking a probiotic supplement without having adequate fiber to promote their growth is not likely to be very effective. "Magic applesauce" made by adding psyllium or other fiber powder and probiotics mixed into standard applesauce can be a good combination to get a child's pooping back on track.

It is worth noting that certain unfriendly bacteria, specifically ones that produce methane (methanogens) can be associated with difficult-to-treat constipation. These bacteria can be increased in the intestines if the microbiome gets altered by any number of insults. In severe, treatment-resistant constipation, gastroenterologists should consider these methane producing bacteria might be a contributing factor.

### 3. Hydration

As a society, we don't drink enough water. Many of us walk around in a perpetual state of mild dehydration, which is not optimal for health. One of the ways this can show up is having hard poops, since 100 to 200 ml (4 to 6 oz) per day of water is excreted in our stools. Soda and milk are not acceptable substitutes for water, although the breast and formula-fed infant should be getting all the hydration they need from their milk and not need extra water. Especially in the summertime, encourage constipated kids to drink water, but make sure it is clean, filtered water (See Chapter 7).

Total fluid intake guidelines from the Institute of Medicine recommend that children ages one to three drink four cups (about a liter) of fluid daily. Increase this amount by one cup (8 oz) of water per year of age up to a maximum of 64 to 88oz per day for older teens. A four-year-old child should then be getting about 32 oz of water daily (but not 32 oz of juice, milk, and certainly not soda).

### 4. Activity

An inactive child is more likely to have an inactive colon. Sometimes this is an inevitable part of a medical condition like cerebral palsy or other neuromuscular disorders. But mostly, inactivity is a product of our modern electronic video game society. If the child is a couch potato or a gamer who doesn't get much exercise, their colon can get slow and lazy. Gamers are also some of the worst stool withholders I have come across in my practice as they get too distracted by the video game to listen to the body's signals that it is time to poop. Some would rather poop their pants than interrupt their game (I wish I were kidding). Physical exercise stimulates proper motility of the colon and is a natural part of overall health.[32,33] Increasing exercise and decreasing video games in a sedentary child will often improve their stooling habits.

### 5. Good bathroom habits.

There is a reason that two common ages of onset of constipation are potty training and starting school: It is called "World Class Poop Withholding" or "The Battle of Wills." A defiant child or one who is constipated during potty training will learn quickly that pooping isn't fun, it hurts, and they just don't want to do it. And as many distressed parents have found out, if they don't want to, you can't MAKE them do it. The two things a toddler can control to some degree are their poops and what they eat.

Signs of stool withholding can include:

+ Standing "tippy-toe" (the poop withholders ballet)
+ Holding on to furniture and getting red in the face
+ Whole body stiffening and leg stiffening
+ Hiding when it is time to use the bathroom
+ Frequent "tummy aches" when it is time to use the bathroom
+ Stool leakage in the undergarments

Taking extra care to make sure toddlers have soft, easy to pass, non-painful stools during potty training will make parent life a lot easier. Also, making potty training a more laid-back, low-pressure situation to minimize anxiety can benefit everyone. Make sure they have a potty seat that fits their little bottoms so they don't feel like they will fall into the toilet. The small floor potties are great starters because they are down on the child's level, have a correctly sized seat, and it puts them in a better pooping position. Humans were designed to squat when pooping (does the phrase "taking a squat" ring any bells?), so having a high-off-the-ground toilet with their little legs dangling in the air is not an optimal pooping position. Older kids can use a "Squatty Potty" or other footstool to help them assume a better potty-posture.

When the body signals that it has to poop, it is essential not to delay or hold the poop excessively. The longer a child holds the poop, the more water their body reabsorbs, making the poop get harder and larger. A world class withholder will often go days between passing stools, then pass the ungodly mother of all poops that clogs the toilet and causes them (and the parent) significant distress. *"How did THAT come out of YOU?"* Gamers and children with ADHD often are notorious stool withholders and need a disciplined poop routine to keep them on track. Scheduled toilet sitting for five minutes after meals can sometimes be a game-changer as this is when the body's poop machinery activates in a process called the "gastro-colic reflex." Kids eat, then poop, like other mammals. Using a "poop calendar" and putting stickers on the calendar for days with a good poop in the potty and rewarding recurring potty successes can be a positive incentive to help reduce withholding.

## Other Factors Involved in Constipation

*Emotional trauma*
Emotional trauma and a history of abuse can certainly lead to significant stooling issues warranting professional help from a pediatric mental health specialist. Toilet phobias are among the most common childhood phobias and need to be worked through with a qualified child psychologist.

*Autism*
For an autistic child, pooping is often overstimulating and can lead to significant withholding. A low fiber diet combined with low muscle tone and sensory issues frequently affects children with autism, resulting in a large proportion of these kids becoming constipated.

*Food allergies and intolerances*
As mentioned previously, food allergies and intolerances can result in significant constipation, with dairy and **gluten** being top on the potential list of suspects. Celiac disease can cause constipation that is difficult to treat and should be on the radar if a child has significant stool difficulties that aren't responding to standard interventions. Multiple studies in the medical literature also link intolerance to cow's milk protein and constipation.[34–37] The child who had to be on special formula as an infant or wasn't tolerating mom's breast milk while eating dairy products may not have outgrown that milk protein sensitivity after all—the same sensitivity just changed presentation and is now sabotaging their poop routine.

Unfortunately, the blood and skin tests for milk allergy are often negative because the milk protein intolerance is not an **IgE-mediated** process. *Elimination of dairy products for a four-week trial is the only way to tell if the child is sensitive.* In addition, it has been demonstrated in previous research studies that intake of milk above 200 ml per day (6 oz) in many younger children is associated with constipation.[38] If a child is a heavy milk drinker, cutting back on dairy intake could reduce pain associated with passing hard stools.

*Magnesium*

Magnesium is an important mineral that is often deficient in the diet. Insufficient dietary magnesium can affect the body in several ways, one of which may be chronic constipation. However, correcting a dietary deficiency either by incorporating more magnesium-rich foods like leafy green vegetables, nuts and seeds, or supplementing with magnesium may help stool output.[39,40] Despite not being as well researched, specific forms of magnesium are often used as a treatment for constipation, such as magnesium hydroxide (milk of magnesia) or short-term use of high dose magnesium citrate often used for a "bowel clean out." Recently, a beneficial effect of magnesium rich mineral water on stool output was shown in several studies.[41] A recent study showed that an infant formula with extra magnesium was safe and effective for treating infant constipation.[42] For a chronically constipated child, make sure they are getting adequate magnesium, preferably through diet, but also consider a lower dose supplement to correct a dietary deficiency. (See common nutritional deficiencies in Chapter 12.)

*Neuromuscular issues*

For a child with spina bifida or cerebral palsy, spinal cord injury, certain genetic disorders or altered colorectal anatomy there are often other considerations that must be made in order to maintain proper stool output. These are special cases that are typically followed by a pediatric gastroenterologist.

Increasingly it is being recognized that milder issues with the functioning of the nerves and muscles of the pelvis can lead to constipation and stooling difficulties in both children and adults. There are diagnostic tests used by trained gastroenterology physicians to try and pinpoint the problem areas, but physical therapists specializing in **pelvic floor therapy** can be essential in treating these cases where there is "**pelvic floor dysfunction**" and "pelvic dyssynergia." In my practice we work closely with a number of physical therapists who specialize in this area to treat children with significant constipation.[43] Pelvic physical therapy should be considered for a child suffering from long-term constipation.

# NUTRITION R$_X$

**1** Any infant with constipation and significant difficulty passing stool, having tummy distention and recurrent blowouts, needs to be evaluated by their PCP and possibly a pediatric gastroenterologist.

**2** It is OK to ask the healthcare provider questions if they seem over-reliant on prescribing high dose or chronic laxatives without looking for the underlying causes of the child's constipation.

**3** If a child follows the "Five Things We Need for a Good Number Two" and the constipation is not improving, talk to the PCP and consider asking for a referral to a pediatric gastroenterologist who can decide if screening for celiac disease or another underlying disorder, such as milk protein intolerance, may be warranted.

**4** Consider a four-week trial of a very low or no dairy diet, which is usually enough time to tell if they respond with improved stool frequency. This means avoiding all dairy, including milk (even lactose free), cheese, ice cream, yogurt, and foods with high milk content to see if milk protein is causing constipation.

**5** Don't forget that pediatric gastroenterologists are the poop experts (a badge we wear with honor), so a doctor within this specialty should evaluate any persistent or severe constipation.

# CHAPTER SIXTEEN

# PEDIATRIC FEEDING DISORDERS, FEEDING TACTICS, AND STRATEGIES

## CREATING A GOOD EATER OR REHABILITATING A BAD ONE

Is your child super picky, eating only the same five foods over and over again? Are they well into their toddler stage but still mostly drinking formula or milk? Are mealtimes a daily struggle that completely stress you out? These could all be signs that your child has a pediatric feeding disorder.

A critical developmental window for adding solid foods into the child's diet occurs during later infancy and toddlerhood that spans from roughly age 6 to 18 months. During this time, the brain and nervous system work to coordinate the act of chewing and swallowing. The child's brain learns to integrate all the sensory input involved with eating, including hunger cues, smells, tastes, and textures.

The emotional context of eating is also crucial during this time. Are mealtimes fun and enjoyable, or are they rushed, stressful, and anxiety-provoking? The act of eating incorporates all five senses simultaneously, and some neurodevelopmental specialists feel that eating is more neurologically complicated than walking! If something disrupts this process during the critical window, and the child does not or cannot develop the skills to tolerate solid foods well before their second birthday, that child can become exceedingly difficult to feed.

Serious food aversions, sensory issues, and maladapted feeding behaviors can develop during this early toddler period. For these and other concerns, it is crucial to *get help early* if there are feeding issues with an infant or toddler! Prevention is always easier than treatment, and early treatment is better than undoing years of disordered feeding. This chapter will discuss common feeding issues in children and when to seek help from the child's medical provider, a pediatric gastroenterologist or a specialist trained in pediatric feeding, such as a **speech-language pathologist (SLP)** or occupational therapist (OT), hereafter referred to for our purposes as a "Feeding Therapist".

## PEDIATRIC FEEDING DISORDERS (PFD)

Pediatric feeding disorders (PFDs) are becoming both more prevalent and well defined.[1-3] *Feeding disorders* are very different from *eating disorders*. Eating disorders result from psychiatric body image issues in older children that lead to conditions like anorexia and bulimia. Feeding disorders are a different beast. PFDs tend to develop in young children and are defined as a difficulty or inability to eat age-appropriate food, which is associated with physical or psychological dysfunction.

| Problem Area | Cause |
|---|---|
| Inadequate eating skills | Chewing, swallowing difficulties |
| Psychosocial issues | Food avoidance |
| | Negative social interactions during mealtimes |
| | Refusing to eat, throwing food, emotional outbursts during meals |
| Medical issues | Genetic syndromes |
| | Gastrointestinal problems |
| | Heart, lung, or other conditions that make eating difficult |
| Nutritional Problems and deficiencies | Insufficient calorie, vitamin, or mineral intake from dietary restrictions or severely picky eating |

PFDs are incredibly common. At least 15% of all children have some type of feeding issue and about 5% qualify as having a more serious PFD. This means feeding issues are more common than asthma, yet until recently have received very little attention. These disorders are even more common in medically complicated kids. Up to half of the children with chronic medical conditions like heart or lung diseases, and up to 80% of children with autism and developmental delays may have feeding disorders.

Historically there has been a significant lag in diagnosis and treatment of these disorders, with most children going two to four years before a PFD is officially recognized. This long delay makes these problems very difficult to reverse. However, good progress has been made in the identification of feeding disorders. A broader assessment of these children is helping sculpt earlier diagnoses and more effective treatments. *Early recognition is vital.* Based on recent research, clinics are using multidisciplinary teams to achieve promising improvements in the feeding abilities of these children. These teams include **speech-language pathologists (SLP)**, occupational therapists (OT), registered dieticians (RD), physicians (including pediatric gastroenterologists), and behavioral child psychologists.

If a child is unwilling or not able to eat a regular age-appropriate diet or if mealtimes are overly time-consuming and stressful, share these concerns with the child's PCP. Consider taking a simple feeding survey on the Feeding Matters website (https://www.feedingmatters.org/what-is-pfd/is-it-pfd/ ).

Feeding Matters is an organization "uniting the concerns of families with the field's leading advocates, experts, and allied healthcare professionals to improve the system of care for pediatric feeding disorder through advocacy, education, support, and research." This organization aims to improve awareness and early recognition of feeding problems. Feeding Matters and the Pediatric Feeding Disorders Alliance have also developed a basic questionnaire called the ICFQ (Infant Child Feeding Questionnaire) to identify children with potential feeding disorders earlier. Below, find the questionnaire, with language slightly adapted for this book.[8]

The following are key questions that a parent can ask to identify feeding problems:

| Question | Score |
| --- | --- |
| Does the baby/child indicate when they are hungry? | If no, score 1 |
| Do you think your baby/child eats enough? | If no, score 1 |
| Do you feel that it takes too long to feed your infant or child? | If yes, score 1 |
| Does your baby/child require anything special to help them eat? | If yes, score 1 |
| Does your baby/child make it clear when they are full? | If no, score 1 |
| Based on these questions, are there concerns about feeding your baby/child | If yes, score 1 |

Any score of 2 or greater warrants a discussion with the child's primary provider and likely an evaluation from a trained pediatric feeding therapist.

Other specific red flag behaviors during meals that need to be promptly evaluated by the PCP and may warrant referral to a specialist:

+ Coughing, gagging, or choking on food
+ Persistently vomiting while eating or after eating
+ Refusing to swallow solid foods
+ Breathing loudly while eating, or face turns blue or gray
+ Persistently falling asleep while eating
+ Persistently screaming or crying when fed
+ Persistently arching or turning away from food or the breast

> *"If you are worried about your child's feeding, listen to your gut!*
>
> *It's ok to ask for help and to advocate for your child.*
>
> *You know your child best."*
>
> – Jaclyn Pederson, CEO of Feeding Matters

*Having a child with a pediatric feeding disorder does NOT mean you are failing as a parent*. On the contrary, recognizing your child has an issue and advocating for the child is precisely what a good parent should do. Get the right help to build skills that allow you to work with your child and improve nutrition by reducing the stress associated with feeding.

What are the more common feeding issues we see in young children? Here we will discuss a few of the notorious players: *The Picker, the Puker, the Grazer, and the Drinker*. To me, these sound like a Steve Miller Band song from the 1970s (which I guess means I am getting old).

### "The Picker:" Picky eaters and food refusers

A common complaint I hear from parents in my clinic is *"My child is super picky,"* and *"They don't like anything I offer."* Probably the most common feeding disorder, picky eating can run the full spectrum, from the child with a mild resistance to new foods and textures to one who only eats the same five to ten unhealthy foods day after day. The picker may be labeled as having "sensory integration disorder" or be on the autism spectrum, but many kids who are developmentally normal are picky eaters as well.

*The picky eater and growth*

Picky eaters may or may not be growing adequately along the growth curve. Children who do not track on this curve are often given the label "failure to thrive." These children tend to receive more attention than their normal weight counterparts, but either picky eater can be at risk for nutritional deficiencies and poor health. It is essential to know if the child is truly failing to thrive because this diagnosis can be overcalled if the child is small but proportional and is holding to their growth curve.

## TWO GROWTH CURVES

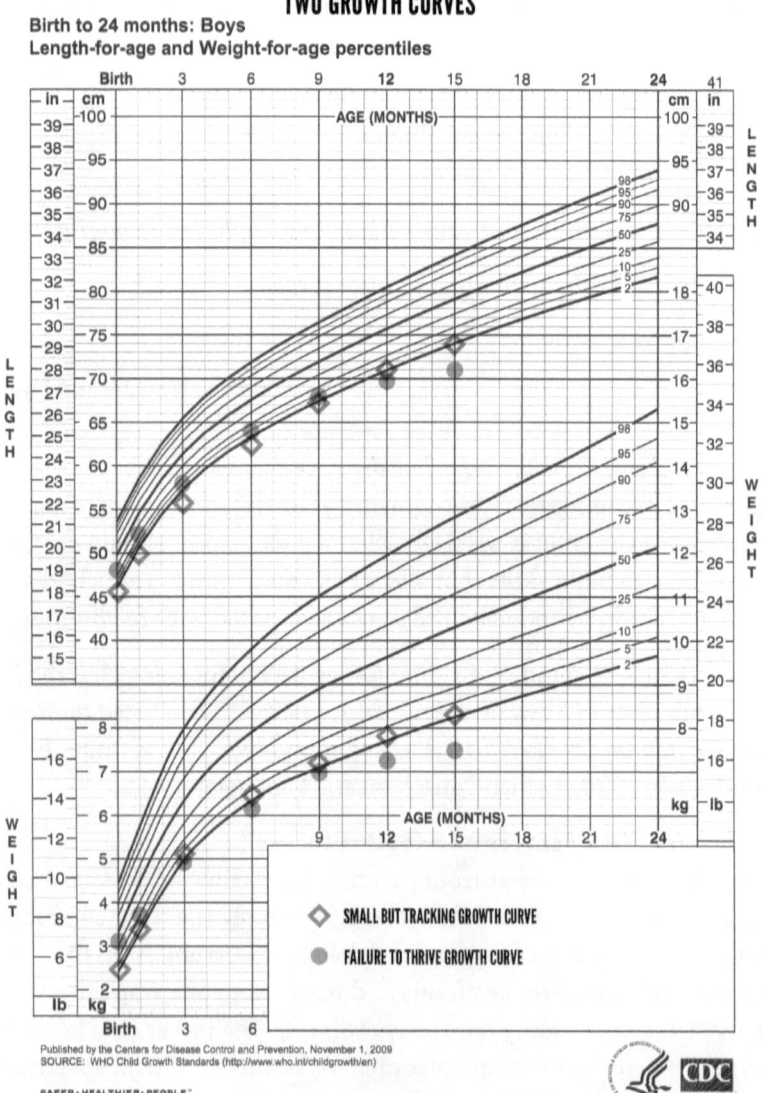

Birth to 24 months: Boys
Length-for-age and Weight-for-age percentiles

◇ SMALL BUT TRACKING GROWTH CURVE

● FAILURE TO THRIVE GROWTH CURVE

Published by the Centers for Disease Control and Prevention, November 1, 2009
SOURCE: WHO Child Growth Standards (http://www.who.int/childgrowth/en)

SAFER · HEALTHIER · PEOPLE™

CDC

Children diagnosed with failure to thrive are often started on some type of calorie supplement, the most common of which is PediaSure, but there are several calorie boosters for toddlers and children on the market.

There is commonly a sense of failure among parents when their child is not gaining weight, and a sense of panic sets in when the growth curve falters. Unfortunately, this can create a vicious cycle, as the young child picks up on parental stress and anxiety at mealtimes, which can worsen their feeding behaviors.

However, do not ignore, blow off, or disregard the picky eater! This child can be at risk for multiple nutritional deficiencies and poor growth and needs to be assessed by a medical provider with nutritional knowledge. Knowledge is power, and the more a parent knows about the causes of a certain behavior, and tools to deal with it, the less stress these behaviors will cause.

*What is Avoidant Restrictive Food Intake Disorder (ARFID)?*
**Avoidant Restrictive Food Intake Disorder (AFRID)** is a severe version of picky eating.[4,5] The American Psychiatric Association now officially defines ARFID as "An eating or feeding disturbance as manifested by persistent failure to meet appropriate nutritional and/or calorie needs associated with one (or more) of the following:"

+ Lack of interest in eating or food
+ Avoidance of certain foods based on the sensory characteristics (too slimy, too chunky, too green, etc.)
+ Concern about the adverse consequences of eating ("It will make me puke," or "It will make my tummy hurt.")
+ Weight loss or failure to achieve expected weight gain (falling off the growth curve)
+ Nutritional deficiency of essential vitamins, minerals, fiber, etc.
+ Dependence on enteral (tube) feeding or oral nutritional supplements like PediaSure
+ Unhealthy and difficult psychosocial interaction and functioning around mealtimes with behavioral issues and outbursts.

*ARFID is NOT*
+ Explained by lack of available food (food scarcity) or by an associated culturally sanctioned practice
+ Occurring with anorexia or bulimia nervosa or associated with a disturbance in the way in which one's body weight or shape is experienced
+ Attributable to a concurrent medical condition or mental disorder, or if it is, the severity of the eating disturbance exceeds that routinely associated with the condition or disorder

Many kids with ARFID and other PFDs out in the community are currently undiagnosed. If a child starts falling off the growth curve, they are more likely to be picked up during screening at a primary care visit. But picky children who are maintaining their growth curve or even growing excessively on the curve are often missed, yet still at risk for nutritional deficiencies. We need to pay attention to these kids, too. These nutritional shortcomings may potentially hurt brain development, school performance, and weaken the immune system's ability to fight off infections. Most of the time, the picky eater is only eating hyperpalatable or highly processed foods that are programming their body for obesity and early **type 2 diabetes** and promoting harmful bacteria in their gut. Understandably, parents of picky eaters are often so relieved when their child finally eats *anything,* they stop caring what it is. A common misconception with both parents and healthcare providers is that as long as children are on the growth curve, then everything is fine. I do not subscribe to this mindset.

ARFID is a difficult situation for sure, but we know that high-calorie malnutrition is the root cause of the leading killers in the Western world: heart disease, diabetes, and certain cancers. Lack of key nutrients, especially in the **first thousand days**, can have serious negative consequences on brain development. What we feed our children MATTERS! It needs to be taken seriously. The exceptionally picky eater needs evaluation and intervention with a pediatric dietician and feeding therapist *early in the game* before patterns are set. Early action is required so that the child will not continue on a path to poor school performance, a weakened immune system, and development of type 2 diabetes, heart disease, or other chronic debilitating conditions. It is much easier to correct unhealthy eating patterns when children are young, but picky eaters of all ages can be helped. Get help sooner rather than later!

*Autism and PFD*

The autistic picky eater is often a class unto themselves.[2,6,7] An estimated 60% of children with autism eat fewer than 20 foods: most of them are starchy snack foods, processed foods, sweets, with very few vegetables and minimal color (a.k.a. the "white foods" diet). Knowing this, we can advance our protocols for treating children with autism and *automatically* enroll them in feeding programs where the parents are trained to improve their children's diets by understanding their sensory issues and fear of new foods.

If the child is an exceptionally picky eater, first seek evaluation by the child's pediatrician, and then potentially by a licensed pediatric trained **speech-language pathologist** or occupational therapist who specializes in feeding. Consider a visit with a pediatric gastroenterologist if there is suspicion of an underlying GI disease such as EoE. Don't wait! The earlier the child is assessed, the better. Even for kids with ARFID, there are effective techniques and trained experts willing and able to help. See the list of additional resources at the end of the chapter.

## "The Puker:" Frequent vomiters and gaggers

The "Puker" frequently chokes or gags on foods or seems like they are *always* throwing up. The mountain of laundry seems endless, and the car may smell like something died in it. This behavior is not normal and is cause for concern. The Puker can progress to develop ARFID if this issue is not addressed. Pay attention if these problems occur weekly or more frequently. A few instances of gagging when the child takes too big of a bite or when they are trying a new texture for the first time is not a cause for concern. However, if this is continually happening, it *must* be evaluated by their pediatrician or primary provider, and potentially a pediatric gastroenterologist.

New abrupt onset of choking or gagging with food could represent a foreign body stuck in the esophagus (kids put many things in their mouths that they shouldn't). This is a fairly common occurrence in a toddler, and they need *immediate* medical evaluation and an X-ray. Objects or food stuck in the esophagus require prompt removal. A swallowed button battery (those thin coin-shaped batteries in remotes or garage door openers) *can be fatal* if not removed immediately.

Other causes of frequent choking, gagging, or vomiting can be:

+ Swallowing disorders
+ Certain types of food allergies (eosinophilic esophagitis, referred to as EoE)
+ Infection of the stomach with *H. pylori* bacteria
+ Celiac disease
+ Large tonsils that are partially blocking the back of their throat
+ Significant tongue-tie
+ Chiari malformation (where the bottom of the skull is squeezing the back of the brain)

These issues warrant medical evaluation.

Some kids may just have a sensitive gag reflex or sensory issues that lead to frequent vomiting. Still, it is wise to let the healthcare provider determine there is nothing more serious contributing to ongoing symptoms. Prompt evaluation is important. Most of the feeding specialists I know work closely with a pediatric gastroenterologist. They may perform a swallow evaluation under X-ray (a video swallow-esophagram) and the gastroenterologist may consider endoscopy (viewing the interior of the esophagus and stomach with a camera) to evaluate these children more fully.

### "The Drinker:" The child who drinks most of their calories

This is the child with a heavy reliance on milk or PediaSure for the bulk of their calories. They may not eat much during mealtimes but willfully drink multiple servings of PediaSure or large bottles of milk every day instead of eating. This can occur because the child has mechanical swallowing issues and needs feeding therapy to train them on how to eat solids. Frequently kids with developmental delays will fall into this category. Some kids unknowingly have eosinophilic esophagitis (EoE) or other esophagus issues where it hurts to swallow solid foods, so they default to drinking their calories.

Some kids are otherwise developmentally normal and do not have an underlying disease but were not introduced to foods at the proper time or in the appropriate manner. The child and the parent have fallen back on a default mode of filling up bottles with milk or cracking open containers of PediaSure as the quick fix. Granted, some children need to be on supplemental formula under medical supervision to gain weight. However, the goal for most toddlers should be to eat a regular diet unless there is a valid reason why they can't.

Except for children with a neurological disorder, developmental delay, or other significant underlying conditions, *relying on a toddler formula or milk for the bulk of their calories is not a great long-term approach*. Milk is not nutritionally complete and overreliance in a child will result in iron and zinc deficiency as well as serious constipation. Toddler formulas are more nutritionally complete but lack adequate fiber and **phytonutrients** for the **microbiome**, and typically don't contain **omega-3** fats like EPA and DHA which are important for the growing brain. The longer a child is on a liquid diet without learning to eat real food, the more difficult it becomes to establish normal eating patterns.

### "The Grazer:" Snackers and nibblers

This is the child who refuses to eat at mealtimes and prefers to snack all day. This maladapted eating pattern seems to be common in kids with ADHD but can occur whenever there is a lack of discipline around set mealtimes. We see many kids with failure to thrive who fall into the grazer category, as they are not getting enough calories this way to support proper weight gain. Especially early in the feeding game, when the child is "learning the ropes," it is essential to set boundaries, especially around meals. Three set meals and two set snacks at predictable times are a good starting point. At these times, it's essential to have everyone sit down together when possible, without distractions, blaring TV, smartphones, or tablets. Everyone should be focused on the meal, and interactions with parents should be positive. Grazers can be reformed with some work and help from dieticians and feeding therapists.

### "The Withholder:" Poop refusers

While not a Feeding Disorder per se, it is well recognized that extremely constipated children, especially those that are stool-withholding can have a high incidence of feeding disorders. If their belly is full of poop and there is no room for the meal, how can they be expected to want to eat? A large intestine full of poop sends signals to the stomach to slow down and not be hungry. I call this the "No Vacancy" rule... if there is no room at the inn (the colon), one cannot accept new guests (food that will make more poop). These kids often improve after the colon is cleaned out (with medical supervision) and we get them pooping daily. Significant constipation should be addressed by the child's PCP or a pediatric gastroenterologist (the poop doctors).

# GETTING HELP FOR PICKY AND POOR EATERS

If there are feeding concerns regarding the child after taking the quiz at the beginning of the chapter, then don't wait—seek help. Bring these issues up with the child's primary care provider and ask for an evaluation by a licensed speech-language pathologist (SLP) or occupational therapist (OT) who has pediatric feeding disorder experience. For the child with major feeding issues, multidisciplinary feeding disorder clinics can get to the root of the child's problem and develop a personalized plan to help them get back on track with expertise from SLP, OT, dieticians, pediatricians, pediatric gastroenterologists, and child psychologists. Unfortunately, these clinics fill up quickly and may have an extensive waiting list. Call the nearest children's hospital to see if they have an established multidisciplinary feeding program.

### Preventing Problem Eaters: Behavioral Modification

What are the best ways to *prevent* Feeding Disorders in children and create healthier eaters for life?

*Set an example*

Ghandi said "Be the change you wish to see in the world." This can apply to a great many situations in life, including parenting and promoting healthier eating—"Be the change you wish to see in your child." The mindset of "do as I say, not as I do" does not help any toddler or child. If children see that the parents aren't eating vegetables, they will not eat their vegetables either. If the parents are eating junk foods, they will also eat junk foods. Children's health and lives depend upon the example their parents set. Explore different ways of preparing vegetables listed in Chapter 11. *Everyone's diet in the home needs to be cleaned up if having healthier children is the goal.* The child mimics the behavior of the parent or caregiver—this is genetically encoded in us as a survival mechanism in our brains with something called "mirror neurons." These **neurons** were first discovered in primates; hence the old adage "monkey see, monkey do."

*Be a salesperson*

Parents have to be effective salespeople and talk up how yummy healthy food is. A sincere effort must be made to demonstrate how good it tastes and how good it makes us feel (even if you aren't so sure at first). With our own kids, we often talked about how good the vegetables were for our belly bugs (probiotic bacteria) and how those belly bugs and all the vitamins were going to keep us healthy and strong. Children can grasp this concept, and the children's book *Buddies in My Belly* by Sarah Morgan and Henry Bell can be a hit and get them on the right track.

If parents or family members are grumbling and complaining about eating vegetables and creating a negative experience surrounding the mealtime, this can have a long-term negative impact on the child's health. The environment created around food and mealtimes is *crucial*! Children are far more likely to develop unhealthy eating behaviors if parents are stressed and distracted during mealtimes or sucked into their smartphone and not paying attention to their child. It is vital to set the example of family-centered meals free of distractions. A positive mealtime environment is critical for creating a healthy eater for life.

### Do not use dessert as a reward
Using dessert as a reward sets a bad precedent. "Here Jimmy…. suffer through this ordeal of having to eat your vegetables, and I'll give you a hit of this sweet treat that is the real payoff." The goal is to have the child enjoy the healthy meal itself, without the need for some external reward. I don't believe in desserts except for special occasions. Having a treat once in a while is OK. When trying to save our kids from a life of obesity, type 2 diabetes, and chronic disease, does it make sense to make sugar at the end of every meal a ritual? The dangers of excessive sugar consumption and epigenetic programming are real. Sugar buzzkill, I know, but this is the reality of the situation. Watch the "Sugar is Killing Us" video for a concise, powerful, and entertaining explanation: https://hypoglycemia.org/sugar-is-killing-us/.

### Mom and dad are not short-order cooks
Making special meals for younger children is a trap that many parents fall into. It's time to dig out of that trap. Everyone should eat the same healthy meal at the same time to foster family bonding and healthy eating patterns.

### Set mealtimes and snack times—no grazing!
Have set times for breakfast, lunch, and dinner, with a set snack mid-morning and mid-afternoon for younger children. Eliminate free access and grazing. This practice will help children regulate their appetite and eat better at mealtimes when it is appropriate, and the food is healthier and more nutritionally complete. Set a minimum of two hours between meals and snacks to allow for digestion and hunger cues to set in. If a child is melting down before dinner, it is OK to offer some sliced veggies with

or without a healthy dipping sauce to bridge the gap, but do not give them the processed starchy snack foods that will fill them up with empty calories and kill their appetite for good food. They may whine a little at first but remember that *parents* (not children) control the food in the house.

### No distractions

Talk to any qualified feeding specialist, and they will say the same thing. Get rid of the TV, cellphones, tablets, games, or any other electronic devices during mealtime. Except in rare circumstances in kids with major sensory disorders, these distractions during mealtime contribute to poor eating, as the attention is not on the food or the family. Expect some grumbling and eye-rolling (especially from tweens and teens), but it is essential to make this a hard and fast rule. Kids with significant behavioral issues may need to be weaned off-screen time at meals but going cold turkey will work for most others.

### Make meals a ritual

Studies show that when a family eats together at set times, there is a positive influence on the child's emotional health and behavior. There is a reduction in teenage eating disorders, as well as other disordered feeding behaviors. It is a time to connect and check-in as a family, even when the rest of the day is crazy. Create positive rituals in the home around mealtime, even if starting with just a few dinners a week. Start with a prayer or blessing or a few words of gratitude. It is time to find out what is going on in our kids' lives. Decades later, children will remember this as a special time.

### Making foods fun, engaging, and exciting

Another part of creating a healthy eater is to make healthy food fun, engaging, and exciting for the child. These are new experiences for them! They are interested in what mommy or daddy is doing in the kitchen. Kids also love to garden, and a family garden, even a tiny herb garden, can be a great learning experience for them. Having the child involved with growing some aspect of their food is immensely valuable.

The more the child is involved in all steps of food preparation, the more they are likely to develop a healthy relationship with food. Take them shopping, so they can help pick out the fruits and vegetables. Let them watch the preparation of the meals and share the process with them. Try cutting fruits and vegetables into fun shapes; there are special cutters for doing this that are very affordable. Appeal to their senses—sight, smell, touch, and taste. Let them nibble on some of the vegetables while preparing the meal if they are at a stage to tolerate raw veggies.

Make fun games out of eating healthy food—let them pretend they are a brontosaurus, and the broccoli is a tree. Eating the rainbow of colorful fruits and vegetables appeals to children's senses. It ensures that they are getting a wide variety of the healthy compounds from fruits and vegetables called phytonutrients. Make some healthier "dipping sauces" that can increase the appeal of vegetables. Don't rely on the chemical-laden ranch dressing from the store; make them from scratch or purchase a cleaner, less processed dressing. Consider hummus, guacamole, almond butter, or natural peanut butter as well.

### Making change and overcoming resistance

If the family is accustomed to poor dietary habits, making changes can be challenging. It is essential to get everyone on board with the *Why, How,* and *What* of healthy eating. Include grandparents, babysitters, and the daycare or school. *Why* are we doing this? *How* do we start eating less junk, and *what's* in it for me? People are motivated by different factors and concerns.

In her book *The Four Tendencies*, Gretchen Rubin lines out four distinct personality types and what each finds motivating. The four personality types are the upholder, the obliger, the questioner, and the rebel. Take the online quiz or get the book to see which personality your family members have.

+ **Upholders/Obligers:** Need defined expectations and accountability. Laying out clear rules for what is acceptable in their diet may be all that is needed to make behavioral changes.

+ **Questioners:** If they are a questioner (like me), they *always* need to know WHY. Explain a bad diet's effect on their belly bugs, brain, and body. Explaining that the new healthier eating plan will make them feel, act, and perform better may motivate these kids or their family members.

+ **Rebels:** Need freedom to choose. The more rebels are pushed, the more they will push back. They will have to accept the change to a healthier diet on their own accord; or by default, if parents are willing to purge the house of unhealthy processed food and provide only good choices.

Try to frame changes in a positive light. Remember that we are making these changes to help the child perform at their best and be healthier for the rest of their life.

*Avoid grandparent sabotage*
Many grandparents love to spoil their grandchildren and indulge them in sweets, treats, and other foods that may not be on the healthy eating plan. It's one thing if this is a holiday or birthday, but another if it is happening daily or multiple times weekly. It is essential to lay ground rules that candy, ice cream, or soda must be reserved for *truly special occasions*. There are plenty of other ways to show children love that don't promote obesity, cavities, and diabetes.

*Other quick tips*
+ Be Persistent. A new food may need to be offered 10 to 20 times before some children will accept it.
+ Offer one new food at a time and consider "pairing" new items with familiar favorites. For example, prepare and offer a new vegetable cut into an attractive shape alongside their personal "faves."
+ Offer the new (healthier) food first, when children are hungriest, and they are more likely to accept it.

### RECOMMENDED READING

1. Nimali Fernando and Melanie Potock, *Raising a Healthy, Happy Eater: A Stage-by-Stage Guide to Setting our Child on the Path to Adventurous Eating (Expermiment LLC, 2015)* This book is a step-by-step guide on how to feed the child at developmental stages.

2. *Feeding Guidelines for Infants and Young Toddlers—A Responsive Parenting Approach*, published by the Healthy Eating Research panel of experts. https://healthyeatingresearch.org/

3. Feeding Matters (Feeding Matters resources are included in this chapter for families and healthcare professionals as a resource to support PFD identification and treatment, but does not imply official endorsement of "Feeding Our Children."). www.feedingmatters.org

# NUTRITION R<sub>X</sub>

**1**  If there are concerns about a child's feeding behaviors, take the ICFQ quiz in this chapter. If they score high, talk to the child's primary healthcare provider and ask about a referral to a pediatric speech-language pathologist or occupational therapist trained in feeding disorders.

**2**  Children's feeding disorders can be corrected with the appropriate therapy and training for the parents.

**3**  Creating a healthy eater takes work and leadership by example. Have set mealtimes and ban electronics at the table. Repeatedly offer healthy foods and explain why they are essential. These practices will help turn children into healthy eaters for life.

**4**  Get help and support; making changes can be challenging. Refer to the resources above. Qualified feeding therapists, and other medical/behavioral professionals can help make positive changes.

# CHAPTER SEVENTEEN

# METABOLIC HEALTH AND THE DANGERS OF SUGAR

Metabolically, our country is a disaster. Epidemic conditions like heart disease, **type 2 diabetes,** and obesity are all symptoms of a dysfunctional and imbalanced **metabolism. Prediabetes**, type 2 diabetes, and obesity are affecting increasing numbers of children. The rate of increase in diabetes and obesity demonstrates that our current diet and lifestyle is out of balance with how we were meant to live, leading to metabolic dysfunction and disease.

This imbalance is created when the body is not able to burn the correct fuels in the correct amounts. Unfortunately, most Americans and escalating numbers of people worldwide are in this state. Over time, this imbalance manifests in a host of damaging pathways affecting almost every organ in the body, especially the heart, liver, blood vessels, and brain. This compromised **metabolism** also contributes to the number of overweight and obese individuals by causing the body to make and store too much fat instead of burning it. This fat can be visible on our bellies and thighs, but the internal or *visceral* fat stored deep inside is the most dangerous. People with metabolic imbalance may have trouble regulating glucose levels in the blood, which are tightly regulated under healthy conditions.

Metabolic imbalance requires the body to produce more **insulin** than it should to keep blood sugar levels in the normal range, leading to the onset and progression of *insulin resistance, metabolic syndrome*, *prediabetes*, *and type 2 diabetes*. These medical problems, traditionally appearing in middle-aged adults, are now being found in children with increasing frequency. Over the past thirty years, the explosion of these diseases shows us that these are not "genetic disorders" in the conventional sense. Instead, they represent a mismatch between our genes, the environment we live in, and the processed food diet too many of us are eating.

The good news is that we are rapidly advancing our knowledge about the preventable factors leading us down the road to chronic metabolic "diseases of Western civilization" that now plague the entire world. We know how to detect the markers for these diseases earlier and make changes before irreversible damage is done. We can make changes *right now* that decrease the chances a child will suffer from these disorders. Let's go over the nuts and bolts of how we got into this mess, and how we can protect our children and ourselves from the epidemic of diabetes and metabolic syndrome. We need to take a good look at the underlying causes of these disorders of the modern diet, and why they are now occurring in children.

Let's start by reviewing sugar metabolism and defining some important terms.

### Blood sugar regulation

The pancreas is an organ right under our stomach that monitors and regulates the amount of glucose in our blood as well as producing digestive enzymes to break down our food. Dietary carbohydrates (starches, grains, potatoes, vegetables, and most sugars except for fructose) stimulate insulin release from the pancreas in a normal biological process. The pancreas senses when blood sugar (glucose) rises and produces the hormone insulin. Insulin's job is to get the glucose into the cells, where it is either burned for energy or stored for future use. Typically, in a healthy diet with vegetables, whole grains, quality proteins, and fats, the rise in post-meal blood glucose is steady and controlled. Only a moderate amount of insulin needs to be produced to get the glucose where it needs to go in the body. The cells in a healthy body listen closely to the instructions that insulin tells them and brings glucose into the cell to be metabolized, so that the pancreas can speak in a whisper, not a shout. Blood glucose fluctuates in a predictable, controlled manner.

In contrast, compared to a whole-food-based diet, the highly processed starches, sugars, and lack of fiber in the modern diet (referred to as high **glycemic index** or **glycemic load**) tend to spike blood sugars after a meal.

Subsequently, insulin levels rise much higher after eating this type of diet, as the body works hard to get things back under control. This aggressive insulin response does more than just try to control blood glucose. Insulin as a side job also promotes fat synthesis by the liver (called **de novo lipogenesis**) and fat storage in fat cells. When excessive, insulin shuts down fat burning, increases fat storage, stimulates inflammation in the body, and drives our blood lipids (triglycerides and "bad" cholesterol) in an unhealthy direction.

### Insulin Resistance (IR)

Insulin resistance is a state in which the muscles and liver aren't listening very well to the signal (insulin) being sent by the pancreas.[1-5] Our modern diet and sedentary lifestyle over time make it harder for the cells in the muscle and liver to listen to the insulin signal, increasing the demand on the pancreas to produce more insulin to get the job done. The pancreas now has to shout to be heard. After years of bad dietary and lifestyle choices, the pancreas has to work really hard to keep glucose under control, and chronically high levels of insulin are needed to try to keep things in balance. In this cycle of dysfunction, the pancreas struggles to get the cells to listen by pumping out lots of insulin to keep blood sugar in the normal range of 70 to 100 mg/dl (3.9-5.4 mmol/L). The pancreas does this because the cells in the human body are damaged by high blood glucose levels, and the body will do what it can to try to restore balance. This situation is referred to as *insulin resistance* and *hyperinsulinemia*: the on-ramp for the diabetes highway.

Insulin resistance is associated with obesity but may occur in non-obese individuals as well. Chronically elevated insulin levels in the blood (hyperinsulinemia) in someone with insulin resistance is damaging to the body even when blood glucose is normal. This excessive insulin contributes to the development of metabolic syndrome, high blood pressure, heart disease, fatty liver disease, PCOS, and development of type 2 diabetes. Although the pancreas does what it can to restore balance to the system, ongoing poor dietary and lifestyle choices eventually cause blood sugar levels to rise over time. When the body can no longer keep fasting blood glucose below 100 mg/dl, it becomes known as prediabetes, and eventually, type 2 diabetes develops unless something changes to halt this progression. A crucial point to keep in mind is that *insulin resistance and hyperinsulinemia damage the body well before developing type 2 diabetes*. Insulin resistance is rampant in today's children but is reversible with diet and lifestyle changes. It can be detected with tests such as the Oral Glucose Tolerance Test (OGTT) or HOMA-IR discussed in the next chapter that utilizes fasting insulin and glucose levels to determine insulin sensitivity.

Eventually, the pancreas gets tired of shouting and cannot keep up with demand. Blood sugars start to rise from a safe fasting level of 70 to 100 mg/dl into the 120s, 130s, and beyond, accelerating damage to the heart, eyes, kidneys, blood vessels, and brain.

As with many medical conditions, early detection is so important. We need to catch people when insulin resistance symptoms first present because it is easier to reverse metabolic dysfunction early versus waiting for full-blown type 2 diabetes. Eventually, when the pancreas gives up, the fight is over. The type 2 diabetes patient may become dependent on external insulin injected under the skin, similar to a person with **type 1 diabetes.** (Type 1 diabetes is an entirely different disease than type 2 diabetes and develops when the body's immune system attacks and destroys the insulin-producing cells of the pancreas, most often in childhood. Type 1 diabetes is also on the rise, but for a different set of reasons.)

Waiting until the lab results indicate type 2 diabetes has emerged is not practicing smart preventive medicine. Why wait until chronic disease is present when it is possible to intervene early to prevent insulin resistance from evolving into type 2 diabetes? To use an old analogy, don't wait until the diabetic horse is out of the barn and running across the field to try to catch him. Massive numbers of children are becoming insulin resistant and prediabetic. Prevention is optimal. The time to act is now—when our children first become insulin resistant. The next chapter will focus on methods of early detection and prevention.

### Prediabetes

Prediabetes is a state of insulin resistance and hyperinsulinemia that leads to "impaired glucose tolerance" (IGT) but not full-blown diabetes.[6,7] This is the stage when the pancreas starts to show signs of stress and fatigue, leading to more difficulty keeping blood sugar levels where they should be. IGT means the fasting blood glucose starts to creep up but has not reached the 126 mg/dl cutoff for type 2 diabetes. The body is also having a more challenging time controlling blood sugar after meals (*postprandial hyperglycemia*). The increased insulin production and higher blood sugars damage the body's organs even before diabetes is present.

Prediabetes is a huge warning sign of impending pancreatic (beta cell) failure and imminent diabetes. Increasing numbers of children are prediabetic without anyone being aware of it, and damage to their bodies is already well underway. According to new guidelines, at least one in four children in the US meet the criteria for prediabetes and diabetes screening. Prediabetes is detected in a blood test when the hemoglobin A1C (HbA1c) is mildly elevated from 5.7 to 6.4%, and fasting blood glucose is between 100 to 125 mg/dl (5.6-6.9 mmol/L).

88,000,000 adults in the US and 500,000,000 adults worldwide have *prediabetes;* the majority will develop diabetes in a few years unless they change course.

Almost 50% of American adults are now diabetic or prediabetic.

1 of 3 *normal weight (non-obese)* adults are prediabetic, and 90% are unaware of it.

More than 20% of teens are now prediabetic; many more are insulin resistant but not yet prediabetic.

### Metabolic syndrome

Metabolic syndrome affects 25% of the adult population and an increasing number of children in the US. Metabolic syndrome, while not full-blown diabetes, represents a state of ill health that may include insulin resistance, prediabetes, elevated **triglycerides,** unfavorable levels of cholesterol (low levels of **HDL** and high levels of **LDL** cholesterol), and high blood pressure.[1,8] Metabolic syndrome is a major cardiovascular disease risk factor and is associated with polycystic ovarian syndrome (PCOS) in females, excessive inflammation, and often, *but not always,* obesity. Plenty of non-obese people have metabolic syndrome, as I will highlight further in the coming section.

### Type 2 diabetes mellitus

The person with consistently *high fasting blood glucose* (>125 mg/dl) or HbA1c (>6.5%) is said to have type 2 diabetes.[9-12] This is a dangerous medical condition where the body can no longer make high enough insulin to keep most of the sugar in the cells and not in the bloodstream. The pancreas is exhausted from years of insulin resistance and just can't keep up with the demand. Blood sugar levels continue to rise, causing damage to almost every organ in the body. Type 2 diabetes in a child is even more damaging than the adult version, with faster pancreatic failure and onset of complications. By the time they are diagnosed, many children with type 2 diabetes have already experienced damage to their heart, blood vessels, kidneys, and eyes. Never before in recorded history have we had to worry about type 2 diabetes in children, but now 6,000 children per year are diagnosed in the US with this deadly disease. If current trends continue, the number of children with type 2 diabetes may quadruple by the year 2050.

No one gets type 2 diabetes overnight. The process of insulin resistance progressing to prediabetes and type 2 diabetes typically takes *a decade or more* to develop but is taking place in our children every day with increasing frequency. This means that *the teenager with type 2 diabetes likely was becoming insulin resistant in grade school, and nobody noticed or did anything to stop it*! It is vital to address this problem early and prevent a life marred with needless suffering and chronic disease. If we allow it to progress, we rob children of years of life and, worse yet, quality of life. The younger a child is diagnosed with type 2 diabetes, the more years of life will be lost. Living with a chronic disease such as type 2 diabetes robs them of leading productive lives and guarantees a life of suffering, costly medical expenses, and uncertainty.

34 million people in the US have type 2 diabetes.

40 million people in the US will have type 2 diabetes by the year 2030.

The percentage of US adults with diabetes tripled between 1980 to 2014.

Children of color, especially Native Americans, indigenous peoples, Hispanic and non-Hispanic Black youth, are at exceedingly high risk for developing type 2 diabetes

Type 2 diabetes was relatively unheard of in children until the past 20 years. Now this disease (previously called adult-onset diabetes) is skyrocketing with a 30% increase in kids from 2001-2009, and rates continue to increase steadily.

1 out of every 4 US healthcare dollars is spent caring for diabetes.

Having type 2 diabetes cuts an average of *10 years* off a child's life.

Having type 2 diabetes doubles the chance of death from any cause.

Hospitalization and death rates for heart attack are doubled among adults with type 2 diabetes.

Medical care costs are more than doubled for those with diabetes.

Heart disease and type 2 diabetes are no longer adult diseases; they start in childhood.

## Non-alcoholic fatty liver disease (NAFLD)

**Non-alcoholic fatty liver disease (NAFLD),** sometimes called fatty liver disease, is directly related to both sugar intake and insulin resistance.[13-17] As a pediatric gastroenterologist, I see this *all the time*. It is an epidemic. This condition is set to be the top cause for adults needing a liver transplant in the next few years. It is also a risk factor for liver cancer, so everyone had better be taking this seriously. It is called NAFLD because when examining a small sample of the liver under a microscope and comparing the liver of an alcoholic with the liver of someone who is insulin-resistant and consuming excessive sweetened beverages, they appear identical. As the name suggests, NAFLD is characterized by an excessive buildup of fat in the liver leading to inflammation and liver damage. Just as long-term alcoholism leads to severe liver damage (referred to as "cirrhosis of the liver"), so can long-term NAFLD. **Cirrhosis** can be irreversible, leading to end-stage liver disease, which is fatal without a liver transplant.

Chronic fatty liver disease from poor diet now affects almost *one in three* members of the US population, totaling 100,000,000 people! It is difficult to get an entirely accurate sense of how many children currently have fatty liver and NAFLD. It is estimated that roughly 10% of the general pediatric population has fatty liver disease, which increases to 35% in obese children. Some studies suggest that up to 70% of obese children may have some degree of NAFLD. In America today, if a child has elevated liver enzymes in a blood test (more than 30 U/L), fatty liver is the most likely reason. Interestingly, elevated liver tests (from fatty liver) are so common that they changed the "normal" lab values for AST/ALT (the main liver tests we look at), so that today's acceptable levels are higher now than those from 30 years ago. (I did not realize this until I attended a lecture from Dr. Robert Lustig, a top expert in this field).

All persistently elevated liver tests need to be evaluated by a qualified healthcare provider. A liver ultrasound can also provide evidence of a fatty liver, although it can also miss some cases, so it is not the best screening tool. A liver biopsy may be required to confirm NAFLD and assess the degree of damage to the liver.

NAFLD is closely linked with obesity and type 2 diabetes, as 70 to 80% of adult obese and diabetic patients have fatty liver disease. However, plenty of non-obese people are developing fatty liver as well. The first step towards a fatty liver is a high sugar diet, which leads to elevated fat production in the liver and contributes to insulin resistance. As we already discussed, insulin resistance is the on-ramp to the diabetes highway. Excessive intake of fructose is directly implicated in the development of fatty liver, as will be outlined below. Other factors that increase fatty liver include systemic inflammation in the body and an altered **microbiome**.

## The Obesity Epidemic

*Obesity as a symptom*
While obesity is arguably one of the *symptoms* of metabolic imbalance (versus the cause), it is one of the most serious. It is interrelated to the other commonly associated health issues, such as insulin resistance, metabolic syndrome, and type 2 diabetes. The vast majority of children with type 2 diabetes are also obese. Obesity is also the symptom that the media and we as a society seem most focused on, perhaps for the wrong reasons. Before you think this chapter is a discriminatory rant or "fattist" diatribe, let me plainly state again that *obesity is another symptom of a*

*dysfunctional metabolism, even if it is technically classified as a separate disease!*

This symptom is the most obvious and can be measured by comparing weight and height in a metric called **Body Mass Index** or **BMI**. The definition of "pediatric overweight" is a child with more than 85th percentile BMI for age. Obesity is defined as greater than 95th percentile BMI for age. This is a rudimentary but generally effective screening tool. In pediatrics, we also watch the *rate of rise* as much as we watch the overall BMI as an indicator of potential trouble in younger children. (see the BMI chart in the following chapter)

Obesity is a signal that all is not right in the metabolic and regulatory pathways in the body. As with all dangerous health conditions, the *root cause* must be identified and treated. I agree that blaming, shaming, and stigmatizing have gotten us nowhere. We need to ferret out the underlying problems and expose them, so that we can address them openly and work to make lasting changes. Obesity is an obvious sign that the body is not metabolizing the correct fuels and is storing fat instead of burning it. It is also an indicator that there are likely other damaging processes going on in the body at the same time.

*The scale of the problem*
What do we know about the current obesity epidemic? A quarter of four-year-old kids are currently overweight or obese, and rates of adult obesity in the US increased from 13% in the 1970s to more than 40% today. If we do not change the way we eat and live, by 2030, there will be 40,000,000 Americans with type 2 diabetes, and 50% of the population will be obese. *Half of our citizens will be obese* and potentially looking at an early grave as unsustainable healthcare costs bankrupt the individual and the nation.

> We cannot afford to provide health care for 40,000,000 Americans with type 2 diabetes; it is an expensive disease. One hundred percent of tax dollars will be needed to provide health care for these people, leaving none for national defense, infrastructure, or education.

The obesity epidemic has become an urgent national and international security threat with the potential to destroy this country and many other countries worldwide. The military is increasingly concerned,[18,19] as are the **World Health Organization** and the folks at the Center for Disease Control. There is an enormous iceberg dead ahead, and we need to take action on *every* level of society, from family and schools to the government and food industry. If we don't all help to turn the rudder, we are headed to the bottom of the cold, cold sea. (Deep breath and cue up the Celine Dion "Titanic" soundtrack.) *It does not have to end this way for your children or mine.*

The rates of increase in obesity and diabetes starting after the 1970s indicates this is an *environmental* issue, NOT a *genetic* problem (our genes don't change that quickly). It is also likely an *epigenetic* issue where obesity genes are getting turned on in our infants and young children by certain foods and environmental factors starting in the womb. I previously discussed avoiding the prenatal epigenetic programming for obesity and diabetes in the chapter on diet during pregnancy, so please refer to that chapter regarding early programming for later disease in the **first thousand days** of a child's life. These first thousand days set the blueprint for health or disease, fitness, or obesity in the child and are among the most significant influences on a child's health—present and future.

As we explored earlier, **epigenetics** refers to environmental factors that have the power to "turn on" or "turn off" a variety of genes in our bodies. It is now thought that epigenetics and environmental factors likely play a more important role than genetics in determining childhood obesity. While many of the epigenetic changes that favor obesity occur in the womb (maternal diet, maternal obesity, **gestational diabetes**, maternal stress, chemical exposures), others continue to go on throughout life. What we feed our children and what they are exposed to in their environment will continually impact the genes that code for obesity, inflammation, and disease. All is not lost if the child has been epigenetically programmed in the womb to be metabolically unhealthy and gain excessive weight. However, it may mean that that the parents must be more vigilant and ensure that the child sticks mostly to whole unprocessed foods. There may be less metabolic wiggle room without some negative consequences. It is probably even more critical that these kids significantly limit the sugar and processed foods earlier in life (something we should all do anyway).

## The main epigenetic factors that foster an unhealthy metabolic profile in children

+ Excessive sugar (especially fructose)
+ Damage to the microbiome
+ Stress
+ Poor sleep
+ Lack of exercise
+ Constant exposure to obesogenic endocrine-disrupting chemicals (EDCs)

The main suspects in this crime against our metabolism are hiding in plain sight in our modern diet—too much sugar (especially fructose), much of it hidden in everyday foods, too many highly processed convenience foods, and additives and chemicals in our environment that are increasingly recognized to be "**obesogens.**" Obesogens are endocrine-disrupting chemicals that alter hormone regulation. They act as **epigenetic modifiers** that turn on the genes that contribute to obesity. Undoubtedly, physical inactivity plays a large role, but not in the way that most people think. Increased stress and inadequate sleep are also important lifestyle factors in the obesity epidemic that increase a child's risk.

### Microbiome and obesity

Like most of the other major health conditions we discuss in this book, there is an interesting relationship between diet, inflammation, obesity, and the gut microbiome.[20-25] The Standard American Diet and certain environmental exposures also damage our children's microbiome, which may have already been compromised by early life events including mode of delivery or antibiotic exposure. In many ways, the microbiome controls the metabolism, and researchers have identified both an "obese microbiome" and a "thin microbiome." The microbiome likely plays a crucial role in obesity, insulin resistance, NAFLD, and cardiovascular disease.

What do gut bacteria have to do with weight gain? In animal models, it has been shown that the gut bacteria in an obese individual can harvest up to 20% more calories from their food as compared to a thin individual. That is like eating a whole extra meal every day! Obesity and type 2 diabetes are also associated with inflammation, which makes the body insulin resistant and store more fat. One source of the inflammation may be from abnormal gut bacteria (**dysbiosis**). Researchers have argued over which came first: did obesity alter the microbiome, or did the microbiome shift contribute to obesity?

> In animal models, transplanting the microbiome from an obese mouse into a thin mouse made the thin mouse gain a lot of weight and become obese. The opposite in mice was also true—putting a thin mouse microbiome into an obese mouse made that mouse lose weight and become more metabolically healthy.
>
> To take this to the next step, researchers are trying this in humans, transplanting the microbiome from a thin individual into the intestines of obese individuals. Preliminary studies have not shown earth-shattering results, however.

There is increasing interest in how overexposure to antibiotics, both through the overprescribing of antibiotics in children, as well as low-dose antibiotic exposure in food (commercially-raised animals like chickens and cattle) and the water supply, alters the gut microbiome, makes people more "susceptible" to becoming overweight. We have already discussed how C-section births and formula feeding can alter that baby's gut bacteria and make them more likely to become obese.

We also know that a person's diet is the largest determinant of their microbiome. This is yet another reason why "a calorie is not a calorie." If the child eats a diet high in processed foods and fructose, the microbiome shifts to favor obesity. Conversely, if they eat a diet high in vegetables containing prebiotic fiber and **phytonutrients**, the microbiome shifts to support health. Taking steps to incorporate foods that contain **probiotic** bacteria (fermented vegetables, high-quality yogurt) or in some cases a probiotic supplement may also potentially help make this favorable microbiome shift. Remember that the first thousand days represent the period when the child's microbiome is the most malleable and can be shaped to a healthier profile by making the right dietary choices. However, improving the diet at any age can help shift the gut bacteria to a healthier less inflammatory profile. Interestingly, recent studies suggest that probiotic supplementation may impact weight loss and a healthier metabolic profile in adults.[24,25]

## A Review of Carbohydrates and Sugar

As we started to explore earlier in the chapter, the *form* in which we ingest calories has an enormous impact on how they are metabolized, and nowhere is this truer than with dietary carbohydrates. Dietary carbohydrates can be further classified into several groups:

*Simple Carbohydrates*
Sugars such as sucrose, lactose, glucose, and fructose are either single sugars (monosaccharides) or two sugars bonded together (disaccharides). All have four calories per gram but very different effects on our bodies and metabolism. These are referred to as simple carbohydrates or simple sugars.

*Complex Carbohydrates*
Chains of glucose bonded together make up starches such as those found in grains and vegetables. Depending on the pattern and food matrix they are found in, these can be further divided into high glycemic index and **low glycemic index** carbohydrates described below..

*Non-digestible Carbohydrates*
This refers to many types of fiber and **resistant starches** found in whole foods that cannot be digested by humans but pass through the GI tract and act as fuel for the microbiome. The most important value of these non-digestible carbs is not the heavily marketed calorie reduction, or reduction in "net carbs," but rather this fiber's value to the gut microbiome. This fiber serves as the ecosystem for growth of beneficial bacteria in our intestines. It is essential to understand the key components of carbohydrates and their nutritional values and not succumb to marketing hype, which often clouds the true values of foods.

*Metabolism of Carbohydrates (Carbs)*
We are told that our bodies need sugar; is this true? Yes and no. The primary fuels that our bodies run off are glucose and fat (lipids). If the body's metabolic machinery is working efficiently, the body will largely rely on fat-burning processes to make its energy. **Ketones** are an energy molecule made in our liver that can also be a useful fuel for our bodies. As we talked about earlier, the brain tends to run on glucose but can also use ketones quite efficiently, especially in a baby. To clarify, glucose is the *only* type of sugar that human cells can use for energy. All other forms of calories need to be converted to glucose or into fat or ketones to be used.

Complex carbohydrates such as vegetables or grains contain chains of glucose stuck together by special links called *covalent bonds*. When the digestive process breaks down the carbohydrates, these covalent bonds are broken to release glucose into the bloodstream. How quickly these bonds are broken to release sugar into the bloodstream is referred to as the **glycemic index.**

High glycemic index foods (a.k.a. "fast carbs," like white potatoes and foods made from processed flour such as regular pasta, crackers, white bread) are metabolized into glucose quickly upon entering the intestines, rapidly driving up the blood sugar. The **glycemic load** includes both the glycemic index (how rapidly foods turn into sugar) and the *total amount of carbs* that will turn into sugar. This is likely a more accurate measure of what that food is going to do in our bodies.

A food that has a high glycemic index but a low glycemic load is not a threat, an example being whole fruit. Foods that have a high glycemic load drive up blood sugar and insulin levels. The body has to pump out a lot of insulin fairly rapidly to counteract this load, potentially causing a subsequent sharp drop in blood sugar in a susceptible person (like a crazy roller coaster). If the pancreas overshoots the mark and pumps out too much insulin after a high glycemic load meal, it can drive the glucose too low in a condition referred to as "reactive hypoglycemia" but commonly referred to as "bonking" or "crashing."

When blood sugar drops quickly during reactive hypoglycemia, it is possible to become jittery and experience brain fog, irritability, anxiety attacks, and intense sugar cravings.[26-29] The hypoglycemic person may then experience the need to binge on high glycemic index carbs again, only to repeat the cycle and push them further down the diabetes and brain dysfunction highway.

While still a controversial idea, behavioral issues in some susceptible children have been linked to bonking and reactive hypoglycemia, impacting ADHD and school performance (see Chapter 19 on diet and the child's brain). A potential link with high glycemic index diets and depression is also still under evaluation.[30] This blood sugar rollercoaster also puts a strain on the pancreas over time and damages the metabolism.

Low glycemic index or glycemic load foods (a.k.a. "slow carbs" like vegetables, 100% whole grains like brown rice, quinoa, steel-cut or rolled oats) refer to slow-release carbohydrates with intact fiber that take longer to metabolize into glucose and do not cause a big insulin surge or bonking after eating them. Too many high glycemic index or glycemic load carbs and dietary sugars are likely contributing to insulin resistance, metabolic syndrome, and type 2 diabetes. Treat the pancreas well, and it will last a lifetime. Abuse this vital organ with excessive sugar and high glycemic load carbohydrates and then pay the price. We don't get a second pancreas (not yet anyway, although someone with a 3D printer is probably working on it).

The body can store a limited amount of glucose in chains called glycogen. This storage form of glucose is packed away in the liver and muscles, but because it is big and bulky, the body can only store a few hours' worth of glucose in the tissues and uses it sparingly, mostly to feed the brain. Fat, however, is a different story. The body can store weeks and weeks of energy in fat cells. Metabolically healthy people maintain what is called **metabolic flexibility,** meaning their body can shift back and forth from fat and ketone-burning to carb-burning but are not overly reliant on carbs (like the person with metabolic dysfunction or diabetes). *The benefit of regular exercise is not the calories that are burned immediately.* The benefit of exercise is that cells and **mitochondria** (the little energy factories in the cells) learn how to metabolize fat more efficiently, be more metabolically flexible and insulin sensitive, and reduce the load on the pancreas.

### Metabolic difference between glucose and fructose

Fructose is a sugar that naturally occurs in fruits, honey, agave nectar, as well as sugar cane and beets used to make table sugar. Fructose makes up half of the molecule sucrose (table sugar), which is one molecule of glucose and fructose bonded together. High fructose corn syrup is a common sweetener added to foods made up of a free solution of (unbonded) glucose and fructose. *Fructose is a metabolic **toxin** at the amounts we are currently eating.* The excessive fructose in our drinks and foods is slowly poisoning us. How?

We never evolved to handle as much fructose as we are getting in the modern diet. From an evolutionary standpoint, we ate a higher amount of fructose in the fall when most fruit was ripe, and we gorged on it to fatten up in order to survive the winter, like a bear. Except now, it is like fall all year long. We are fattening up for the winter all the time. Dr. Richard Johnson from University of Colorado and Dr. Robert Lustig from University of California San Francisco, two of the leading experts on fructose metabolism agree that fructose should be viewed mostly as an *energy storage* molecule rather than a clean fuel source for the body. They are also in agreement that excessive fructose in our diet is in no small part driving most major diseases of modern society.

Fructose intake *per person* increased from half a pound to more than one hundred pounds annually in the past fifty years, with an *average* daily intake of over 80 grams (320 calories), mostly from high fructose corn syrup and sucrose (table sugar). This overload is contributing to metabolic syndrome, diabetes, obesity, and fatty liver disease. There is also mounting evidence that excessive fructose also contributes to heart disease and Alzheimer's.[31-33] The potential indirect effects of sugar on brain function and behavior in children will be explored in the final chapter of this book.

Fructose and glucose are not the same, even though they are both simple sugars. Unlike glucose, which is used by every cell in the body, *the cells in our body cannot burn fructose directly for energy* and the liver must convert it to other forms of energy like glucose or fat (triglyceride). The modern liver has quite a burden to bear, processing all the fructose currently in our diet, and converting what it can to glucose, then converting the rest to store as fat. With all the fructose we are eating, the liver is required to work really, really hard, and the liver cannot keep up.

To process all the fructose in our current diet, the liver must convert it to fat (triglycerides). And if you are the liver, making all this fat quickly to get rid of the potentially toxic fructose, where is the easiest place to store this fat? Right in the liver's backyard. Remember what we talked about with fatty liver disease? We pack the liver full of the fat until it chokes on it, and develops liver inflammation (hepatitis) and eventually liver damage and death (cirrhosis). Dr. Robert Lustig published a journal article entitled "Fructose; it's alcohol without the buzz," which says it all. Fructose in high doses has a host of unfavorable metabolic effects, not dissimilar to alcohol.[32,39]

Let's take a deeper dive into the science that illuminates the damaging effects of fructose.

*Why is a high fructose diet detrimental to health?*[13,33-42]
+ Fructose bypasses the typical regulation that governs glucose metabolism. It can only be metabolized in the liver, and to a lesser degree, the small intestine. High amounts of fructose place significant stress on the liver.
+ Unlike all other forms of calories, fructose *depletes* the energy (ATP) inside of our liver cells. (In contrast, glucose and fat burning *generate* ATP in our cells.)
+ This ATP depletion makes the body think it is starving when it is not, *causing metabolism to decrease* while a potentially toxic metabolite called uric acid is increased.

+ When the liver is overloaded with fructose, it converts it to fat (triglycerides) for storage.

+ High fructose intake is said to increase **de novo lipogenesis**, which is the liver making new fat. This process increases the fats that are packed in the liver, potentially causing hepatitis, but these fats are also implicated in heart disease and are known as VLDL, triglycerides, and small particle LDL

+ Therefore, fructose promotes energy storage, not energy production.

+ Fructose directly promotes fat storage, especially types like **TOFI** (**Thin Outside, Fat Inside**), a common condition where people store their fat around their vital organs rather than their bellies and thighs. These people are at high risk for heart disease.

+ High fructose intake increases *uric acid*, a chemical produced in the body which has a host of damaging effects at high levels:

  – Decreases the production of nitric oxide, driving up blood pressure, damaging the blood vessels, and promoting heart disease.

  – Crystallizes in the joints causing gout.

  – Contributes to insulin resistance and directly contributes to the development of fatty liver disease, metabolic syndrome, and the development of type 2 diabetes.

  – Promotes oxidation and inflammation.

  – Damages the vital **mitochondria** that make our energy.

+ Fructose accelerates cellular aging by promoting *oxidation* and the formation of nasty substances called **AGE's (advanced glycosylation end products)**.

> Fructose in the blood sticks to proteins in a process called **glycosylation** or **fructosyla-tion**. This is similar to the process in diabetes, where excess sugar sticks to red blood cells (glycosylated hemoglobin). This is the basis of the test hemoglobin A1c that shows average glucose levels in the blood. A high HgbA1c indicates lots of glycosylation going on in the body with potential damage to the kidneys, eyes, blood vessels, and heart. Unfortunately, this process is *considerably more likely to happen with fructose than glucose.*

+ The oxidation products from a high sugar diet and AGEs directly stimulate inflammation in the body. Excessive inflammation is linked to every degenerative disease of Western society, including heart disease, diabetes, Alzheimer's, and cancer. This chronic low-grade inflammation also contributes to further insulin resistance in a vicious cycle.

+ High fructose intake stimulates pro-inflammatory **gene expression** (epigenetic modification), further promoting inflammation in the body.

+ In animal models, a high fructose diet causes inflammation in the brain, leading to brain cell dysfunction and death. It may increase the potential for a host of neurological conditions like depression, ADHD, autism, and Alzheimer's.[31,43]

+ Increased fructose in the diet is implicated in insulin resistance and elevated insulin levels in the blood. (Insulin resistance > hyperinsulinemia > diabetes)

+ A high fructose diet alters the bacteria in the gut microbiome and promotes dysbiosis, which may be another part of the pathway leading to metabolic syndrome (these gut bacteria control almost every aspect of our life!)[44]

+ Excessive fructose also contributes to a **leaky gut,** leading to systemic inflammation, partly by a process called **endotoxemia,** and is thought to be linked to many diseases, including metabolic syndrome and heart disease.[44-47]

Here's the real kicker. Sugar in and of itself is also addicting like a drug. It stimulates the reward pathway in the brain and *creates addiction and food-seeking behavior* in a susceptible person.[39,49,50] Sugar meets every medical definition of a substance of abuse:

+ Sugar stimulates the brain's pleasure center (the ventral tegmental area, which is rich in dopamine—the pleasure neurotransmitter).

+ Tolerance builds over time and more and more sugar is needed to "scratch the itch."

+ Withdrawal symptoms develop when it is absent, including mood swings, headaches, and altered behavior.

+ Withdrawal symptoms lead to a sugar binge (we have all seen someone's candy wrapper pyramid of shame).

+ There is a desire to quit or cut back. "I really should stop drinking soda and eating candy...but I can't!"

+ Craving and seeking behavior. People feel that they can't control themselves around sweets.

+ Clearly negative consequences result from this abuse: metabolic syndrome, obesity, diabetes, heart disease, etc.

## What the heck is leptin, and who is ghrelin?

Evidence exists that the rising level of fructose in our diet alters our appetite regulation, leading to overeating and excessive cravings.[39,48-50] Fructose decreases the brain's ability to feel satiety (feeling full after meals) and leads to overeating. Fructose does not suppress hunger signals such as the hormone grehlin as most meals do, but it does suppress the fullness signal (leptin) that tells the brain to stop eating. This combination leads to overeating, increased calorie intake, and fat storage.

**Leptin** is the hormone produced by the fat cells to tell the brain that they are full. Leptin tries to tell the brain to decrease appetite and food-seeking behavior. Become *leptin resistant*, and guess what? You become *Always Hungry* (the name of the highly informative book by Dr. David Ludwig from Boston Children's Hospital that describes this metabolic conundrum in detail).

In a nutshell, the brain interprets a decrease in leptin signaling (leptin resistance) as starvation, driving the body to eat to survive. In obesity, a state of leptin resistance develops so that the brain doesn't receive the leptin signal that the fat cells are full. Leptin resistance may parallel insulin resistance. Hunger continues, the metabolism decreases to conserve energy, but the brain still thinks it is starving.

Leptin can be blocked by many factors, including increased insulin, stress, inflammation, high triglycerides, high fructose, and quite possibly by environmental toxins (endocrine disruptors known as "**obesogens**," such as BPA and phthalates in our foods and plastics). Welcome to the modern world! This system of metabolic dysfunction linking hormones and weight is diabolical—as if designed to do the most harm in the modern world we are living in!

In a pre-diabetic or insulin-resistant person with chronically increased insulin and leptin resistance, we get the following:

+ Signals in the brain drive an appetite for highly processed "comfort" foods full of high glycemic index carbohydrates and obesogenic chemicals while in constant starvation mode.
+ The body fights weight loss by decreasing metabolism and decreasing the urge to be active, so fewer calories are burned.

As outlined in the next chapter, the first step in breaking this cycle is decreasing the sugar and highly processed food in the diet!

**How much sugar are kids eating? How much should they be eating?**
Children currently get 16% or more of their daily calories from *added sugar.* This does not refer to total carbohydrates from vegetables or grains or sugars in fruit; this is looking at extra *added* sugar not naturally found in the food supply. The estimated average intake of added sugar for children in the US is 80 grams, far exceeding the recommended upper limit. According to the American Heart Association and the American Academy of Pediatrics, the goal for children is less than 25 grams daily, or less than 5% of daily calories from added sugars.[51]

### TABLE 17.1 RECOMMENDED UPPER LIMIT OF ADDED SUGAR (5% DAILY CALORIES)

| Age of child (years) | Grams of sugar |
|---|---:|
| 0-2 | 0 |
| 2-3 | 15 |
| 4-8 | 18 |
| 9-13 | 25 |
| 14-18 | 25-32 |

The average child gets 20 tsp (80 grams) of added sugar daily. If we look at what is contained in sweetened beverages, we can see why so many people exceed these recommendations.

### TABLE 17.2 GRAMS OF SUGAR IN COMMON BEVERAGES

| Beverage (12 oz) | Grams of sugar |
|---|---:|
| Soda | 35 |
| Sweet tea | 35 |
| Grape juice | 56 |
| Apple juice | 36 |
| Sports drinks | 21 |
| Chocolate milk | 16 (plus natural lactose) |

Even though the sugar in the fruit juice is "naturally occurring," it is super concentrated and not how mother nature packaged it, so I would consider it added sugar. The American Academy of Pediatrics and other health organizations tell kids to *ditch the sweetened drinks*! Ditch the soda, sports drinks, and chocolate milk. Limit juice. Kids should drink mostly water.

Revealing these facts about the increasingly common metabolic "diseases of modern civilization," we should be much more interested in what our children are eating. If a child eats the **Standard American Diet (SAD)**, their future health is in peril. However, this does not have to be. How do we protect our children and ensure they live a life of optimal metabolic health? The next chapter provides a metabolic recovery plan for a child at risk.

### RECOMMENDED READING

1. Hypoglycemia Foundation: https://hypoglycemia.org/info

2. Robert Lustig. *Fat Chance: Beating the Odds Against Sugar, Processed Food, Obesity and Disease,* (Plume, 2014). www.robertlustig.com

3. David Ludwig. *Always Hungry? Conquer Cravings, Retrain Your Fat Cells, and Lose Weight Permanently,* (Grand Central Publishing, 2018).

## NUTRITION $R_X$

1. Obesity, prediabetes, and fatty liver disease are increasingly common in today's children, and are a health crisis.

2. The modern diet contributes to the progression from insulin resistance to prediabetes and eventually type 2 diabetes, even in children.

3. Main contributors to this progression are diets containing excessive sugar (fructose) and highly processed foods, as well as inadequate sleep, excessive stress and lack of exercise.

4. Fructose in high amounts is damaging to the body and promotes obesity, inflammation, diabetes, fatty liver disease and heart disease.

5. Most kids are getting far above the recommended intake of added sugar on a daily basis.

# CHAPTER EIGHTEEN

# METABOLIC HEALTH: THE RECOVERY

## THE COMEBACK KID: A PATIENT'S STORY

There are children in all of our communities who are only a few years away from becoming type 2 diabetic, and they do not even know it (nor do their parents). Unfortunately, neither do most of their healthcare providers. However, having concrete evidence of their impending risk can be the turning point in a child's health.

I recall a patient who we will call Brendon (not his real name). Brendon was 16 years old, 6 foot 2 inches tall, and obese, although his height helped him hide it better than some. He came to me with elevated liver enzymes in his blood, with an ALT over 200, indicating a damaged liver from excessive fat storage (fatty liver disease). Normal ALT levels should be optimally less than 30. An ultrasound showed that his liver and spleen were moderately enlarged, and his liver showed signs of fatty liver disease, which is a cardinal sign of metabolic dysfunction. His labs also showed that his fasting glucose and his hemoglobin A1c were "borderline normal," so, by current standards, he did not yet have diabetes and was initially thought to be doing OK—except that he wasn't.

Brendon was at risk of his fatty liver disease progressing to more serious liver disease like **cirrhosis** (think long-term alcoholic). We discussed the role diet and exercise could play in reversing this. Despite this conversation, I could tell he wasn't "getting it" or taking the matter seriously, or very willing to make significant changes at that time. I sent him home with some lab orders for fasting **insulin** levels along with a repeat glucose and a cholesterol/lipid panel and had him come back to my clinic in a few weeks. The results were shocking.

His fasting insulin was close to 200, over 10 times the normal upper limit, indicating major **insulin resistance.** Despite the high insulin levels, his fasting glucose was starting to become elevated, just over 100. His **LDL** (the supposed "bad cholesterol") wasn't excessively high, but his triglycerides were shooting up to 250 (healthy values are less than 100). His **HDL** "good cholesterol" was low in the mid-30s (healthy values are greater than 50). Also, his blood pressure was starting to rise to a level that bordered on hypertension. All evidence indicated serious metabolic dysfunction.

We talked about what this meant for Brendon's body and how he was dangerously close to becoming a type 2 diabetic in a few years and having an early heart attack unless we changed course. I let him know in very clear terms that I wasn't concerned about his weight per se. This wasn't about his weight; *this was about the substantial evidence of metabolic damage to his body.* At that moment, he had likely already sustained early damage to his blood vessels, eyes, and kidneys. I also let him know that we still had a chance of reversing it if we started making changes without delay. After some additional discussion, Brendon told me that he had an uncle with **type 2 diabetes** who was deteriorating before his eyes, with failing kidneys and heading towards a second heart attack. When this young man had concrete proof that he was heading in the same direction, it hit him like a ton of bricks: there in black and white, with no denial, his lab report showed that he was prediabetic with **metabolic syndrome.** He began to take immediate action.

After six months on a low sugar diet with no sweetened drinks and fewer processed-foods, combined with weight training and cardiovascular exercise, the turnaround for Brendon was remarkable. He dropped 35 pounds and his liver tests normalized. Most importantly, his fasting insulin dropped to 30, his **triglycerides** were down to 130, and his fasting glucose was safely in the low 90s!

Brendon, his mother, and I were ecstatic. He was no longer prediabetic or significantly insulin resistant; he no longer had evidence of fatty liver disease, and his heart disease risk was plummeting. When he walked into my clinic, even before I saw the lab results, his skin looked better, he had an energy I had not seen before, and his eyes shone brightly. He admitted that he felt better than he had in years, and his brain was functioning at a level higher than any time in recent history. This young man had fundamentally changed and upgraded to a new version of himself – 'Brendon 2.0.'

This should be the legacy we leave our children: a life characterized by vibrant health and the ability to access their full potential. When children are young, they are resilient, and they can make remarkable turnarounds. They can make changes that will profoundly affect the rest of their lives.

In this chapter, I want to give parents real, actionable steps to help reduce children's risk of falling victim to the epidemic of "non-communicable diseases" such as heart disease, type 2 diabetes mellitus, and metabolic syndrome; conditions that are associated with the majority of deaths in modern industrialized society. I will not offer some "quick fix" or "hack" that sounds too good to be true (and generally is). The real-life solution is not sexy or flashy and is not always *easy*, although it is relatively *simple*. Making positive changes as early as possible is essential to fostering life-long health for our children. It is never too early or too late to make positive change and turn a child's health in the right direction. These changes can save a child's life – not just the *years* of life lived, but the *quality* of life lived.

I have heard tales of physicians who tell their insulin resistant and predia-betic adult patients:

+ "This is genetic,"
+ "Nothing can be done."
+ "Diabetes is inevitable."
+ "Come back when you have diabetes, I'll prescribe medication."

This attitude is dangerous and counterproductive.

It has been *proven* that some cases of type 2 diabetes can be reversible with the proper diet and exercise.[1-3] It is therefore negligent to say that nothing can be done for a prediabetic patient until the disease has progressed.

An inspiring example of a paradigm shift in diabetes treatment is Virta Health. Virta Health offers a program to potentially reverse type 2 diabetes in adults. Many of their patients achieve blood sugar control while removing medications *in as little as a few weeks*. (See https://www.virtahealth.com/). Such programs are proving that there are remedies for metabolic syndrome, insulin resistance and **prediabetes**, and type 2 diabetes, even in relatively advanced stages. Even though reversing type 2 diabetes is possible, some patients may be trapped in self-destructive behaviors or have given up on taking control over their health.

However, with kids, the story is different. We can't give up on them. Are we going to tell our children, "Ahh, you're only insulin resistant! There is nothing we can do. Come back after you progress to type 2 diabetes, and then we will explain how you will likely have ten years less to live and face possible blindness, kidney failure, and amputated limbs"? Hell no. *We must fight for our children and their right to lead healthy lives.*

Good health isn't rocket science or a medical miracle. Fundamental, reproducible changes can alter someone's health destiny, perhaps your own child's health destiny. *In a nutshell, reduce the sugars and the processed carbs in the diet and start a regular exercise program to improve the body's insulin sensitivity and fat-burning machinery.* As a result, the body's insulin levels are lowered, applying the brakes on fat storage and inflammation, while removing the brakes on fat burning. The fat then starts to leave the liver and other storage sites and gets burned for energy. This way, metabolic balance is restored. I use these metaphors as a simple way of describing the principal changes that are needed. I have seen this approach work first-hand in my medical practice; it can work for almost any child. Let's take a deeper dive into this process.

## EARLY DETECTION

How do you know if your child is approaching the on ramp to the diabetes highway?

Increasingly, it has become paramount that the children who are at increased risk for metabolic dysfunction, insulin resistance, and development of type 2 diabetes be seen and diagnosed early by a pediatrician or primary healthcare provider. If rates of type 2 diabetes in teens are on the rise and it takes up to ten years of silent insulin resistance to get to full-blown diabetes, this would indicate that there are large groups of younger children who are already insulin resistant and on their way to diabetes. Early screening tests to verify insulin resistance and other risks will allow earlier changes in diet and lifestyle to prevent a lifetime of ill health and an early demise. What are some of these clues ("canaries in the coal mine") that tell us that a child is at risk?

### Start with family history

A strong family history of type 2 diabetes, obesity, and early heart disease should raise some red flags that this child could be genetically and epigenetically predisposed to suffer the same conditions. Was the child born to a mother with obesity or **gestational diabetes**? This could further increase the risk. Are they a person of color? We know that people of African and South Asian descent, Native American and Pacific Islanders, and those of Hispanic heritage are at increased risk of developing type 2 diabetes and metabolic disease. However, Caucasian children are not exempt by any means.

### Diet and sugar-sweetened beverages

It has been suggested that the intake of sugar-sweetened beverages (SSB) such as soda, sweet tea, or sweetened fruit drinks could be an additional vital sign to screen for potential health issues at every primary care visit. Evidence is mounting that even in non-obese children, a high intake of sugary beverages is an independent risk factor for developing insulin resistance, metabolic syndrome, and type 2 diabetes.[4-8] The same is true for a diet high in **ultra-processed foods** and low in fruits, vegetables, and whole grains. A poor diet with a high intake of sugar-sweetened beverages should be considered a risk factor for insulin resistance, **non-alcoholic fatty liver disease (NAFLD)**, and metabolic syndrome. In fact, just one sugar-sweetened beverage per day increases risk for type 2 diabetes, according to research.

### Body mass index, weight, and body composition

**Body Mass Index** is calculated by a child's weight in kilograms divided by height in meters squared. ($kg/m^2$). This value should be part of every child's growth chart. The goal is for children to be less than the 85% BMI for their age. For children, the overweight BMI range is 85 to 95%, and above 95% is considered obese. BMI is a decent screening measure, but some very muscular older children and teens have a higher BMI and are metabolically healthy. There are also examples of children with a normal BMI who experience profound metabolic derangement and insulin resistance. However, a rapidly rising BMI percentile should be cause for concern. An excessive increase in a child's BMI is a metric that should raise a red flag to indicate that a child's metabolic health may be poor. Any child with a BMI above 95% should be considered at high risk.

## RISING BMI GROWTH CHART

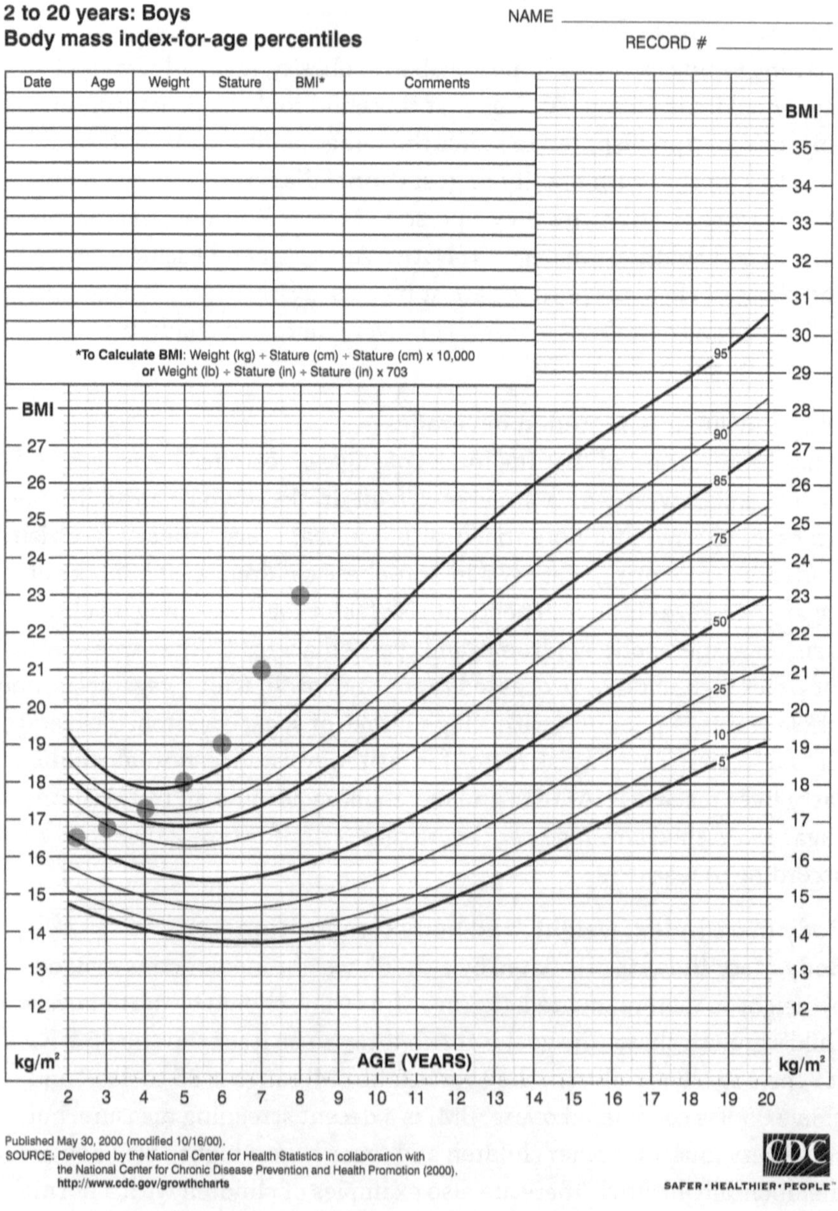

**2 to 20 years: Boys**
**Body mass index-for-age percentiles**

NAME _____

RECORD # _____

| Date | Age | Weight | Stature | BMI* | Comments |
|------|-----|--------|---------|------|----------|
|      |     |        |         |      |          |
|      |     |        |         |      |          |
|      |     |        |         |      |          |
|      |     |        |         |      |          |
|      |     |        |         |      |          |
|      |     |        |         |      |          |
|      |     |        |         |      |          |

*To Calculate BMI: Weight (kg) ÷ Stature (cm) ÷ Stature (cm) x 10,000
or Weight (lb) ÷ Stature (in) ÷ Stature (in) x 703

[BMI-for-age growth chart for boys, 2 to 20 years, with plotted data points]

Published May 30, 2000 (modified 10/16/00).
SOURCE: Developed by the National Center for Health Statistics in collaboration with
the National Center for Chronic Disease Prevention and Health Promotion (2000).
http://www.cdc.gov/growthcharts

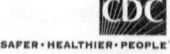

SAFER · HEALTHIER · PEOPLE™

Another illuminating tool in use at some clinics but often not widely available is a bio-impedance scale, which uses electricity to measure muscle mass, bone mass, intracellular/extracellular body water, body fat (and locations of the fat), among other metrics *in addition to total body weight*. Such measurements can be quite revealing, as it is possible to gain weight that is muscle mass while at the same time losing body fat. A simple scale and the BMI ratio will not account for this.

## Blood pressure

High blood pressure, also known as hypertension, is associated with obesity and insulin resistance and metabolic syndrome and is often missed in children in a primary care office. Properly screening using the correct sized blood pressure cuff for a pediatric patient is crucial because of the association with high blood pressure and blood vessel damage leading to heart and kidney disease and stroke. Measuring hypertension in children can be challenging. The thresholds are not standardized like they are for adults. Whether a child has hypertension depends on how the patient's blood pressure compares to that of peers, factoring in gender, height, and age. Blood pressure should be below 120/80 for teens and below the 90th percentile for age in younger children.[9] Detection of hypertension in younger children is made simpler by an online calculator created in conjunction with the AAP, which can be found at https://www.mdcalc.com/aap-pediatric-hypertension-guidelines.

Excessive fructose intake independently causes elevations in blood pressure; blood pressure may normalize by simply removing sugary beverages from the child's diet. Repeated elevations in blood pressure should warrant a referral to a pediatric cardiologist and further screening tests.

## Acanthosis nigricans

**Acanthosis nigricans** is the darkening of the skin around the neck and armpits, typically in an overweight child that is a strong indicator of insulin resistance and poor metabolic health. It is easily picked up on a physical exam and should be a giant red flag to the provider that further workup is warranted.

## Important lab tests and metrics for metabolic dysfunction

Suppose a child is at risk for insulin resistance, metabolic syndrome, or type 2 diabetes, based on these screening parameters, overall history, and physical exam. In that case, some of the blood tests I highlight below can provide more information on the nature and degree of a child's metabolic dysfunction. Not every child requires these labs, but they may be useful and sometimes very motivating. The child's medical provider should determine whether these are clinically useful, based on the clinician's experience and level of concern.

*Liver enzymes (LFT)*
Elevations in ALT (alanine aminotransferase) can indicate fatty liver disease secondary to metabolic dysfunction. ALT should be below 40, optimally below 30. By far, the most common cause of elevated liver enzymes in a child is from non-alcoholic fatty liver disease (NAFLD), typically caused by excessive fructose intake and other components of the Western diet. Any persistently elevated liver function tests should be investigated by the child's primary care provider and potentially a pediatric gastroenterologist to rule out other causes and for long-term monitoring. This is not to be taken lightly as NAFLD can progress to cirrhosis and irreversible liver damage, eventually requiring a liver transplant.

*Fasting insulin and glucose*
Fasting glucose, (measured in the morning after eight hours of nothing other than water to eat or drink) should be below 100 mg/dl, optimally less than 90. Fasting glucose between 100-125 mg/dl (5.6-6.9 mmol/L) may signal impaired glucose control and prediabetes. Fasting glucose above 126 mg/dl on several occasions is a diagnostic criterion for type 2 diabetes.[10] This is a late finding on the path from insulin resistance to type 2 diabetes.

Signs of insulin resistance and potential prediabetes are apparent earlier when the blood's *fasting insulin* level starts to creep up. This is an easy, relatively inexpensive test to perform. For a child, the goal is to have a fasting insulin less than 15 in the prepubertal period and less than 30 in the pubertal period. Teenagers are naturally insulin resistant during this growth phase, which unfortunately puts them at even higher risk for prediabetes and diabetes. The fasting insulin may be more useful in the context of calculating a HOMA-IR (described next) using concurrent fasting insulin and glucose levels. I test children and teens in my clinic who come in for concerns about fatty liver and obesity and have been shocked at the number of kids who have significantly elevated fasting insulin levels, well above 100, and some even closer to 200 and beyond! These children are pulling onto the diabetes on-ramp without even knowing it.

*HOMA-IR score (HomeOstatic Model Assessment of Insulin Resistance)*
HOMA-IR is a metabolic screening tool calculated from fasting insulin
and glucose levels. Universally accepted HOMA cutoff levels that determine insulin resistance lack expert consensus and are to some degree a
subject of controversy. Overall, cutoffs HOMA levels less than 3.4 have
been proposed in recent studies but vary depending on puberty status.[11-15]
Children are naturally a little insulin resistant during puberty, so higher
cutoff values during this period are acceptable. (For example, some
studies allow up to 5.2 in pubertal boys; the UCSF obesity clinic allows an
overall cutoff of 4.3).

## HOMA-IR SCORE

Calculated by fasting plasma glucose (nmol/l) x fasting plasma insulin (mU/l) divided by 22.5

Or alternately:

Fasting plasma glucose (mg/dl) x fasting plasma insulin (mU/ml) divided by 405

Calculations can also be performed using computer modeling (HOMA calculator), some of which
are available online.

In my opinion, the HOMA score is an underutilized tool to screen at-risk
children for potential insulin resistance before things get out of hand.
While not perfect, it is a valid screening tool, inexpensive and non-inva-
sive. As long as a child is genuinely fasting for 8 to 10 hours before the
test and is not in advanced stage diabetes, the HOMA score has been
shown to have a reasonable correlation with some of the other insulin
resistance testing methods. Obese (or non-obese) children who are more
insulin resistant are known to be at greater risk for developing type 2
diabetes and cardiovascular disease as well as polycystic ovary syndrome
(PCOS) and NAFLD. Many experts feel insulin resistance is the best predictor of type 2 diabetes development.[12,16] An overweight or obese child
who is metabolically healthy and not insulin resistant may not have to
be followed as closely or managed aggressively by a healthcare provider
because they are at significantly lower risk for complications. Insulin and
HOMA are also excellent benchmarks and a way to tell if the treatment
being implemented by the healthcare team is effective in improving
insulin sensitivity, regardless of what their weight is doing initially. If
the dietary changes and activity program are effective, we should see a
steady improvement in the fasting insulin and HOMA-IR score. Checking

HOMA-IR remains somewhat controversial in the pediatric clinic setting despite being well described in the medical literature.[17-20]

These markers are more sensitive than isolated fasting glucose or the hemoglobin A1c which tend to only identify patients with pre-diabetes or type 2 diabetes, *not* those with insulin resistance but who still have adequate glucose control. Recall that elevated insulin levels can cause damage even before blood glucose starts to get out of control. An even more sensitive way to detect insulin resistance is with an oral glucose tolerance test (OGTT). This test checks the body's response to an oral glucose challenge every 30 minutes for two hours to see what the insulin and glucose levels in the blood are doing and accurately tells if someone is insulin resistant; however this test is more involved and more expensive than a HOMA score.[21,22]

*Hemoglobin A1c (HbA1c)*

HbA1c is a marker of *average* blood glucose levels in the preceding three months. Chronically elevated blood sugar levels and poor blood glucose control will result in more glucose getting "stuck" on the red blood cells, which is detected by this test. Elevations in HbA1c mean the child is developing diabetes, and we want levels optimally below 5.5%. HbA1c of 5.7-6.4% is consistent with prediabetes but may not be the optimal screening test for children. Some experts caution against using HbA1C as the only prediabetes screening tool for children, as this test in children has been shown to have inferior sensitivity for detecting prediabetes.[23] An HbA1C of more than 6.5% indicates type 2 diabetes and is one of the diagnostic criteria.

There are some caveats with the HbA1C. An excess of highs and lows in blood sugar is referred to as "glycemic variability" and is harmful to the body but may not be reflected in the HbA1c, which only detects the *average* glucose. The roller coaster effect in someone with poor glucose control can damage the heart and blood vessels and exacerbate other serious health concerns. Since this test represents average blood glucose without taking into account glycemic variability, it is possible to have a normal HbA1c *yet still have significant metabolic imbalance*. That is why a fasting insulin, HOMA score, or an oral glucose tolerance test in addition to HbA1c may be more accurate indicators of metabolic imbalance, insulin resistance, and prediabetes.

*Uric acid*
Uric acid is a natural compound created by the liver during specific metabolic processes and ordinarily present in small amounts in a healthy individual, as the kidneys excrete the excess. However, levels can rise in people with an excess of fructose in the diet, insulin resistance, metabolic syndrome, cardiovascular disease, and an adult condition known as gout.[24-27]

Initially thought to be an innocent bystander to other liver processes, a growing body of research suggests that elevated levels of uric acid may be a central player in the damage caused by metabolic syndrome, fatty liver, and cardiovascular disease. In fact, according to some experts, "Today there is overwhelming epidemiological evidence that shows that hyperuricemia (elevated uric acid) both presents and predicts the development of insulin resistance and type 2 diabetes."[25]

Elevated uric acid has also been shown to be an independent risk factor for the development of fatty liver disease.[26] If elevations in uric acid predict the development of insulin resistance, type 2 diabetes and can be used as a marker of fructose-related damage to the body, it may have an essential role as a screening tool and for monitoring children at risk for fatty liver, metabolic syndrome, and type 2 diabetes. High uric acid levels also correlate with increased blood pressure and increased inflammation in the body, both of which are associated with metabolic syndrome. Levels of uric acid should be below 6 mg/dl. If someone is metabolically unhealthy, decreasing their sugar intake may be the only thing they need to do to get their uric acid levels back in the normal range.

*Fasting lipids (cholesterol and triglycerides)*
Metabolic syndrome is characterized by high triglyceride levels and low **HDL** levels (the "good" cholesterol). Triglycerides in children should be (optimally) below 100 mg/dl and HDL more than 50 mg/dl. I monitor but don't focus as much on total cholesterol (the goal is less than 200) and LDL (the goal is less than 130, optimally, less than 100).

I would rather check an **apolipoprotein B (ApoB)** level in my older kids and teens, which tells me if there are a lot of small dangerous cholesterol particles in the blood. In cases of insulin resistance or metabolic syndrome, this may be a more accurate risk marker for cardiovascular disease than total LDL.[28-32] The goal is an ApoB level that is less than 80 mg/dl optimally. Unfortunately, we need to start thinking about cardiovascular disease risk in children, as the process that leads to an eventual heart attack starts in childhood and is markedly accelerated in someone with insulin resistance and metabolic syndrome or type 2 diabetes, all of which are on the rise in children.

Work with the child's healthcare provider if there are metabolic concerns. If a child is at risk for diabetes/prediabetes, or fatty liver, or has a rising BMI that is concerning, their provider may want to monitor some labs to check their progress. I have found it more helpful to focus on other markers of metabolic dysfunction and not weight initially if I am seeing an overweight child with fatty liver. *The main emphasis should be on improving their insulin sensitivity, metabolic health, health of their liver, and avoiding type 2 diabetes*. Weight is a secondary marker in my opinion. Use whatever motivators work for both the child and family. Labs can be rechecked, as well as BMI and blood pressure, in six months to see if they are on the right track. If possible, incorporate qualified health coaches and qualified dieticians to develop a support team. However, if these people start touting low-fat diets, significant calorie restriction, or pre-packaged foods, run the other way.

## FOUR OBESITY MYTHS

Part of the problem that has contributed largely to the ongoing epidemic of metabolic diseases is the pervasive misinformation that has persisted in the public consciousness. Let's break down some of the myths and fallacies that are consistently disproved by science but nonetheless bombard us in marketing and in the media. With a better understanding of the mechanisms that contribute to metabolic related disease, we can be inspired to make better choices for ourselves and our children.

### Myth #1: Eating fat makes us fat; therefore, a low-fat diet is the healthiest.

Wrong! Fat does NOT make us fat and, in general, does not cause heart disease! This huge myth keeps getting recycled over and over. Yes, fat has nine calories per gram versus four calories per gram of carbohydrate, but so what? If fat makes us fat, why do people tend to lose more weight and keep it off on a lower carbohydrate and higher fat diet, as multiple meta-analyses have shown?[33-38] Side by side in research studies, people tend to do better on a diet that is higher in (healthy) fat, but lower in sugar and high-**glycemic index** carbohydrates (food made with processed flour that turns to sugar instantly in the intestines). Sugar and highly processed foods are the real culprits.

Done correctly, a higher fat diet *does not* raise the risk of heart disease (a prime example is the Mediterranean diet). Modern science is proving that a *higher fat* Mediterranean style diet (with extra fat from olive oil and nuts) is better for the heart and lowers all the markers that are known to be linked with increased risk of heart disease, including inflammation.[39] There is also mounting evidence by some of the top lipid (fat) researchers in the world that the link between **saturated fat** and heart disease is not as strong as the mainstream media would have us believe.[40] Olive oil may contain up to 20% saturated fat, yet higher intake of olive oil is associated with lower risk of heart disease. This is an interesting paradox.

An outline of early nutrition research that led us astray was published in the respected medical journal JAMA Internal Medicine as well as the New York Times "How the Sugar Industry Shifted the Blame to Fat" Sept 12, 2016, and was brought to light thanks to scientists' fearless work at University of California, San Francisco (UCSF).[41] These articles revealed documents confirming that scientists receiving funding from the sugar industry conveniently "discovered" that sugar was healthy, and that dietary fat was causing the increase in heart disease seen in this country. One of the researchers implicated in the original scandal who claimed that dietary fat was driving heart disease went on to become the head of nutrition at the United States Department of Agriculture (USDA), where the federal government's misdirected low-fat dietary guidelines were created.

In a related finding, Dr. David Ludwig and colleagues from Boston Children's Hospital published a paper in 2007 showing the strong bias in published research funded by the food industry. These industry-funded studies were 760% more likely to be favorable to a food product compared to non-industry funded studies.[42] Again, this is not a conspiracy theory, but the unpleasant facts suggest that the people who previously dictated our health policy may not have been the most scrupulous, fact-driven, or objective reporters of truth. Based on recommendations from scientists who touted a low-fat, low cholesterol diet as the way to prevent heart disease, the US embarked on a 50-year journey down the wrong path. The assertions that *"Fat makes us fat"* and *"dietary cholesterol plugs up the arteries"* are not based on hard science. These badly constructed narratives aligned with, and even fostered, the advent of highly processed foods in our diet, and are leading culprits in the current explosion of type 2 diabetes, obesity, insulin resistance, and *increased* heart disease.

We are in the process of coming out of the dark ages of politically and commercially influenced nutrition science. Research-driven advisory committees are in the process of lifting limits on total fat and have removed restrictions on dietary cholesterol.[43] Science is showing, again and again, that fat is not the enemy; it is excessive sugar and highly processed foods. However, the message still needs to be carried further. A 2014 Gallup poll showed that most US residents are still trying to reduce fat in their diet, and the 2015 to 2020 Dietary Guidelines for Americans still recommends limiting calories from saturated fats to less than 10% of the total calories we eat each day.

There are multiple reasons why low-fat and low-calorie diets generally don't work in the long haul. Millions of years of evolution have enabled the human body to fight starvation and survive times of feast and famine. *No one* has the power to fight this system and win in the long run. If the brain thinks it is starving (even when the body has more than enough calories), it will fight back with everything it has, resulting in fat storage, unstoppable cravings, and food-seeking behavior. Conversely, if we sculpt the right diet (with adequate fiber and moderate amounts of healthy fat and high-quality protein), we can shut off cravings and promote a healthier **metabolism**. *For a dietary plan to work and be sustainable, we need to allow our brain and fat cells to feel satisfied, not starved, and allow the fat cells to release stored fat for energy production.* The bottom line is that low-fat diets are unnecessary in most cases, especially for children. Don't be afraid of dietary fat, just make sure it is the right kind.

### Myth #2: A calorie is a calorie
WRONG! All calories are not created equal.[44-49] Some, like those created from fructose, are more likely to be stored as fat, raise insulin, and cause inflammation. Others are burned more efficiently. Some feed a healthy gut **microbiome**, while others feed **dysbiosis** and a pro-obesity population of gut bacteria. The type of calories and the downstream metabolic effects dictate largely whether those calories are stored or burned. Broccoli and soda are both carbohydrates. They are not the same metabolically.

## Myth #3: It doesn't matter what we eat—we can just "burn off" excess calories with exercise.

Yes...but no. There is a great deal more to maintaining a healthy weight than just *"Calories in = Calories out."* This overly simplified mantra insinuates that all dietary sins can be absolved through exercise. On the contrary, it has been stated previously by cardiologists and exercise physiologists that *you can't outrun a bad diet!*[50]

Physical activity is critical to maintaining metabolic health. However, the value of exercise is not in the calories burned during the activity; it is in the teaching and the training of our cells and **mitochondria** (the cells' powerhouses). Physical exercise leads to improved insulin sensitivity and better glucose clearance from the blood into our cells. By teaching the body to metabolize both fats and carbohydrates more effectively and easing the burden on the pancreas, we can help prevent the metabolic abnormalities associated with insulin resistance, obesity, and diabetes. Regular exercise is no doubt crucial for staying metabolically healthy.

However, if exercising while continuing to give the body the wrong fuel and contaminants (such as excessive sugar and processed food), it is impossible to maintain good health indefinitely. A high level of physical activity can buy us some time, but sooner or later, the chickens come home to roost. (Ask any mechanic what happens to a lawnmower or boat motor when cheap low-octane, high-ethanol gas is used over time.) Teaching the body to metabolize fat the way it was designed to and choosing a healthy whole food diet, one does not have to count and cut calories to maintain a healthy metabolism. *Counting calories does not work unless one is a specimen in a metabolic lab.* The best way to sustain metabolic health is to focus on the *quality* and the *pattern* of the diet. Making food choices that support overall well-being and incorporating physical exercise allows the body to burn the right fuels.

## Myth #4: Some people can eat whatever they want and get away with it.

Most people who think they can eat whatever they want are not getting away with it. Just because someone is not obese, they can be (and often are) a ticking time bomb that would be detected with the right tests. Contrary to common thought, obesity is just one possible result of metabolic imbalance. Researchers at the University of North Carolina at Chapel Hill's Gilling's School of Global Public Health found that more than 80% of American adults are metabolically compromised.[51] Since the current estimate is that 40% of Americans are obese, *that means up to 40% of those with sub-optimal metabolic health are non-obese.*

Today's average human body struggles to metabolize the constant flood of sugar calories, so it converts the excess to fat (triglyceride) and stores them through a process known as **de novo lipogenesis**. *This doesn't always show up as obesity.* The metabolic imbalance may show up in other ways, such as another common phenomenon known as **TOFI** ("thin on the outside, fat on the inside," an actual clinical term).[52,53] What is TOFI? This can be a person who appears relatively thin but eats poorly: guzzling soda or wolfing down fast food at every turn while touting that they "burn it off"–perhaps to the envy of their overweight peers. Then one day, they "surprisingly" drop dead of a heart attack. Not surprising given what we now know.

When radiologists look at special magnetic resonance imaging (MRI) of TOFI patients, they find these people don't have the kind of excess fat stored just beneath their skin (making them appear thin), but the kind of fat that cakes the internal organs–a dangerous condition known as "visceral adiposity." If the correct labs are performed on these patients, we may find out that they are ticking metabolic time bombs. With proper analysis, chances are we will find markers such as insulin resistance, high inflammation and triglycerides, and a cardiovascular risk profile that makes a cardiologist shiver.

Is this rare? Hardly. As shown in the study just mentioned, *forty percent of "normal weight" adults* have some degree of metabolic syndrome and TOFI. Conversely, twenty percent of obese individuals have a healthy metabolism and are not as high risk as one would think based on appearances. In our modern but often misinformed society, there is a false sense of security and even superiority by those who do not carry their fat externally. This can be a fatal trap. Revealing markers such as fasting insulin and glucose, liver enzymes, fasting lipids with triglycerides and an ApoB, and inflammatory markers (high-sensitivity CRP) can tell the real story. If these all look good, they may be in the clear. If not, 'buyer beware' the next time they pass the donut shop! While these TOFI folks may not be obese, they may well have all the other signs of metabolic imbalance. This is the silent and unseen driving force behind many health issues such as type 2 diabetes and early heart disease.

Now that we have dispelled some metabolic myths, let's look at what a basic metabolic recovery plan should look like.

# A METABOLIC RECOVERY PLAN

### Step #1: Ditch the Sweetened Drinks!

The absolutely vital first step for every child (especially any child with a rapidly increasing BMI, who has evidence of fatty liver, or signs of insulin resistance or metabolic dysfunction) is to **remove sweetened drinks from their diet.**[19,54,55] It doesn't matter if it is juice, sweet tea, sweetened coffee drinks, chocolate milk, energy drinks, or soda. *To have a healthy child, sweetened drinks must be eliminated as a regular part of their diet.* Pediatricians and primary care providers need to start using sweetened beverage intake as a vital sign like blood pressure and heart rate. We must ask, "How many sweetened drinks per week is the child getting?" The goal is close to zero sweetened drinks except for rare, special occasions. Get rid of all of them and keep them out of the house. This is the low-hanging fruit (pun intended). This change alone can start children on their way to metabolic recovery, as has been shown in some of the studies mentioned in this chapter. Don't buy sweetened drinks or keep them in the house, and make sure the child's school does not allow open access to sweetened beverages.

An epidemiologic study in a 2015 issue of the highly respected medical journal *Circulation* stated that 25,000 deaths per year in the US are attributed to sweetened beverages.[56] This statistic quite likely grossly underestimates the situation. This figure may be significantly less than the 450,000 deaths attributed to smoking, but the loss of this many lives is completely unacceptable. Another study in 2015 published in the *British Medical Journal* calculated a nearly 20% increased risk of developing type 2 diabetes from just *one serving* of sugar-sweetened beverage, such as soda, per day.[57] (Interestingly, diet drinks also presented a significantly increased risk for diabetes, but this finding is highly controversial.) However, these epidemiologic studies look at large populations of people and their self-reported intakes of food items and disease incidence. The researchers then draw conclusions based upon this subjective recall versus actual physical evidence. For the average person, these studies may be interesting but not provide very compelling proof. For that reason, let's look at some more direct experimental data that show a potential link between sugar, heart disease, and diabetes.

A study in 2011 compared the effects of consuming three drinks per day containing glucose, fructose, or high fructose corn syrup on top of a regular diet to measure the impact on health markers for heart disease risk. For two weeks, 48 healthy adults consumed this diet, then had their blood drawn. The results were startling. The group drinking pure glucose had no significant increases in their heart disease risk markers (triglycerides, LDL cholesterol, and ApoB), but the fructose group had significantly increased markers, and the high fructose corn syrup group had the highest risk increases overall.[58] All calories do not have the same metabolic impact, and fructose at these levels (after two weeks) showed signs of damaging the body.

In a human intervention study in 2011, the researchers looked at the effects in healthy young men from drinking just one 20 oz soda per day and found evidence suggesting a significant increase in cardiovascular disease risk.[59] After only three weeks of drinking one soda per day, their inflammatory markers went up, they started showing signs of mild insulin resistance, and their small dense LDL (the dangerous cholesterol that sticks to the arteries) started to increase. Imagine what might happen after three years or thirty years of daily soda intake.

In 2015, Stanhope et al. performed a nonrandomized, double-blinded intervention study in which adults were divided into groups and consumed beverages sweetened with varying amounts of high fructose corn syrup (HFCS). These participants consumed HFCS as 0% (aspartame-sweetened), 10%, 17.5%, or 25% of their daily calories over a two-week period.[60] Daily blood collections were taken during the baseline and throughout the study. Their results showed that consuming beverages with 10%, 17.5%, or 25% of calories from HFCS produced a **linear dose-response** increase of triglyceride and cholesterol risk factors for heart disease as well as uric acid. A linear dose-response provides concrete evidence that the substance being studied is the driver for the marker being tested. The more HFCS they drank in this study, the higher the risk factors for heart disease, metabolic syndrome, and fatty liver.

A strong link between sweetened beverage consumption and NAFLD development is demonstrated in a meta-analysis published in 2019. The authors gathered data on 35,000 people from 12 different studies consuming varying amounts of sugar sweetened beverages. Yet again a linear dose-response was found, which showed the higher the intake of sweetened drinks, the higher the risk for fatty liver disease.[6]

These results support the findings of prior epidemiologic studies that suggest the risk of cardiovascular disease, fatty liver disease, and type 2 diabetes is associated with the consumption of increasing amounts of added sugars from sugar-sweetened beverages. Limiting sugary drinks is one of the most essential health measures we can make for our children.

### Step #2: Reduce the amount of added sugar in the diet!

The next step is to start reading labels to decrease a child's daily sugar intake. Hidden sugar is everywhere, with many names, and a parent's job is to detect and minimize it (most of the time) as much as possible. This may mean cleaning out the pantry and the freezer and doing a complete overhaul on the foods that were once regulars on the shopping list. Often, we have to find substitutes and healthier versions for some foods with less or no sugar added. Desserts and sugary treats should be reserved for special occasions and not become a nightly ritual, or just because it is someone's birthday (every day of the year is someone's birthday). Excuses for consuming large amounts of sugar and processed food can happen all year-round if we let them.

Based on compelling data, cutting most sugar out of the diet is essential for the metabolic health of the child—not what many parents want to hear, I know. Call me Dr. Killjoy. However, sugar isn't "joy" or "love." In fact, evidence indicates that excessive sugar consumption decreases serotonin, the brain chemical associated with true happiness. There is no quick fix, no magic bullet, no pill we can give anyone to reverse the effects of excessive sugar. Get the sugar out. The evidence is too strong, and the implications are too severe to ignore. Excessive sugar is a killer. The **World Health Organization** knows it, the American Heart Association knows it, the American Academy of Pediatrics knows it, and it's time you did as well.

The goal is for children (two and under) to have *zero grams added sugar* in their diet and for older children a maximum of 5% of their calories as added sugar (an average of 25 grams daily).[19] More accurately, using age-based recommendations for daily caloric intakes in a reasonably active child, 5% of calories as sugar would amount to a **maximum** of:

### TABLE 18.1 MAXIMUM GRAMS OF ADDED SUGAR BY AGE

| Ages of children (years) | Maximum grams of added sugar |
| --- | ---: |
| 0-2 | 0 |
| 2-3 | 15 |
| 4-8 | 18 |
| 9-13 | 25 |
| 14-18 | 25-32 |

*Performing the Sugar Scan*

Unfortunately, once we eliminate sugar-sweetened beverages, there is still a TON of *added sugar* and high fructose corn syrup sneaking in the food supply in a wide variety of foods, many of them targeted towards kids. ("Ton" is used lightly here: in 2017, over 11 million metric tons of sugar were consumed in the United States. Roughly 34% of this were in sugar-sweetened beverages, so that leaves more than 7 million metric tons of sugar consumed from other sources.) Parents need to start reading labels on cereals, yogurt, "fruit snacks," breakfast bars and snack bars, bread, and even lunch meat that may be adding tremendous amounts of sugar to the total daily load. Refer back to the 3 sample diets in Chapter 12. The preschool and school-age child can easily get over 70 to 150 grams of added sugar daily if parents are not paying attention. That's three to six times the upper recommended limit for children.

I encourage all parents to periodically do a "sugar scan" of their child's diet. Take one or two days (a weekday and a weekend are useful to compare) and write down everything they eat and drink for those days. Then look up the labels for these foods and drinks and jot down the amount of *added sugar* for each of the foods listed under the nutrition information. Consider the serving size carefully—many children eat more than one serving of hyper-sweetened foods when they are available. How many ounces of sugar-sweetened drinks are they consuming daily? At the end of the day, tally up the total grams of *added sugar* consumed. Odds are most parents will be unpleasantly surprised at how much sugar their children eat. Understanding the scope of the problem can be eye-opening. *What do we need to do to get a child's added sugar intake under 25 grams per day?*

+ Become aware of all the different names for added sugar and start reading labels.
+ Choose better breakfasts and skip the sugar-laden cereals, breakfast bars, and pastries.
+ Switch to the lowest added sugar options for sauces, salad dressings, condiments, snack foods, and bread. Be cautious of baked goods that tend to be loaded with added sugar. It all adds up!

Paying more attention to the added sugar and making healthier choices can put a child well on their way to metabolic recovery, as was proven by the following study.

A 2016 paper published in the journal *Obesity* described a study led by Dr. Robert Lustig. In this study, obese African American and Latino children with metabolic syndrome were recruited.[44] *Without reducing their daily calorie intake*, dietary sugar was reduced from 28% to 10% of calories, and starch (think pasta or bread) was substituted. Fructose intake was reduced to 4% of daily calories. It was an "isocaloric study," so no change in total calories was made, just a reduction in the amount of sugar, specifically fructose. The average diet was 50% carbs, 33% fat, 16% protein. Weight loss was not an intended part of the study. However, *after ten days*, the children lost on average 0.9 kg (2 lbs), their blood pressure decreased, their glucose tolerance and insulin levels improved (indicating improved insulin sensitivity), and there was evidence for increased fat burning. Fasting insulin and insulin resistance *decreased by more than 50%*. Fasting triglycerides were also reduced by 46%. After ten days the researchers saw profound improvements with the only change being reduction of sugar and fructose! That is pretty compelling evidence.

Refer to the Added Sugar Repository: https://hypoglycemia.org/added-sugar-repository/ that lists more than 250 names for sugar currently in the marketplace.

### Step #3: Work on smart choices and overall dietary and lifestyle patterns

I don't focus on strict portion sizes and counting every calorie or fat gram because the overall pattern of the child's diet matters most. Decrease the sugar intake and decrease a child's reliance on highly processed foods. Prepare as many meals at home as possible from simple, healthy ingredients. Increasing vegetables is going to be necessary. Learning to cook is going to be essential for regaining control over what our children are eating. Choose 100% whole grain, high fiber options whenever possible. These high-fiber, slower-release carbohydrates are better for our children's microbiome and put less strain on the pancreas. Reduce foods with enriched, bleached white flour. Look for labels that say 100% whole grain and ask for whole grain options while dining out whenever possible. Increasing fiber should be primarily through high fiber diet choices, but supplemental fiber such as psyllium may also hold benefits.

Finding ways to increase dietary fiber is going to be crucial for several reasons:

+ Fiber feeds the microbiome. A healthy microbiome is associated with improved metabolism, decreased inflammation, and improved insulin sensitivity decreasing risk for type 2 diabetes.[61,62]
+ Fiber supports the production of SCFA by the intestinal bacteria that have beneficial metabolic and epigenetic effects.
+ Fiber promotes a feeling of fullness and promotes appetite regulation.
+ Fiber effectively lowers the glycemic index of foods, slowing the absorption of carbohydrates and decreasing the post-meal insulin surges seen with low fiber processed food diets.

Don't underestimate the role of *high-quality protein* in the diet. Eating plans that incorporate good quantities of protein mainly in the form of meat, poultry, fish, or eggs have been shown to have several advantages. Some of these benefits may be possible with high protein plant-based foods as well. Higher protein diets help people feel more satisfied after a meal. If they do not immediately feel hungry again, they can stick with the diet more easily. Higher protein meals stabilize blood sugar levels after the meal, lowering insulin surge and helping prevent the roller-coaster effect. Proteins boost the metabolism after the meal by a process known as the *thermogenic effect of food,* which is highest with protein foods. They also support growth of lean mass (muscle), which is the most metabolically active tissue in the body.[63–66]

Combining a diet that contains healthy amounts of protein foods with high fiber foods may provide the best of both worlds, providing for a both better metabolism and a diet that is possible to maintain without feeling hungry.

Consider a diet like the Mediterranean diet with proven health benefits, but any vegetable and fiber-heavy diet will be far better than the **Standard American Diet (SAD)**. Many resources are available for eating a whole food diet.

### Step #4: Ditch low-fat or calorie-restricted diets
Significantly calorie-restricted diets do not work in the long run. The body is too smart for this, knows when it is being starved, and shuts down the metabolism, conserving fat stores. These very low-calorie diets also tend to lead to starvation mode in the brain, causing intense cravings and binging, which leads to even more weight gain (the yo-yo dieting that we have all seen).

To be metabolically healthy, especially for a growing child, we need to have the body in metabolic balance and not starvation mode. Counterintuitively, a person may need to *increase* the good fats like olive and avocado oils, nuts, and **omega-3s** to become more metabolically healthy. Having good fats in the diet is beneficial because fat does not stimulate insulin, and fat stimulates the fullness signals in the brain. We cannot forget that a child's brain needs fat to grow and function and that the brain is 60-70% fat. Cooking with avocado oil and olive oil, which are monounsaturated and have a higher smoke point, are recommended. Even some saturated fats like butter, palm, or coconut oil that have less chance of oxidation can be used healthfully *if not excessive*.

However, minimize deep-fried foods, especially from restaurants where they may use the same frying oil for days or weeks, which gets heavily oxidized and damaged from the heat. These fats can be hazardous to the body and brain and should be avoided when possible. Most vegetable oils and seed oils like sunflower, safflower, corn, soybean, and vegetable oils should also be used somewhat sparingly. Too much **omega-6** oil can promote inflammation and crowd out the essential omega-3 fats that are anti-inflammatory. Recall that inflammation is directly linked to obesity, insulin resistance, and type 2 diabetes.

Switching from a processed food diet, which is high in sugar and **oxidized oils**, to a whole foods diet with healthy fats and oils will provide many metabolic benefits. Based on the science, both for improving metabolism and reducing the risk of type 2 diabetes and heart disease, emphasis should be placed on *reducing the sugars and processed and refined carbohydrates*, not decreasing the fat content of the diet. This is not to say someone should go out of their way to gorge on lard, and especially not on trans or hydrogenated fats, but all this low-fat nonsense continues to steer us in the wrong direction. For the real goals of making someone more metabolically healthy and less at risk for developing heart disease and diabetes (with better blood lipids and lower insulin levels), a diet low in processed carbohydrates wins out over a diet that is low in fats and high in carbohydrates.

I am not suggesting all children should be on a very low carbohydrate diet, although obese or prediabetic children in some circumstances may benefit from one. Low carb diets are being examined in research studies, but they should only be undertaken with the guidance of a qualified physician or pediatric dietician. On the contrary, I think that improperly done a very low carbohydrate diet could be dangerous for a child. However, more children would benefit from a *high fiber, whole food diet with healthy fat*. Reducing the amount of sugar and highly processed carbohydrates and fats will hold immense long-term benefits for most.

### Step #5: Make sure children stay active

To improve insulin sensitivity in a metabolically compromised individuals, their bodies must be retrained to listen to the insulin signals and to burn fat as a preferred fuel source. Remember, the main benefits of exercise are not in the calories burned during the activity, it is the boost to our metabolism, specifically by improving our mitochondria. The mitochondria are the cells' power plants, and when they are not functioning correctly, things fall apart. Exercise and activity teach our little power plants to burn more fat at rest and even while we are sleeping. The high sugar, highly processed food diet full of **endocrine disrupting chemicals** has likely damaged many people's mitochondria to some degree, but this is recoverable.

By improving the body's insulin sensitivity, we decrease the need for the pancreas to keep pumping out high levels of insulin. Insulin levels drop, which helps stop the excessive production of fat in the liver and allows fat to be released from storage in the body to be burned for energy. Decreased insulin also helps lower body-wide inflammation, which helps to get our metabolism back on track, as inflammation derails many normal biological processes. Regular physical activity combined with a diet lower in sugar and processed food will help prevent the development of NAFLD, metabolic syndrome, obesity, and type 2 diabetes in children.

Find any way possible to get children active every day! Start small, with 30 minutes of walking, riding a bicycle or stationary bike, or just playing outside with other children. Swimming can be an excellent activity for overweight and obese children as it gets them moving without as much stress on their joints. Look into local programs at youth centers or fitness centers that may offer discounts or scholarships for kids. If located near a large city, there may be hospital-based multi-disciplinary programs that focus on metabolic health for obese and diabetic children.

### Step #6: Minimize exposure to obesogenic chemicals

Aside from the hidden sugar, the high glycemic index carbohydrates, and the lack of fiber, another damaging aspect of highly processed and packaged foods is the increased amounts of endocrine-disrupting chemicals

(EDCs) that may act to disrupt metabolism. Some of these chemicals are being labeled "**obesogens**," as they seem to promote fat storage in the body and derail our normal metabolism. BPA, phthalates, persistent organic pollutants (POPs), along with pesticide and antibiotic residues in our food may all be acting to decrease our metabolism and increase fat storage.[67-69] By cutting back on the packaged food, not microwaving in plastic containers, not eating or drinking hot foods or beverages in plastic, filtering our water, and paying attention to other sources of contaminants in our food and cosmetics, we can start cutting back on some of these chemicals entering our children's bodies. (Refer to Chapter 7 for more details).

### Step #7: Make sure children are getting adequate sleep. Be mindful of their stress levels

Take the situation of a child with a poor quality, high sugar diet, and combine that with a stressful environment (e.g., the modern world, especially in a financially disadvantaged home) and sleep issues (an American epidemic) and we really throw the metabolism a knockout punch.[70-73] Lack of sleep or disruptions in the sleep-wake cycle, like staying up late playing video games or having sleep apnea, totally derails the body's regulatory system and almost instantly makes a person become more insulin resistant, crave processed carbs, and have dysregulated hunger and satiety signals. *Chronic sleep issues can make a person prediabetic very quickly.* Getting 8 to 10 hours of *quality* sleep improves appetite regulation and improves the body's sensitivity to insulin, helping to stave off prediabetes.

Chronically elevated stress in children and adults increases the stress hormone cortisol, contributing to insulin resistance and increasing the phenomenon of "stress eating" highly processed carbs. Elevated cortisol levels from stress also increase visceral and central (abdominal) fat storage.

> Stressed spelled backwards = Desserts

For more details on sleep hygiene and stress mitigation, refer to the "Six Pillars of Health" in Chapter 1.

### Step #8: Make sure children are getting adequate amounts of key nutrients

Assuring that our children receive all their essential nutrients promotes insulin sensitivity and a healthy metabolism, but fiber, magnesium, vitamin D and dietary antioxidants and **phytonutrients** may be especially important.

The importance of dietary fiber for maintaining a healthy metabolism was discussed earlier. We know that most children in the US and many other industrialized countries are not getting adequate fiber in their diet, so this is a vitally important nutrient to boost in their diet, mostly through food. However, supplements can be helpful as well.

Magnesium is required for proper carbohydrate metabolism, insulin action, and entry of glucose into the cells. Magnesium is also anti-inflammatory and protective of the heart. In earlier chapters, we discussed that **subclinical** magnesium deficiency is rampant in the US and other industrialized countries, likely contributing to insulin resistance and the development of heart disease, type 2 diabetes, and NAFLD. People with diets higher in magnesium appear to be protected somewhat from the development of cardiovascular disease and type 2 diabetes and several studies have linked low magnesium intake with insulin resistance in children.[74,75] Other studies have shown improvements in insulin sensitivity and glucose control with magnesium supplementation in insulin-resistant or diabetic individuals.[76–79] Especially for children who are obese or at risk for insulin resistance and development of diabetes, focus on magnesium-rich foods and consider a magnesium supplement of 100 to 200 mg daily to help with insulin sensitivity and glucose control. Discuss this with their healthcare provider to make sure it is safe to do so. Refer to Chapter 12 on common nutrient deficiencies in children for more information on magnesium.

Recently, vitamin D deficiency has also been associated with insulin resistance and the development of type 2 diabetes.[80–83] Low vitamin D levels are common in obese individuals, but it is unknown if this is harmful or just an association (bystander effect). Some studies have shown an improvement in glucose control in people with diabetes who were given vitamin D supplements while others have not shown a beneficial effect. Given the myriad important effects of vitamin D in the human body, efforts should be made to correct a low vitamin D in a child, especially one who is obese or at risk for developing insulin resistance and metabolic syndrome. The goal for blood levels is greater than 30 nmol/l.

We know that there is a damaging role of **oxidative stress** in developing insulin resistance, metabolic syndrome, NAFLD, and cardiovascular disease.[84–88] Therefore, dietary components (a.k.a. **antioxidants**) that help protect the body against *oxidation* are also likely to protect against the development of these "diseases of Western civilization." However, rather than megadosing on vitamin C, we should incorporate foods with naturally occurring antioxidants and phytonutrients that decrease oxidative stress in the body. "Eating the rainbow" of multiple colorful fruits and vegetables ensures that we are getting a host of protective compounds in our bodies that help to shut off inflammation and the genes that code for inflammation. It also helps to ensure that we are getting other important micronutrients like chromium that directly help with insulin sensitivity, and selenium, which is a component of several important antioxidant enzymes in the body.

As we stated earlier, making positive changes in our diet is relatively simple, but not always easy. Old habits die hard, individual and family patterns can be resistant to change. Add to this the addictive properties of sugar and hyperpalatable junk foods and it is easy to see why not everyone is jumping at the opportunity to get healthier. But at the end of the day, all those excuses are not going to save your child. It is not an exaggeration to say that your child's life depends on making these changes. As parents, schools, governments and corporations, we need to do better for our children.

> *It's ok to start small. One better choice leads to another and can start reversing the health tailspin we are in as a nation. And if you ever feel like it is getting too hard to make the right choice or do the right thing, just look at your child. Hug them and ask yourself if there is anything you wouldn't do for them, to make their life better and a little bit healthier. That love more than anything else will fuel positive change.*

## SCHOOL BREAKFAST AND SCHOOL LUNCH PROGRAMS; THE ROLE OF SCHOOL SYSTEMS

For any of the teachers, school administrators, or parents on the school board or PTA who happen to be reading this book, your attention and help are desperately needed. What use is trying to make positive changes at home if the child's diet is undermined at their school? If we want to see test scores improve, behavioral issues decline, attendance and a child's overall health improved, the school food system needs to do its part. Working to improve the quality of the food offerings at our schools and daycares will pay significant dividends down the line. Starting *real* nutrition education early and reinforcing positive choices throughout a child's growth and development is imperative.

I realize budgets are tight, and in some cases, the system is set up against us, but forward-thinking people across the country are making an impact and implementing changes in their local school systems for the better. Governmental systems and subsidized nutrition programs will have to change under pressure from the **World Health Organization, American Academy of Pediatrics,** The US Military (who are *very concerned* about lack of eligible recruits due to the obesity epidemic), and We the People. Do not underestimate the power of local activism and involvement with local school boards and politicians to reverse the harmful effects of years of sugar and food industry lobbying and manipulation. Get educated, get mad, connect with the inner mama/papa bear, and *demand* positive change for your children and all the children in our communities. Below are listed some ideas for action items to improve nutrition in our school systems.

Potential Action Items for the US School Systems

+ School Breakfast Program- Restrict/eliminate high sugar cereals/breakfast bars/pastries/juices
+ Offer healthier whole food meals for breakfast and lunch and limit added sugars.
+ Eliminate high sugar chocolate milk as an option
+ Eliminate access to soda and sugar-sweetened beverages on all campuses
+ Provide child/parent education on the dangers of sugar much in the way of the DARE program and drug abuse prevention
+ Restrict the practice of giving out candy as rewards in the classroom
+ Get more schools working with local agriculture and ranching to provide farm-to-school meals
+ Involve students in food growing, preparation, and cooking to increase practical knowledge of food and nutrition. Some schools are creating their own on-campus gardens as part of the curriculum.

+ Incorporate age-appropriate nutrition education throughout the school system- K-12.
+ Consider screening for nutrient deficiencies by performing a three-day diet analysis on at-risk children, which can then be used to target dietary change or supplementation of the deficient nutrients.
+ Have **reverse osmosis** water filters installed on campus to ensure easy access to clean lead/arsenic-free water is provided for hydration without plastic bottles.
+ Reinstate physical education as a mandatory core of the education curriculum in all schools.

## NUTRITION R$_X$

**1** Early identification of a child who is at risk for insulin resistence and development of type 2 diabetes is crucial so that the problem can be addressed early.

**2** A rapidly rising BMI, acanthosis around the neck and armpits, and high intake of sugar-sweetened beverages are all signs that the child could be headed for trouble.

**3** Discuss with your child's PCP whether any further testing is warranted. Elevated liver enzymes, uric acid level or a HOMA-IR score can sometimes provide more insight into metabolic damage that is occurring and may be a better metric than just focusing on the scale.

**4** The first step in metabolic health is to minimize a child's exposure to sugary beverages, including soda, sweet tea, fruit juice, and chocolate milk. Then start reducing the added sugar in the food.

**5** Emphasize a whole food eating plan, with plenty of fiber and magnesium rich foods while reducing reliance on fast food and packaged foods.

**6** Keep your child physically active

**7** Ensure adequate, good-quality sleep, which is crucial to healthy metabolism.

# CHAPTER NINETEEN

# DIET AND THE CHILD'S BRAIN

Can the diet that we are feeding our children be damaging or impairing their brains? ADHD, behavior problems, anxiety, and depression are the most commonly diagnosed mental disorders in children. How much of this is nutrition related?

We already discussed the impact of prenatal nutrition and early life feeding on the infant's brain. How we feed our children as they grow and develop later in childhood may have a lot more to do with their mood, behavior, and academic performance than we previously realized. This chapter will look into ways to support our children's brains as they move beyond the critical **first thousand days** and into the school years.

Even though the school-aged child is well past those critical first thousand days of life, diet still plays an essential role in health and academic performance. This is not the time to give up. Sound diet rules still apply. We need to give growing children foods that:

+ support the ongoing growth, development, and health of their brain
+ support the healthy gut microbiome
+ limit epigenetic programming for chronic disease

It is imperative to remember that just because most parents feed their kids a certain way doesn't mean that the average child's diet is healthy or safe. The **Standard American Diet (SAD)** is damaging and dangerous no matter how many people we know are eating this way. Look around. There are life-long ramifications of a suboptimal diet for our children.

When we look at the common dietary deficiencies discussed in Chapter 12, it is like reading a "Who's Who" of essential brain nutrients that are lacking in many children. The typical Western diet also alters the gut **microbiome**, disturbing the **brain-gut-microbiome axis** and promoting inflammation throughout the body and brain. We are learning more every year about the roles of critical nutrients, epigenetic programming, and the microbiome and their profound effect on a child's learning, behavior, and mood.

According to the **CDC**:[1]

9.4% of children aged 2-17 years (approximately 6.1 million) have received an ADHD diagnosis.

7.4% of children aged 3-17 years (approximately 4.5 million) have a diagnosed behavior problem.

7.1% of children aged 3-17 years (approximately 4.4 million) have been diagnosed with anxiety.

3.2% of children aged 3-17 years (approximately 1.9 million) have been diagnosed with depression, which is likely significantly underdiagnosed and underreported.

Depression and anxiety have increased over time. Among children aged 6–17 years, these disorders increased from 5.4% in 2003 to 8% in 2007 and to 8.4% in 2011–2012.

Worldwide, 20% of children and teens experience a mental, behavioral, or **neurodevelopmental disorder**. As mentioned previously, 3.5 million children in the US are presently on ADHD medication, compared to 600,000 in 1990. It was reported in 2014 that 11% of US kids have been diagnosed with ADHD at some point in their lives, an increase of 42% from 2003. The worldwide prevalence is estimated to be somewhere in the neighborhood of 5 to 7% of all kids having ADHD.[2]

Why are the rates of these brain issues rising in our children? While there is some evidence to suggest that we are doing a better job of screening and therefore increasing the diagnosis of these conditions, there is also evidence that these brain conditions continue to increase in the general population. Again, despite a strong family link with a few of these disorders, such as ADHD, we cannot blame genetics. In my opinion and that of a growing number of scientists, these are primarily environmental disorders. The obesity epidemic and the surge of pediatric cognitive and mood disorders are an overlapping phenomenon. It is well documented that obese and overweight children overall do not perform as well academically, and that obese children are at increased risk of ADHD.[4-6] It is also becoming abundantly clear that sugar and processed food play a role in the obesity epidemic. Is there a way to link diet, inflammation, and brain dysfunction?

A staggering number of US kids are medicated for ADHD. More than 30% of those treated are still symptomatic despite the medications. Many children experience medication side-effects, including headache, abdominal pain, loss of appetite, and sleep disturbance.[2,7] This is a significant issue, as ADHD is associated with lower academic performance, behavioral outbursts, increased risk-taking behavior, and even all-cause mortality (risk of death from any cause). ADHD, at the very least, can severely impact the child's quality of life and leads to overall increased stress on the child, school, and the family. Unfortunately, 50% of children with ADHD will continue to battle this disorder into adulthood. Taking the long view on ADHD, the brutal reality is that research shows stimulant medications may help initially, *but there is a very real possibility that the effects will eventually wear off.* In most children, medications either lose their effectiveness or the side effects increase to a point where they must be discontinued. Then what? What are we going to do when we can't medicate our way out of this?

Increasingly, evidence shows that many brain disorders may be:

+ Inflammatory in nature
+ Triggered by environmental exposures that may be contributory or causative
+ Associated with and perhaps partially caused by nutrient deficiencies in the diet
+ Associated with alterations in the gut microbiome
+ Associated with **leaky gut** and leaky **blood-brain-barrier**

All of these factors are directly affected by what the child eats. Multiple studies show that children with ADHD have a much more nutrient-deficient diet than children without this disorder. Most children with ADHD consume less nutrient-dense foods such as vegetables, meat, fish, and eggs and consume more nutrient-poor **ultra-processed foods** high in sugar and salt. This may lead to a vicious cycle where the poor diet worsens the ADHD, and the ADHD changes the brain to crave addictive unhealthy foods.[8-11]

The cycle can be broken. Dietary therapy and nutritional supplementation may prevent or improve symptoms of common brain disorders such as ADHD, potentially reducing the need for escalating doses of medication (and possible side effects) and prolonging the benefits. Why not use nutritional therapy as a strategy? If improving our children's diets can decrease the risks and severity of neurological disorders like ADHD and improve cognitive and academic performance, this additional strategy could have far-reaching benefits, both socially and financially.

How can we ensure that we are nutritionally supporting optimal brain function in our children? How can we best prevent or treat brain disorders like ADHD, depression, and anxiety in our children? These are questions that every primary care provider, parent, school, daycare, and government regulatory agency should be asking. This chapter will review some of the evidence supporting the link between diet and a child's brain.

# HOW CAN DIET AFFECT CHILDREN'S BRAINS, LEARNING, MENTAL HEALTH, AND MOOD?

Diet can directly or indirectly influence brain function and brain disorders like ADHD. By examining these links, we can provide a framework for creating healthier diets for our children's brains. Mechanisms of diet impact on the brain include:

1.  Structural and functional support for **neurons**, **neurotransmitters**, and growth factors
2.  Neurotoxic effects of additives and contaminants
3.  Effects on detoxification pathways in the body
4.  Effects on the supply of energy for the brain
5.  Effects on the Brain-Gut-Microbiome (BGM) axis
6.  Effects on brain inflammation

### Neuronal death by a thousand cuts

One very important point to keep in mind is that the modern diet's impact on a child's brain is rarely caused by one single nutrient deficiency, one isolated imbalance, or one single toxic exposure. This must be made abundantly clear: for most kids, *multiple insults* occur simultaneously–a "death by a thousand cuts." Making one change or adding one single nutrient supplement to a poor diet, is unlikely to achieve anything clinically significant (although sometimes miraculously it does!). Improving the brain health of our children requires a multifaceted and multi-targeted approach that considers all the potential deficiencies, excesses, and toxicities. Making changes in the overall patterns of the diet and supplementing nutritional deficits are most likely to result in clinical benefits.

Research studies in Western medicine are usually designed to only change one thing (variable) at a time. This often results in "reductionist" thinking. However, the human body and brain are too complex to view from a reductionist perspective. Studies that have compared two dietary patterns, if done correctly, (like looking at the Mediterranean diet versus other diets) have shown significant improvements in health while recognizing that it is the overall *pattern* of the diet, not just the olive oil or the red wine, that gave the benefits. This is how we need to view nutrition and child brain disorders (minus the red wine). What is the overall pattern of their diet and exposures? How can we reshape this pattern to be healthier?

## THE MULTIPLE HIT HYPOTHESIS

**System Overload!**
Kids at greater toxic risk than adults:
- Toxic dose per weight is much higher
- Less able to detoxify some chemicals
- Immature brain and rapid growth
- Critical development windows

SAD diet low in vital brain
and detoxification nutrients:
- Iron, zinc, magnesium,
  DHA, folate, choline, B₁₂,
  phytonutrients

INADEQUATE NUTRITION
FOR BRAIN DEVELOPMENT

IMMATURE/
DAMAGED BBB

INADEQUATE
PROTECTIVE NUTRIENTS

INCREASED OXIDATIVE STRESS

LEAD
MERCURY
ARSENIC

DETOXIFICATION
PATHWAYS

BPA
PHTHALATES
PFOS

PESTICIDE
RESIDUES

(DYSBIOSIS)
LEAKY GUT &
ENDOTOXINS

# STRUCTURAL AND FUNCTIONAL SUPPORT

Specific nutrient deficiencies in pregnancy and childhood can leave the young brain structurally unsound and unable to perform properly. Even more subtle **subclinical deficiencies** can have a negative impact on brain performance. The brain is continually reconfiguring itself through the processes of **synaptogenesis** and **neurogenesis.**

*Neurogenesis* is the creation of new neurons. Once thought to be complete by age 2, it is now known that neurogenesis can occur throughout the lifespan, albeit on a much smaller scale than in the **first thousand days** of life.

*Synaptogenesis* is the creation of new connections between existing nerve cells (neurons) in the brain. Synaptogenesis is how learning occurs, and the reinforcement of connections between neurons is thought to be how new information is stored in the brain.

*To support ongoing optimal synaptogenesis and neurogenesis, the proper nutrients must be present, and certain toxins that damage neurons and hinder these processes should be avoided.*

Diet can affect brain chemistry and the production of the chemical signals known as **neurotransmitters** produced by the brain, such as dopamine, serotonin, and **acetylcholine**. A delicate balance of these signals in our brain is needed for a stable mood, sustained attention, and the ability to learn. Disrupting this balance has strong potential to affect mood and the ability to focus and learn. How can we expect our children's brains to work well if we are not supplying them with the necessary components needed to grow, maintain, and protect themselves and manufacture the proper neurotransmitters? It doesn't make logical sense.

## Key Brain Nutrients

Certain nutrients are vital to brain function and commonly low in large numbers of children (especially those with ADHD, neurodevelopmental, or behavioral issues). While this does not necessarily imply causation, there is an association between poor diet and increased risk of deficiency of several essential nutrients in kids with ADHD, including iron, zinc, magnesium, B6, B12, folate, choline, vitamin D, **omega-3 fats**, and high quality protein.[7-20,26-30,43-48] These are reviewed extensively in chapter 12. Selecting a diet rich in these nutrients is important for supporting your child's developing brain.

### TABLE 19.1 NUTRIENTS AND THEIR EFFECT ON THE BRAIN

| Nutrient | Effect on the brain |
| --- | --- |
| Iron | Myelin formation, neurotransmitter formation, oxygen delivery |
| Zinc | Needed for 200+ enzymes in the body, neurotransmitter formation |
| Magnesium | Needed for 300+ enzymes, neurotransmitter formation, calming/neuroprotective |
| B6 | Supports detoxification, neurotransmitter formation |
| B12 | Supports detoxification, neurotransmitter formation |
| Folate | Supports detoxification, neurotransmitter formation |
| Choline | Key component of nerve cell membranes and neurotransmitters; detoxification |
| Vitamin D | Supports nerve growth factors, neurotransmitter formation |
| Omega-3 EPA | Anti-inflammatory, brain protective, stimulates nerve growth factors |
| Omega-3 DHA | Key component of nerve cell membranes, stimulates nerve growth factors |
| Protein | Supplies amino acids to build neurotransmitters |

## Using a multi-targeted approach

We know from studies and clinical experience that the diet of most American children is suboptimal and may be inadequate in several vital nutrients that allow for proper brain functioning. This is especially true for children with ADHD, who often tend to have an inferior diet high in processed, nutrient-poor foods. The million-dollar question is *would a child's behavior and brain functioning improve if we corrected nutrient deficiencies by enhancing the quality of the diet and using safe levels of supplementation of several vital nutrients*, rather than relying on a single nutrient approach? If a child is low in 5 to 10 essential brain nutrients, shouldn't we correct *all* the deficiencies so that their brain has the best chance of functioning properly? Studies looking at isolated supplementation of omega-3, zinc, vitamin D, and magnesium for ADHD have shown positive results for some patients.[21-25,49-55,58-61] Several recent studies using L-methylfolate for depression have also found positive results.[31,32] Research using a multi-targeted supplementation approach containing combinations of the nutrients discussed earlier indicate potential benefits for ADHD, depression, and autism.[7,24,56,62-66] If safe doses are used, nutrient supplementation would appear to have minimal risk and considerable potential benefit.

## REDUCING NEUROTOXIC CHEMICALS

Chemicals, heavy metals, and pesticides in our food and water have the potential to damage or kill brain cells. More than one thousand chemicals commonly used in various US industries are known *neurotoxins*. Deficiencies in crucial protective nutrients like **antioxidants** and **phytonutrients**, magnesium, and folate also lead to suboptimal functioning of detoxification pathways used to rid our bodies of these contaminants. The inability to properly detoxify these items and clear them from the body increases the potential for damage to a child's brain. Remember that a growing brain may be more vulnerable to damage by toxic exposures and inadequate nutrition than an adult brain. **Oxidative stress,** neuroinflammation and a specific neurotoxicity called "**excitotoxicity**" are being looked at as potentially contributing to autism and ADHD, among other brain disorders. The Standard American Diet could be contributing to oxidative stress and neuroinflammation by a growing number of neurotoxic chemicals with insufficient antioxidant nutrients to "quench the fire." Ignoring the effect of these substances on our children is dangerous, and ongoing research is raising red flags on many of these chemicals. As a refresher, here are a few of the items in our food supply that could negatively affect our children's brains. Please refer back to Chapter 7 on **toxins** for more detail.

One of the problems with Western medicine is that it has a reductionist view of human health and disease. It still carries with it the desire to narrow health issues down to a "one disease, one cause, one pill" model. While this model works well for a simple infection, it does not work well for something as complex and nuanced as a neurodevelopmental disorder such as ADHD or autism. In reality, many of these increasingly common brain disorders are likely the result of a number of insults that can occur before and after birth:

- Nutrient deficiencies (overt and subclinical)
- Harmful environmental influences (toxic chemicals and oxidative stress)
- Genetic predispositions that increase susceptibility
- Decreased ability to detoxify harmful compounds in the body
- Damaging epigenetic modifications from environmental exposures
- Impaired energy production by cells in the brain
- Increased inflammation in the brain
- Altered intestinal microbiome

Individual children may have different sets of exposures and predispositions that all end up leading to neurodevelopmental disorders. To borrow an analogy, many roads lead to the same destination. These differences can make it more difficult to study affected children as a group and make it easier to discount the role of diet or toxic exposures. The **Multi-Hit Hypothesis** figure illustrates the variety of potential insults, or "hits," that can occur to the child's brain during the critical early years of development. This book clarifies which steps can be taken to minimize exposure to these threats and supports parents as they strive to protect the development of their children's brains and bodies. This starts on day one, at conception or even prior!

## Pesticides

Growing evidence suggests that exposure to neurotoxic pesticides in pregnant mothers or young children may play a part in the increased rates of neurodevelopmental disorders in children. Because of these risks to our children's brains, the American Academy of Pediatrics and other scientific research groups, as well as the United Nations, have issued position statements and action plans to limit or eliminate organophosphate pesticides in our foods.[67,68] Exposure to increased levels of pesticides via diet, as measured by urine levels of pesticide metabolites, has been associated with double the risk of ADHD.[69,70] However, five days on an organic diet eliminated detectable levels of pesticides in kids' urine.[71]

### BPA and Phthalates

Exposure to both BPA and phthalates has been linked with an increase in ADHD behaviors, and a recent **meta-analysis** links early-life exposure to the development of ADHD.[72-77]

### Heavy Metals

Lead, arsenic, and mercury are all neurotoxic, and all have the potential to damage a child's brain and drop their IQ. There is *no safe level* of any of these heavy metals. Taking steps to reduce a child's exposure is crucial.

### Artificial Food Coloring

See Food Additives in chapter 11. Recent evidence suggests a link between high amounts of artificial food coloring in a child's diet and hyperactive behavior, even in kids without ADHD.[78-82] The European Union requires food products with artificial food coloring to carry a warning label.

## DIET AND BRAIN ENERGY

Recall that an infant's brain uses more than 70% of their total calories whereas an adult brain uses about 20%. A toddler or school-age child is likely somewhere in the middle of these, using a high proportion of daily calories. A steady supply of fuel is essential for a well-functioning brain. Recall that the brain only runs on two fuels—glucose and **ketones**, so one or both of these fuels need to be in steady supply for optimal brain functioning. A proper diet and metabolic machinery maintained by adequate exercise are both essential for continuous energy production in the brain. A diet rich in lower **glycemic index** carbohydrates, healthy fats, and adequate protein is better suited to sustained brain performance by supporting a steady supply of fuel for the brain.

Low blood sugar, inattention, and behavioral issues are related. The brain runs on a steady supply of either glucose or ketones. It cannot use any other fuel. Interrupt the supply chain, and the brain runs out of options. We must look carefully at the substance as well as the timing of what we feed our kids. Food choices and timing can affect whether there is a steady supply of fuel to the brain, what neurotransmitters are being produced, and the ability to maintain sustained attention. Optimally, humans can handle a reasonably long duration of time between meals while maintaining an adequate supply of fuel to the brain, utilizing glucose from its stored form (glycogen) in the muscle and liver, and ketones derived from our fat stores. However, in the modern world, in a somewhat nutritionally compromised child who is not metabolically healthy and perhaps obese, they cannot always access this stored energy between meals. This could lead to impaired mental performance if the correct diet is not eaten.

It has been shown decades ago and confirmed in recent meta-analyses that skipping breakfast (or lack of access to breakfast in inner-city or financially disadvantaged kids) impairs brain and school performance in children.[83-85] This led to the development of the school breakfast program to make sure that all school-age kids have access to breakfast. Unfortunately, many if not most of the original studies justifying this program were funded by the food industry, and some of the foods that are served via this program are suspect.[85] High sugar cereals, chocolate milk with added sugar, pastries, and doughnuts loaded with sugar and unhealthy trans or oxidized fats are not a good alternative to skipping breakfast. These foods promote tooth decay and obesity and may not be the optimal way to fuel brain performance.

As discussed in Chapter 17, high glycemic index foods are the foods that raise blood sugar levels quickly but then can lead to low blood sugar (rebound hypoglycemia or "bonking") when there is an excessive **insulin** response to the rising glucose. These foods have been shown to have a negative impact on the ability to sustain attention in some children. *A high sugar/high glycemic index breakfast may contribute to blood sugar instability, increased stress hormones, decreasing sustained attention, behavioral changes including inattention, fidgeting, anxiety, hunger, and cravings, leading to decreased academic performance.* Let's review some of the evidence.

A study by Dr. David Ludwig at Boston Children's comparing effects of a low, medium, and high glycemic index meal on stress hormones in kids showed a significant spike in blood levels of the stress hormone epinephrine four to five hours after a high carb/high sugar meal.[86] Another recent study in 2013 comparing **low glycemic index** to high glycemic index meal showed a plummeting blood sugar level one to two hours after the high glycemic index meal, with a corresponding significant increase in stress hormones and hunger.[87] More recent research showed that significantly less energy is available for the body and brain several hours after a high carbohydrate versus a low carbohydrate breakfast in overweight adults.[88] Reactive hypoglycemia (bonking) was found to be common in obese adolescent females after consuming a sugar-containing beverage.[89]

Several research studies comparing a high sugar breakfast cereal to a low glycemic index breakfast in school-aged children generally show improved brain performance and memory in the low glycemic index group.[90–95] However, the glycemic effect on brain function in children is not universally accepted and is still being debated. A recent meta-analysis indicated that the data supporting lower glycemic index breakfasts were inconclusive for other cognitive measures besides memory.[95] Study results may depend on whether quick versus sustained attention are being measured. Impact of the diet on school performance may also vary depending on the child's overall metabolic health. A normal weight, metabolically healthy child may not be as affected as a child who is obese or insulin resistant.

Overall, there seems to be a consistent consensus that a high glycemic index breakfast, while supplying a "quick" energy burst, is not as beneficial for *sustained attention and memory* as a low-glycemic index, low-sugar meal with moderate fat and protein. Based on the evidence, what happens to a child mid-morning after a breakfast of sugary cereal or a few pastries? The blood sugar drops, the stress hormones spike, the fuel supply to the brain falls short of demand, and sugar craving signals are sent from the addiction center in the brain. *Imagine how this affects a child's attention, learning, and grades!* A better breakfast has the potential to improve their performance, behavior, and mood.

### Protein
Adequate protein in the diet supplies essential amino acids that support neurotransmitter production in the brain and proper child growth. Estimated minimum needs for school-age kids are just below 1 gram of protein for every kilogram of body weight (for example, a child weighing 70 pounds (32 kg) should get at least 30 grams of quality protein daily or slightly more). If children are addicted to carbohydrates, only eating cereal, pasta, sweets, and bread, and no meat, fish, chicken, eggs, or beans, they may not be getting enough *high-quality protein* to support their bodies and brains. There is evidence that the *quality* of the protein eaten affects neurotransmitter production in the brain.[38–40] Dietary patterns favoring high-quality protein foods like fish, chicken, and pork were shown to be protective against ADHD.[15] Adequate protein and fat in a meal tends to change the glycemic index (how fast the meal raises blood sugar), with evidence suggesting that lower glycemic index meals support more sustained attention in school-age children.[41,42]

Are we feeding our children a diet that supports sustained brain energy and the correct neurotransmitters to help them pay attention and succeed in school? When you eat a meal with high-quality proteins and lower glycemic index carbohydrates like vegetables or salad, how does *your* brain work, and how do you feel? Alternatively, how does *your* brain work after consuming a high carbohydrate/high glycemic index, low protein meal comprised of a hefty serving of pasta or a large stack of pancakes? For me, there is no comparison. High-carb meals kill me every time, and my brain goes into shut down mode as I slide into a post-meal food coma.

If I want to get things done, have sustained attention, and be highly effective, I need a meal with moderate protein from fish or lean meat and some high-quality fat such as extra virgin olive oil or avocado. The same will likely apply to many school-aged children. Make sure to get some high-quality proteins in their diet, especially for breakfast and lunch when their brain can use the protein for "awake and aware" neurotransmitters. Consider a protein shake, eggs, sausage, or full-fat low-sugar yogurt in the morning (rather than skipping breakfast or grabbing a sugary cereal) to boost their intake and their mental performance.

### Effect of Sugar on Behavior

How does sugar specifically affect the child's behavior? Can sugar cause hyperactivity? There is a longstanding controversy regarding the behavioral effect of sugar in children. Dozens of studies have been performed looking for a definitive relationship between eating sugar and objective measures of attention and hyperactive behavior. To date, results have been mixed at best, and meta-analyses (studies that pool together all the results from several prior studies) cannot find a definitive relationship.[96,97] When reviewed, there were many variations between these studies (known as heterogeneity) involving the design of the studies, the patient populations, and the background diets, which sometimes makes it more difficult to prove a relationship.

The current data is not strong supporting a link between sugar and hyperactivity in children *as a population*. However, we can *mechanistically* make a case for why sugar might negatively affect a susceptible child's behavior and learning. Excessive sugar promotes inflammation, leaky gut, an altered microbiome, and unstable blood sugar levels in susceptible individuals. All of these dysfunctions could affect a child's brain.

As a pediatrician, I adhere to the Cardinal Rule of Pediatrics: ***"Listen to the parents."*** If large numbers of parents (or even one) are telling us that when their kids eat sugar or artificial food coloring (or any food for that matter) they have an adverse reaction, our responsibility is to listen to them and take them seriously. This is referred to as the "N of 1" or *personalized medicine* approach. The distinction between *personalized medicine* and *population-based medicine* is important.

As a *population*, giving children peanut butter is safe, as the vast majority of children tolerate this food without issue. Do we roll our eyes and balk when parents tell us their child has an anaphylactic reaction to peanuts? "No, your child can't have a negative reaction to peanuts because the research says most kids have no reaction." That would be ridiculous. Why are other foods held to a different standard? What if some children metabolize sugar differently, or have a different microbiome that causes them to react negatively to high doses of sugar? They might behave quite differently than another child without those factors.

Western medicine can sometimes appear arrogant or at least resistant to evolving science. Some health professionals seem to struggle with the idea that what we feed our children can affect their brains. While the field of nutritional psychiatry is gaining awareness and respect, many medical professionals appear to be utterly unaware of food as psychoactive medicine. They may be more inclined to prescribe a medication than investigate the nutritional basis of a child's condition. Is it that much of a stretch to concede that what we feed our children can influence mood and behavior?

## BRAIN-GUT-MICROBIOME AXIS

With an ever-growing number of studies demonstrating the relationships between our gastrointestinal tract, gut microbiome, and brain, care needs to be taken to support these crucial functions, especially among our children. One of the most exciting areas of research in medicine is the role of the **brain-gut-microbiome axis** in several neurologic and psychiatric disorders, including depression and anxiety, ADHD, even autism.

## BRAIN GUT MICROBIOME AXIS

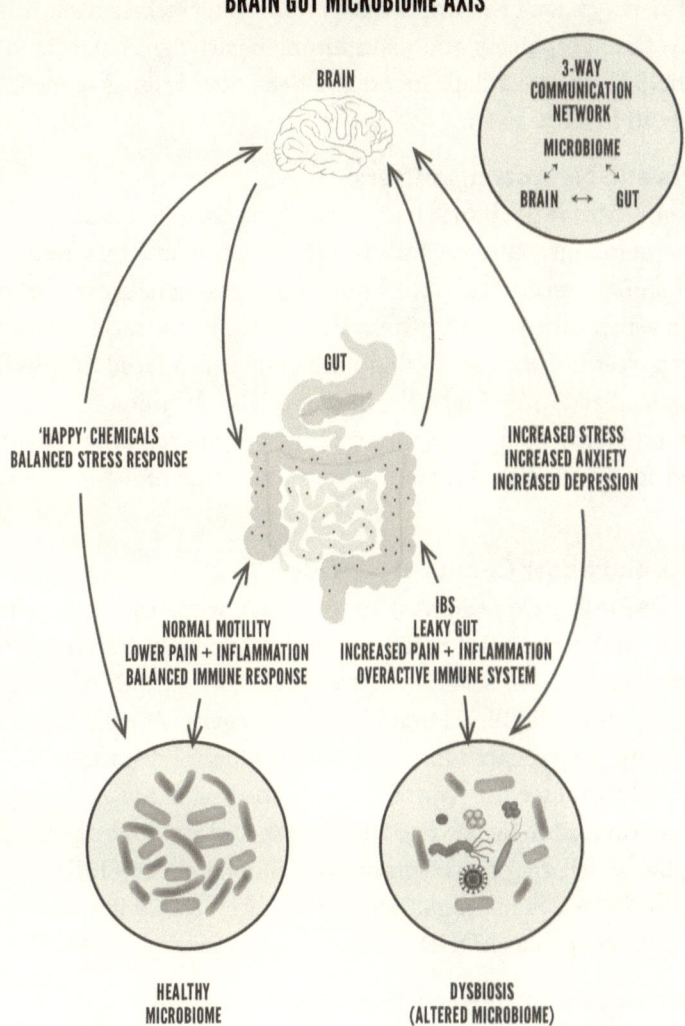

The BGM axis refers to the complex interplay between our brain and the nervous system of the gut (the enteric nervous system, sometimes referred to as the second brain) and the large family of bacteria living in our gut at any time (the microbiome). Having an imbalance of bacteria or overgrowth of "bad" bacteria in the gut (referred to as **dysbiosis**) can lead to the production of bacterial by-products that negatively affect brain and gastrointestinal function and may contribute to neurodevelopmental disorders like ADHD and autism. Conversely, having a healthy gut microbiome promotes brain health and balanced neurotransmitter activity that fosters improved mood and mental performance. Many children's microbiome may have been impacted by numerous factors discussed previously. Could repairing and maintaining healthy gut bacteria in our children help to improve their mood and behavior? Science is revealing the answer to this question.

### Probiotics and Neurotransmitters

Research shows that **probiotic** bacteria such as *Lactobacillus* and *Bifidobacteria* manufacture several crucial neurotransmitters and influence neurotransmitter receptors in the brain. The calming neurotransmitters GABA and serotonin are both heavily influenced by bacteria in the gut.[98–101] Ninety percent of the serotonin in the body is produced in the GI tract, both by specialized intestinal cells, influenced by the microbiome, and by the gut microbiome itself. Disruption of the gut microbiome can affect GABA and serotonin signaling in the brain, affecting mood and brain function.

### Probiotics and Short Chain Fatty Acids

**Short Chain Fatty Acids (SCFAs)** are produced when certain gut bacteria metabolize soluble fiber and **resistant starch** from our diet. Aside from fueling the intestinal cells that help prevent "leaky gut," SCFA are also found to help maintain blood brain barrier integrity. A leaky blood brain barrier is being investigated in a host of neurological disorders. SCFA are potent signaling molecules from the gut to the brain. They increase **brain derived neurotrophic factor (BDNF)** release and support the regulation of microglia, which are primary immune cells that control inflammation in the brain. Excessive microglia activation is implicated in many neurological disorders such as ADHD, autism, and depression.[103–105]

### Probiotics and Brain Derived Neurotrophic Factor

Increasing evidence shows that another mechanism by which the microbiome influences the brain is by promoting the production of support molecules called **neurotrophins**, including the most studied BDNF, which is like is "miracle-grow" for the brain. BDNF is one of the main neurotrophic factors that stimulate new nerve growth and keep neurons alive and healthy as we age. Growing evidence supports a link between gut bacteria and the production of BDNF, both by the production of SCFA by the gut bacteria and direct stimulation.[102,103] Reduced levels of BDNF have been seen in ADHD as well as conditions like Alzheimer's. It is also worth noting that omega-3 (fish oil) intake and intense exercise also boost BDNF levels.

## Probiotics, Leaky Gut, and the Blood-Brain Barrier

Through several mechanisms, including SCFA and epigenetic effects, the microbiome influences both intestine and blood-brain barrier permeability. An intact barrier in both the gut and the brain is crucial to preventing excessive inflammation in the brain from immune cells (especially microglia) that get activated by responding to "bad" gut bacteria, their by-products, and incompletely digested food molecules. Increased permeability (a leaky barrier) leads to increased levels of inflammatory **cytokines** (proteins involved in cell-signaling) being released from the body's immune system. Cytokines can leak into the brain and activate microglia cells, stimulating brain inflammation that may contribute to neurologic disorders. Increased permeability of the gut is being linked to a host of neurological and autoimmune disorders in addition to cardiovascular disease.[98,104,106] Through this process, science suggests dysbiosis leads to a leaky gut, which contributes to a leaky brain and brain disorders.

## Probiotics and the HPA Axis

Our gut bacteria regulate stress hormone production through a system called the *hypothalamic-pituitary axis (HPA)*, which involves the brain and the adrenal glands. A dysregulated HPA that causes an abnormal stress response is thought to be involved in several neurologic and psychiatric conditions, including ADHD, depression, and anxiety disorders. There is a fascinating two-way street with the BGM axis; early life stressors are known to reshape the microbiome, with the microbiome then influencing the body's stress response. There may be a critical window in early childhood during which probiotic bacteria have the best chance at balancing stress response and the HPA axis, stressing the importance of a healthy microbiome in the first thousand days.[98]

## Probiotics and Epigenetics

Our intestinal bacteria have the power to affect our **gene expression** positively or negatively. Substances like SCFA produced by the microbiome affect the expression of genes involved in inflammation and immune activation. Based on our diet, lifestyle, and microbiome, do we express genes that promote inflammation and disorders like depression and ADHD or the genes that suppress them?

## Proof of Evidence for the Brain-Gut link

Proof is growing that alterations in the gut microbiome can lead to changes in behavior, learning, inflammation, and mood. Let's break down a little of the recent evidence pointing to a link between gut bacteria and brain health.

The high incidence of gut issues in children with ADHD and mood disorders (as well as autism), whether that be chronic abdominal pain, "irritable bowel," or constipation, suggests impaired intestinal functioning and a coexisting dysbiosis that may be involved in the process.

In mouse models, germ-free mice (those raised without any probiotic bacteria or microbiome) had exaggerated stress response via the HPA axis, which was reversible by giving probiotics (*Bifidobacteria infantis*) within a critical time window when the mice were younger.[102,107,108]

Depressive symptoms in rats (nothing is sadder than a depressed rat) were transferable to other rats receiving gut bacteria (a fecal microbiome transplant) from the rats with "depression."[109] Similarly, hyperactivity in mice was inducible by transferring the microbiome of hyperactive humans into normal mice, making them hyperactive.[110] These animal models show evidence that the bacteria living in the gut partially control mood and behavior. What if this were true in our children?

A recent study showed that kids with autism were three times more likely to have evidence of a form of dysbiosis known as **small intestinal bacterial overgrowth (SIBO)** on a breath test, at a prevalence of 31%.[111] Several studies showed improvement in symptoms of autism in some of these children when placed on antibiotics, thereby altering their microbiome.

A recent study out of Arizona State University demonstrated that performing a fecal microbiome transplant in a group of children with autism *led to long-term improvements in both their gastrointestinal and autism symptoms*.[112,113]

An early (pilot) study from 2015 showed that infants receiving a probiotic for the first six months of life had a significantly lower risk of having ADHD at 13 years of age.[114]

A recent review paper looked at higher quality clinical trials of pre- and probiotics for the treatment of anxiety and depression. Their conclusion was that while **prebiotics** by themselves appeared to have no significant effect, *every* qualifying study examining the effects of *probiotics or combinations of prebiotics and probiotics* "demonstrated a significant, quantitatively evident decrease or improvement of symptoms and bio-chemically relevant measures of anxiety and depression."[115]

Overall, while solid evidence supports a link between the gut, microbi-ome, and brain, research into diagnosing and treating many brain-related conditions using probiotics or altering the microbiome are still in the early stages. More research is needed using more uniform testing meth-ods and utilizing more uniform probiotic supplements that incorporate multiple species instead of a single species. So far, no convincing evidence has shown that isolated probiotic supplementation improves symp-toms of ADHD or that probiotic supplementation later in childhood will improve cognitive functioning in children. Again, improving the diet with more fiber and phytonutrients to shift the microbiome to a healthier profile should always be the first and most crucial step to a longer-term improvement.

### Small Intestinal Bacterial Overgrowth
**Small intestinal bacterial overgrowth (SIBO)** is an extreme form of dys-biosis and altered microbiome.[116,117] Once thought to be out on the fringe of science by Western medicine, SIBO is now acknowledged as a valid clin-ical condition. Recent research shows that many cases of **irritable bowel syndrome** may be related to this overgrowth of unfriendly bacteria in the small intestine.

The symptoms of SIBO can vary but almost always include bloating, abdominal pain, and pressure after meals, and may sometimes be accom-panied by nausea, constipation, or diarrhea. There is growing interest in the link between dysbiosis, SIBO, and brain and mood disorders such as depression, anxiety, and "brain fog."[118] Just about anyone can get SIBO, but risk is increased in those with a history of multiple antibiotics, intestinal surgery, and underlying motility disorders (where food does not move through the intestines in a normal fashion). Anyone taking long-term acid blockers like proton pump inhibitors (PPI) or eating a diet high in processed foods and added sugar is at increased risk of dysbiosis and SIBO. Although less well defined and researched in younger age groups, kids can get SIBO too, and growing numbers of children are getting tested and treated for this condition.[119-121] Correctly diagnosed and treated SIBO can be a game-changer in the way some kids and adults feel and act.

# BRAIN INFLAMMATION

Multiple links exist between diet, inflammation, and the brain.[122-128] These links may involve both direct and indirect dietary effects on inflammatory chemicals produced by the body, permeability of the intestine and **blood brain barrier**, the gut microbiome, and the expression of pro-inflammatory genes.

The Western diet, environmental toxins, and disturbance of the gut microbiome are all felt to contribute to low-grade inflammation in the brain in a susceptible person. There is mounting evidence that low-grade inflammation and a dysregulated, overstimulated immune system may be involved in multiple diseases, including brain disorders like depression, ADHD, and autism. Studies show that markers of *oxidative stress* are increased in brain disorders, such as depression and ADHD, indicating that the body's protective mechanisms are not fully operational or may be overwhelmed.[129] Oxidative stress and inflammatory chemicals can damage brain cells, contributing to brain disorders.

The diet of the typical American child promotes inflammation in several ways:

### The wrong fats
Historically, the highly processed diet that most kids had been eating contained significant amounts of hydrogenated and artificial **trans fat** (until the FDA finally banned the latter in 2018). Processed foods are often high in oxidized pro-inflammatory **omega-6** vegetable and seed oils and lack anti-inflammatory omega-3s **(ALA/EPA/DHA)**. This shift in omega-6 to omega-3 ratios makes the Western diet very imbalanced and inflammatory.

### Too many refined carbs and sugars
The average child's diet is far too high in sugar and refined grains and flours. These ingredients tend to spike blood sugar levels and cause increased *insulin secretion* by the pancreas and *increased oxidative stress* on the body. High insulin levels and **insulin resistance** are associated with increased inflammation. High amounts of fructose in the diet (from juice, sweetened drinks, added sugar, and high fructose corn syrup) increase free radical formation and markers of inflammation in the human body. High sugar, low fiber diets promote gram-negative bacteria (think *E. coli*) in the gut, producing a chemical called lipopolysaccharide (LPS) which is very inflammatory in the body and brain. In the setting of a leaky gut or

high amounts of these bacteria, LPS can increase in the blood, causing inflammation, even in the brain.

## Not enough antioxidants from fruits and vegetables

Vegetables are the root of a healthy life. Without vegetables, the diet will be low in magnesium, fiber, phytonutrients, and antioxidants, which *decrease a child's ability to buffer inflammation and oxidative stress*. Oxidative stress refers to the damage to the body by free radicals, which are compounds that occur naturally in the body but are kept in balance by antioxidants in our foods and antioxidants produced by our bodies given the proper nutrients. Research shows that phytonutrients are important **epigenetic modifiers**, helping to *turn off* genes that promote inflammation in the body and brain as well as *turn on* genes that quench free radicals.

## Low fiber

A low vegetable/low fiber diet, high in sugar and processed foods, can also lead to a state of *dysbiosis,* with increases in *"bad" bacteria and inhibition of probiotic bacteria.* Fiber feeds probiotic bacteria in the gut, and lack of fiber causes gut bacteria to consume the protective layer in the intestines, potentially leading to leaky gut and inflammation. Probiotic bacteria, fed by dietary fiber, have been shown in multiple studies to have powerful immune-modulating effects. These include protecting the body, preventing leaky gut, and controlling excessive inflammation and overactive immune responses through the actions of T-regulatory cells and other mechanisms.

## High Allergy Foods

Foods with the highest allergic potential (wheat, dairy, and soy) constitute the majority of the American diet, which is bad news if someone has food allergies and intolerances. Undiagnosed **food intolerances** may drive inflammation in some, but not all kids. There is increased risk of ADHD in children with allergies, eczema, and asthma. Some speculation exists that undiagnosed food intolerances could be driving adverse behavior in a subset of these children with ADHD and autism. Eliminating these foods is endorsed as a possible therapeutic measure for ADHD and autism, referred to as the *Few Foods Diet* or the **Oligoantigenic Diet**. We will explore this in some detail later in the chapter.

## Chemicals, pesticides, and food additives

These are described in greater detail in Chapter 7. Conventionally grown produce and highly processed foods may contain increased amounts of chemicals, pesticides, and food additives, which can act as endocrine disruptors, inflammatory agents, and **epigenetic modifiers** turning on genes for chronic inflammation. Growing evidence suggests that inflammatory and immunologic mechanisms linked to exposure to neurotoxic chemicals such as pesticides may raise the risk for brain disorders.

# ANTI-INFLAMMATORY AND ELIMINATION DIETS

Shifting to a whole food diet rich in antioxidants and phytonutrients from fruits and vegetables, with healthier fats from olive oil, avocado, nuts, and fish, can help support the body's protective mechanisms and decrease oxidative stress on the brain. We have reached epidemic proportions of children with ADHD, anxiety, and depression. If we are looking to prevent these disorders, an anti-inflammatory diet is an excellent place to start. Given the growing evidence for the link between a pro-inflammatory diet, altered microbiome, leaky gut, and brain disorders, a dietary overhaul is a potential therapeutic intervention with multiple justifications.

# DIET, INFLAMMATION AND DEPRESSION

Depression is increasingly recognized as a disease related to brain inflammation in some patients, especially those resistant to treatment.[130,131] Environmental risk factors for depression include early life stressors, trauma, obesity, and the Standard American Diet (SAD) full of sugar and processed food. All of these factors stimulate inflammation, as does dysbiosis and an altered microbiome via the mechanisms described earlier. Anti-inflammatory medications are being investigated for their possible roles in treating resistant depression.[132]

A recent meta-analysis of studies looking at the effects of pro-inflammatory versus anti-inflammatory diets on depression found a 40% increased risk of depression among those eating a pro-inflammatory diet.[126] In recent research called the SMILES (Supporting the Modification of Lifestyle in Lowered Emotional States) study, the researchers looked at the effect of placing people with major depressive disorder on an anti-inflammatory diet using a randomized controlled trial, the "Holy Grail" of medical proof. The dietary intervention group following a modified Mediterranean diet with social support showed significantly more improvement in mood and overall symptoms of depression at 12 weeks than a social support group not receiving the diet.[133]

When considering the combined risks and loss of quality of life and health care costs associated with depression, anxiety, and ADHD, adopting a Mediterranean style diet or some other type of whole-food-based diet could save many lives and billions of dollars in the healthcare system. The fundamentals for a brain-healthy diet cut to the beneficial core of what diets like the Mediterranean diet are all about—whole-food, vegetable-heavy, anti-inflammatory, and brain-friendly. The Standard American Diet is SAD for our children's brains and needs to be significantly altered if we are going to pull out of our society's mental health tailspin. Adoption of anti-inflammatory brain-healthy diets can give us happier, healthier, and higher functioning children. What are we waiting for?

### Basics of the Anti-Inflammatory Diet

Based on the research, we can forge a dietary blueprint for supporting healthy brain function in our children. Let's begin by working towards a diet that minimizes the big players in the inflammation game.

Limit the obvious dietary factors promoting inflammation:

+ Added sugars, especially excessive fructose, which directly increase inflammatory markers in otherwise healthy individuals.
+ Highly processed carbohydrates (especially white flour-based products), which are essentially metabolized instantly as sugar in the gut, spiking insulin levels, and promoting dysbiosis.
+ Unhealthy hydrogenated oils and **trans fats** (the worst food industry experiment of all time).
+ High omega-6 fats like corn oil, sunflower, safflower, and vegetable oil, which may get heavily oxidized, act like trans fats in the body, and act as inflammatory precursors.
+ Artificial food additives and **toxicants** such as artificial colors and flavors, pesticide residues, and preservatives that may promote inflammation and act as endocrine disruptors.

Eat more anti-inflammatory, brain-friendly foods with well-documented health benefits, such as

+ Green, nutrient-rich, leafy vegetables (e.g., kale, spinach, mustard, chard)
+ Cruciferous vegetables (e.g., broccoli, cauliflower, brussels sprouts, cabbage)
+ Fresh colorful fruit (e.g., berries, grapes, pomegranates)
+ Cold water fish (e.g., salmon, trout, sardines, and herring)
+ Non-seed oils (e.g., extra virgin olive oil, avocado oil)
+ Nuts (e.g., almonds, walnuts, cashews, pistachios)

Overall, any diet that emphasizes vegetables, fruits, nuts, whole grains, and good fats will be vastly superior to the average Western diet. A brain friendly diet will also contain some high-quality protein sources. These may vary based on any potential food reactions (see below) but may include chicken and turkey, fish and seafood, beef, pork, eggs, and game meat.

### Dietary Elimination and ADHD: The Oligoantigenic "Few Foods" Diet

Growing evidence shows that a number of children with ADHD and autism can react negatively to certain common foods, worsening their behavior. There is also evidence that food *intolerances* (not full-blown allergies) may be stimulating some children's immune systems, causing chronic low-grade inflammation that affects the child's brain. Some of the most common foods in the American diet may partially drive an inflammatory response that affects some children's brains. Once an initial effort has been made to decrease the significant inflammatory agents in the diet and increase the anti-inflammatory vegetables, fruits, omega-3 fats, and probiotic/prebiotic foods, we may also need to consider if there are common foods in the child's diet that could be adversely affecting their mood and behavior.

Unfortunately, there is no blood test for this, no skin test, no "muscle test" that is accurate. The only way to tell if certain foods are a behavioral trigger is to eliminate these foods for several weeks and observe how a child feels and behaves. This is referred to as the "Elimination Diet," the "Few Foods" diet, or the "Oligoantigenic diet." This is not voodoo or witchcraft; this is supported by real science and is backed up by multiple studies and meta-analyses in highly respected peer-reviewed journals starting in the 1980s.[8,134–141] The studies show there are responders and non-responders to the "few foods" diet. According to the research, up to 60% of children with ADHD respond favorably to the diet *with a good number able to discontinue their medication*. Not all studies on elimination diets showed positive results, but the majority did. The collective data from all qualifying studies shows the potential for an elimination diet to improve ADHD symptoms in a significant number of kids.

The naysayers will argue that any positive effect of changing the child's diet is due to the increased attention that a child gets on this diet from parents and teachers versus an effect of the diet itself. I don't buy that argument. There is sufficient probable cause and research into mechanisms for why these diets can and do work. Knowing the failure and side effect rate of ADHD medication, elimination diets and other nutritional interventions mentioned here should be used far more often than they are currently—with medical backing and assistance.

Is an elimination diet going to work for every kid with ADHD? No, but evidence shows a strong likelihood that eliminating certain foods may improve behavior and attention *in more than half of children with ADHD*, especially when other nutrient deficiencies are addressed. Properly guided nutritional interventions are safe, they are backed by science, and they can be used along with pharmacologic therapy to improve the behavior and performance of the child. Why aren't we using these dietary therapies more?

### How to perform the *few foods* elimination trial
The list of foods to be eliminated on the few foods diet may seem daunting. Wheat/gluten, dairy products, soy, corn, eggs, artificial food coloring, sugar, and peanuts are the main items shown in studies to be some of the leading culprits. The proper *few foods diet* used in the most rigorous of these studies temporarily eliminates *everything* except a restrictive shortlist of foods over four weeks. During this period, allowable foods include lamb, chicken, turkey, rice, quinoa, potatoes, banana, apple, pears, broccoli, cauliflower. This diet may be the most effective at looking for a response, but it is very restrictive and not meant to be sustained long term. Once it is determined whether a child responds to the restricted diet, foods can be systematically reintroduced one at a time, monitoring for symptoms, under guidance from healthcare/nutrition professional.

| Allowable Foods on the Few Foods Diet | Foods to Eliminate on the Few Foods Diet |
|---|---|
| Lamb | Wheat/barley/rye |
| Chicken | Dairy products |
| Turkey | Soy |
| Game meat | Corn |
| Rice | Eggs |
| Quinoa | Beef |
| Potato | Pork |
| Sweet potato | Added sugar of any kind |
| Banana | Peanuts |
| Apple | Artificial food colors |
| Pear | MSG (autolyzed yeast/yeast extract) |
| Broccoli | |
| Cauliflower | |

Before looking at this food elimination list and just giving up, let's take a step back for a second and consider a few things. *This is temporary.* The strict elimination period generally lasts 4 to 6 weeks before challenging foods back in. If you discover that a food is a major trigger, you are likely not going to want to feed it to your child and endure the behavioral deterioration. There is *absolutely no harm* in trying a well-planned elimination diet, removing sugar and other common triggers like wheat, dairy, and food coloring. There are no nutrients a child will be deficient in by removing these foods if the proper steps are taken.

Also, if the child on this diet begins to feel and act significantly better, they may not want to go back to their old diet and feel awful all the time. How much easier would life as a parent be if your child's mood and behavior were more stable? If the diet doesn't work . . . no harm, no foul. *But what if it works,* and you suddenly have a different child on your hands with better behavior and attention?

I have lived this. I did an elimination diet over 20 years ago, and it changed my life. I do not have ADHD as far as I know (although I was accused of having it by an attending physician during my pediatric residency after weeks of sleep deprivation, but that is another story). Eliminating problem foods had profound effects on my brain function and gastrointestinal system. The first few weeks were a little rough (food withdrawals are very real). But when I broke through the other side, it was like a fog had lifted. My brain felt like a laser, and my processing speed and information retention skyrocketed. Having my brain in this state allowed me to rock the MCAT (the medical school admission test) and was a turning point in my life. If I had not done this dietary elimination trial, I would likely not be a physician today.

Making change is not easy, especially when it comes to diet. This is even more true with children who have behavioral, developmental, or emotional issues. It may be challenging to pull this off in a house with multiple kids and a crazy schedule, but it is possible. To be successful, *GET SUPPORT* from friends, family members, teachers, online support groups, a good dietician, a nutritionally educated medical provider. Build your team! Make a plan and develop some strategies. With help and support from the proper resources, it is possible to dramatically increase the chances of success. I know this type of change can be hard, and initially, it may be extremely challenging. Nonetheless, if this diet can do for a struggling child what it did for me, I strongly encourage parents to consider this option.

Aside from my personal experience, there is ample scientific evidence that this nutritional approach benefits many children with ADHD or behavioral issues. For these children, are amphetamine-based or powerful psychoactive medications the best answer? I'm not saying these medications don't have their time and place, but medication is *never* the substitute for proper nutrition.

The parent wishing to pursue this nutritional path may get pushback from their child, other parents, or even their health care provider. This diet goes against the societal norm and challenges many widely held beliefs about what is "normal" and "healthy." Despite what others may tell you, this is an evidence-based approach. Feel free to share the references in this chapter with any skeptics to help educate them that science is showing diet can make a difference in a child's mood and behavior.

At the end of the day, I believe in using the "N of 1" approach, which asks the question, "Does YOUR child get better by incorporating some or all of these nutrition recommendations?" As a clinician, that is what I care about. At the end of the day, what matters is the individual, not the population at large. Did I help *that* child who came to my office for help? Your child is not a statistic, they are not a population, they are YOUR child, a beautiful, unique individual. How does their diet affect *them*? The proof is in the pudding so to speak.... A whole new field is emerging called "*personalized nutrition,*" and the "one size fits all" nutrition model is rapidly becoming obsolete. Welcome to the leading edge of nutrition—and the *power of one*.

For a sample menu on an elimination diet, please refer to the website for this book www.feedingourchildren.com, or www.thomasflass.com

# NUTRITION R$_X$

According to the research, a child's diet can impact their chances of academic success as well as protect them from the worst symptoms of disorders such as depression, anxiety, and ADHD. Adopting a healthy brain eating plan should be a consideration for all parents of a school-aged child.

Components of a healthy brain eating plan include:

**1** Starting each day with a healthy breakfast containing *moderate* fat and protein, lower glycemic index carbohydrates, and *minimal* sugars and refined carbohydrates.

**2** Making sure your child's brain has a steady supply of fuel by having a more balanced diet, as described in this chapter.

**3** Doing our best to limit exposure to neurotoxic chemicals/additives/pesticides in the diet and getting children the proper nutrients to support their body's ability to detoxify them.

**4** Supporting proper brain structure and function with proper amounts of essential nutrients like iron, zinc, omega-3 fats, adequate protein, choline, B$_{12}$, and folate.

**5** Removing or limiting pro-inflammatory agents in the diet and following an anti-inflammatory diet as much as possible.

**6** Repairing and maintaining their microbiome to support the brain-gut-microbiome axis

**7** Considering an elimination diet for children with ADHD or behavioral issues to determine if they react negatively to certain foods

# CLOSING THOUGHTS

We have covered a lot of nutritional ground. Peeling back the layers of an unhealthy food system can make us want to crawl under the covers and just give up. *Don't do it. Don't give up the fight.* If not for yourself and your own health, keep fighting for your children, for their future. Because as we just found out, what you feed them may largely determine their future health. Don't look back and get paralyzed by guilt or self-doubt about what you should have done differently. Keep looking forward. Making even small, sustainable changes will add up to a better future for your child.

Simple changes are not always easy. Making the right choices for your child can seem like swimming upstream against a powerful current. I get it, because my wife and I live in those same currents every day, and so do an increasing number of parents. Doing the right thing, making the right choices at the end of the day when you are spent and pulled in a thousand different directions may require you to dig deep. I am hoping that making good choices will become easier for all of us as more people become educated about the dangers in our current food system. The tide is turning. Increasing numbers of parents are, like you, peeking behind the curtain and not liking what they see. Tribes are forming—parents and communities are demanding better for their children, parents who realize the Standard American Diet is not acceptable for their kids or any kids.

Going against the grain can be unpopular. People who challenge the established norm may be attacked, discredited, and slandered for their ideas by forces who would like things to stay the way they are because it benefits them emotionally or financially. That is the way of the world, and the way the game is rigged. For this reason, I included more than a thousand references from peer-reviewed scientific journals that back up the information and recommendations in this book. I'm not saying I have all the answers, but when we compile the research done by thousands of dedicated scientists and physicians, we find clear evidence that the modern diet damages our children, evidence that would be foolish and dangerous to ignore.

As we pull back the curtain on what is happening to our children and their health, I have to ask a question: Do *you* want things to stay the way they are? Or do you think we can do better, as parents, as corporations, and as a nation? And I'm not asking everyone to be an activist for changing the food system (although if you have the gumption that would be fantastic). I am asking us to look at our own diet and what we are Feeding Our Children and do what we can in our own homes to help turn the tide.

Vote with your wallet. They say, "money talks and BS walks," so at the end of the day buying and serving real food makes the difference locally and globally. Start cutting back on the highly-processed garbage that is taking over our supermarkets. If you ain't buyin it, they ain't makin it....

Consumer demand is changing. Do you know who the largest sellers of organic produce in the world are? Walmart and Costco. Farmers markets, community supported agriculture, and urban gardens are popping up even in our big cities. Sustainable ranching and agriculture are rising behind the scenes because people like you realize the way we shop, the way we cook, and the way we are Feeding Our Children impact the health of our families.

But we must work together. We need help from those involved in our daycare and educational systems to provide better food when our children are away from home. We need help from the support systems that supply food to our nation's most vulnerable and financially challenged kids, so that healthy food is available to every child. People far smarter than me have done the math and calculated that by cleaning up our food systems we save *billions* of dollars with decreased health care costs and improved outcomes and achievement in our children. So why aren't we doing more?

As said before, I don't have all the answers. I am just a guy who likes to connect the dots and follow the research to find a way out of our current mess. I am a parent who loves his children more than anything, and who will do whatever it takes to protect them and give them the best, healthiest life possible. I am hoping that you are too.

# GLOSSARY

**A**

**AAP**. An abbreviation for *The American Academy of Pediatrics*, the largest academic governing body that oversees education, policies, guidelines, and recommendations for pediatric medicine.

**acanthosis**. Also called *acanthosis nigricans*; a darkening of the skin, typically around the neck and armpits that is associated with insulin resistance and prediabetes.

**acetylcholine**. An important signaling molecule (neurotransmitter) in the nervous system and brain made from choline.

**adaptive immunity**. The parts of our immune system that "learn" which specific invaders to fight.

**advanced glycosylation end products (AGEs)**. Proteins and other structures in our bodies that get damaged by excessive sugar, altering their structure and promoting inflammation.

**alpha-linolenic acid (ALA)**. An 18-carbon (short chain) omega-3 fatty acid found in plant foods such as flaxseed, canola, and hemp.

**anaphylaxis**. A potentially life-threatening allergic (IgE-mediated) reaction to medication, food, or insect stings that results in hives, swelling, and breathing issues.

**anti-nutrients**. Natural compounds in plant foods, including phytates and lectins, which can block the absorption of certain nutrients such as iron and zinc. These compounds also have some health benefits and are not entirely detrimental.

**antioxidant**. A substance, typically a vitamin, phytonutrient, or enzyme that neutralizes damaging chemicals (free radicals) in the body and helps reduce *oxidative stress* thereby preventing damage to our cells.

**ApoB**. Abbreviation for *apolipoprotein B*, a protein marker that is part of every lipoprotein cholesterol (LDL) molecule produced in our body. The higher the ApoB level, the more lipoprotein cholesterol molecules we have in our blood. Having higher numbers of small dense LDL (as measured by a high ApoB) is more dangerous for the heart than having fewer large "fluffy" LDL (with a lower ApoB). ApoB may be a better marker of cardiovascular disease risk than standard LDL.

**ARA**. Abbreviation for *arachidonic acid*. A long chain polyunsaturated omega-6 fat found in meat and eggs. It is made in our body from omega-6 linoleic acid found in plant oils like corn, sunflower, safflower, and vegetable oil. ARA is vital for the growing child, but too much ARA promotes inflammation in the body.

**ARFID.** Acronym for *Avoidant Restrictive Food Intake Disorder*. A common pediatric feeding disorder and a severe form of "picky eating."

**autoimmune disease.** A disorder in which the body's immune system attacks and destroys its own tissues. Examples include type 1 diabetes, Hashimoto's thyroiditis, and rheumatoid arthritis.

## B

**baby-led weaning (BLW).** A method of weaning infants to solid foods that skips purees and allows the infant to feed themselves from the initiation of solid foods.

**bioavailability.** The amount of a nutrient that is digested, absorbed, and assimilated into the body from foods. A food that has a moderate amount of a low bioavailable nutrient is therefore not a great source for that nutrient, as relatively less is absorbed into the body.

**blood brain barrier (BBB).** The structure of the blood vessels in the brain that acts as a gatekeeper, only allowing in very select nutrients. A leaky BBB is implicated in a number of brain disorders.

**body mass index (BMI).** A metric that looks at someone's weight per height to calculate a proxy for body fatness and obesity.

**brain-gut-microbiome axis.** The 3-way communication that goes on between our brain, the nervous system of our gut, and the bacteria that live in our intestines.

**brain derived neurotrophic factor (BDNF).** A chemical produced by the brain that stimulates growth of new neurons and supports the health of existing brain cells. It is protective of the brain at all ages and helps prevent age-related cognitive decline.

## C

**carbohydrate.** Any number of dietary sugars (simple carbohydrates) or chains of sugars (complex carbohydrates like starch).

**casein.** One of the main proteins in animal milk. Casein is the main protein in cow's milk but is found in lower amounts in human milk.

**CBC.** Acronym for *complete blood count*, a lab test that looks at the numbers of white and red blood cells in our bodies.

**CDC.** Acronym for *Center for Disease Control and Prevention*. The US government's health protection agency.

**chelated.** Minerals such as zinc and magnesium are sometimes bound (chelated) to agents that increase their absorption into the body. These *chelating agents* can include amino acids such as glycine or other organic acids.

**cirrhosis.** Advanced stage of liver disease characterized by scarring (fibrosis) of the liver. Cirrhosis is the final step in liver disease before liver failure occurs.

**complementary diet.** The first foods added to an infant's diet other than breastmilk or formula.

**conjugated linoleic acid (CLA).** A special type of fat in milk that may be protective against heart disease and diabetes.

**cytokines.** Chemical messengers in our bodies that can send signals to our cells to perform certain actions, for example pro-inflammatory cytokines increase inflammation in the body.

**D**

**de novo lipogenesis.** The process of the liver making new fat from carbohydrate or other substrate.

**DHA.** An acronym for *docosahexaenoic acid*, a long-chain omega-3 polyunsaturated fatty acid that is highly concentrated in the human brain. Very small amounts can be made in the human body. Found in the diet in fish and to a lesser degree in eggs.

**dysbiosis.** An imbalance in our intestines with overgrowth of potentially harmful bacteria and too few beneficial (probiotic) bacteria.

**E**

**eclampsia.** Seizures during pregnancy caused by severe high blood pressure (preeclampsia).

**electromagnetic fields (EMF).** The fields emitted by most electronic devices.

**elemental formula.** Infant formula that does not contain any intact protein, only amino acids. These formulas are fully hypoallergenic.

**endocrine disrupting chemicals (EDCs).** Refers to any number of chemicals that can disrupt the hormonal systems of humans.

**endotoxemia.** Potential adverse physical effects from gram negative bacteria such as *E. coli* or their by-products; mainly lipo-polysaccharides (LPS) crossing into the bloodstream from the intestines. Now linked to heart disease and inflammatory disorders.

**eicosapentaenoic acid (EPA).** A long chain polyunsaturated omega-3 fat found in fish oil. Has strong anti-inflammatory effects in the body.

**epigenetic modifier.** Any substance that impacts gene expression, effectively activating or silencing DNA via processes such as methylation and acetylation, without altering the DNA structure.

**epigenetics.** The study of how gene expression is affected by environmental influences like diet, stress, and chemical exposures.

**excitotoxicity.** Overstimulation of the nerve cells in the brain leading to damage.

**exposome.** The sum of all the exposures impacting gene expression and human health.

**F**

**fecal microbiome.** The population of bacteria, fungi, and viruses that inhabit the human intestine and can be analyzed in stool.

**fecal microbiome transplant (FMT).** A medical procedure whereby the microbiome from a healthy person's stool is concentrated and infused into another person's intestine. Most commonly performed for recurrent *C. difficile* infections.

**ferritin.** A sensitive marker of iron stores in the human body, and a laboratory method to screen for iron deficiency.

**First Thousand Days.** The concept that the period of human growth from conception until age 2 is a critical window for rapid brain development, the establishment of the intestinal microbiome, and the highest amount of epigenetic programming.

**FODMAPs.** The acronym for *fermentable oligo and disaccharides, monosaccharides, and polyols,* which are substances in foods that may cause irritable bowel syndrome symptoms in susceptible people.

**food intolerance.** Typically used to refer to an adverse food reaction not caused by the immune system.

**food sensitivity.** A non-specific term often used to refer to any non-classic adverse reaction to foods. Sometimes may be referred to more accurately as a *food hypersensitivity* or *delayed hypersensitivity*.

**G**

**gene expression.** When part of the DNA contained in our genes is translated into a protein, it is said to be expressed.

**gestational diabetes.** A state of glucose intolerance and high blood sugar that occurs only during pregnancy.

**gluten.** The protein in wheat, barley, and rye that gives these grains their elastic properties but can also cause adverse reactions in many people.

**glycemic index.** The measure of how quickly a food can raise blood sugar levels. Pure glucose has a glycemic index of 100. High-fiber whole foods have a lower glycemic index.

**glycemic load.** A measure of the product of the glycemic index (how quickly a food raises blood sugar levels) and total carbohydrate content of the food.

**glycosylation/fructosylation.** Damage to proteins in the human body from excessive glucose or fructose. Most well known as a process in diabetes, excess sugar sticks to red blood cells (glycosylated hemoglobin). This is the basis of the test hemoglobin (Hgb) A1c that shows average glucose levels in the blood. A high HgbA1c indicates increased glycosylation occurring in the body with potential damage to the kidneys, eyes, blood vessels, and heart. This process is *considerably more likely to happen with fructose than glucose.*

**ghrelin.** The hunger hormone that tells the body when it is time to eat.

**H**

**heme iron**. The form of iron found in animal foods like meat, poultry, and fish. It is more bioavailable to the human body than non-heme iron from plant foods.

**hemoglobin**. A laboratory test that is part of the CBC, which measures the protein in the blood responsible for delivering oxygen to the body. A low hemoglobin level is referred to as anemia.

**heterozygous**. Carrying two different copies of a particular gene, which if one copy is "normal" and one copy "abnormal" may not result in clinically significant disease. For example, being heterozygous for the cystic fibrosis gene (delta F508) does not cause the disease, as the person also has one normal copy of the gene but is then labeled a "carrier."

**high calorie malnutrition**. The state of many Americans who consume too much highly processed food, receiving plenty of calories, but lacking several important nutrients. This state leaves people at risk for many of the "diseases of Western civilization" such as heart disease, diabetes, and cancer.

**high density lipoprotein (HDL)**. Often referred to as "good cholesterol," HDL is responsible for bringing cholesterol back to the liver to be processed. High blood levels of HDL may be cardioprotective. Low HDL may be a risk factor for cardiovascular disease.

**histamine**. The chemical released from white blood cells (mast cells) during an allergic reaction. Massive histamine release causes anaphylaxis.

**homocysteine.** A naturally produced amino acid that is damaging to the body at high levels and linked to birth defects, heart disease, stroke, dementia, and several other diseases.

**homozygous.** Carrying two identical copies of a particular gene that may impact the function of certain bodily functions and in some cases leaves the body more prone to certain diseases. For example, being homozygous for the cystic fibrosis gene delta F508 causes the carrier to have the disease known as cystic fibrosis.

**human milk oligosaccharide (HMO)**. The ultimate baby prebiotic in breastmilk that promotes growth of the early beneficial gut bacteria and a healthy infant microbiome.

**hydrolyzed proteins**. Proteins that are partially broken down with enzymes, similar to digestion, making them less allergenic.

**hyperpalatable foods**. Foods that are overly stimulating to the pleasure center of the brain, making them more likely to be overconsumed by susceptible people and potentially contributing to the obesity epidemic.

**hypoallergenic.** A food or substance less likely to trigger an allergic reaction.

**I**

**IgE-mediated food allergy**. "Classic" food allergies that cause immediate reactions such as hives, swelling, and itching.

**immune mediated**. A reaction or physical response that is caused by some part of the immune system.

**immune tolerance**. The state of non-reaction by the immune system whereby it does not view a food, the body's own tissue, or other nonharmful substance as a threat. Loss of immune tolerance is responsible for food allergies and autoimmune disease.

**inflammatory bowel disease (IBD).** Refers to one of several chronic non-infectious autoimmune conditions of the intestines, namely ulcerative colitis and Crohn's disease.

**innate immunity.** As opposed to adaptive immunity, this part of the immune system does not "learn" but is rather programmed to react to certain triggers as a first line of defense.

**insulin.** The hormone released by the pancreas in response to rising blood sugar levels. Insulin acts on many cells in the body to get the glucose into the cell to be metabolized.

**insulin resistance.** The state where the body's cells are not responding to standard healthy levels of insulin, so increasing amounts are needed to maintain blood glucose control.

**irritable bowel syndrome (IBS).** Non-inflammatory, non-autoimmune condition of the digestive system resulting in bloating, cramping, diarrhea, or constipation.

**K**

**ketoacidosis.** A state in which there are abnormally high ketone levels in the body, making the body too acidic and causing adverse physical reactions. Most commonly seen in diabetes.

**ketones.** Small molecules made in the liver from fat that are an alternate fuel source to glucose for the body and brain. Ketones are elevated when fasting or on a very low carbohydrate diet.

**ketosis.** The state of the body when there are elevated ketones in the blood, which are being burned for energy. This is a normal physiologic process as long as the person does not progress to ketoacidosis.

**L**

**lactose intolerance.** Inability to digest and absorb the milk sugar lactose, typically due to lack of the enzyme lactase. Primary lactose intolerance occurs when a person lacks or loses the ability to produce the enzyme lactase for digesting milk sugar. Secondary lactose intolerance refers to a *reversible* loss of the lactase enzyme due to irritation or inflammation of the intestines.

**leaky gut.** A state of increased permeability of the intestines, allowing food particles or bacteria and their by-products into the bloodstream where they potentially cause inflammation and immune system activation.

**leptin.** A hormone produced by our fat cells that signals the brain that they are full. Also called the satiety hormone, this hormone acts to decrease appetite and increase metabolism.

**linear dose response.** A graph which plots the amount of measured response to an increasing dose of a drug or toxin. A linear dose response provides strong evidence that what is being measured is actually causing the observed response.

**linoleic acid (LA).** An omega-6 short chain polyunsaturated fatty acid, found in high amounts in plant oils such as corn, sunflower, safflower, and vegetable oil. Can be converted to arachidonic acid (ARA) in the body.

**long chain polyunsaturated fatty acids (LCPUFAs).** Biologically important omega-6 and omega-3 fatty acids that are 20-22 carbons in length, used in our cell membranes; also used to create signaling molecules called eicosanoids in the body.

**low density lipoprotein (LDL).** LDL is the major transport molecule for cholesterol in our blood. High levels, especially of the small, dense LDL particles, are associated with increased heart disease risk.

**low glycemic index.** Foods that do not cause a rapid rise in blood sugar levels. Mainly refers to carbohydrates that have an intact fiber matrix that slows digestion and absorption of glucose.

# M

**macrocytic anemia.** A state of too few red blood cells in the bloodstream that are larger than normal size. Typically caused by folate and/or vitamin $B_{12}$ deficiency.

**medium chain triglyceride (MCT).** A saturated fat that is shorter length than most typical saturated fats in the diet and is more easily metabolized by the body to create ketones.

**meta-analysis.** A research study which collects data from a group of prior studies and pools the data together to try to reach a stronger conclusion using higher numbers of research subjects.

**metabolic flexibility.** The ability of the body to shift back and forth from fat and ketone burning to carbohydrate burning without being overly reliant on carbohydrate and glucose for energy.

**metabolic syndrome.** A state of ill health characterized by insulin resistance, elevated blood pressure, elevations in blood lipids (triglycerides) that is on the path to development of type 2 diabetes and cardiovascular disease. Most often associated with obesity but may occur in non-obese people as well.

**metabolism.** The functioning of the body's cellular machinery and which fuel is used to keep it running.

**metabolomics.** The study of small molecules (metabolites) in the blood, urine, and stool that indicate what biological processes are occurring in that individual person. Can be used to identify defects or abnormalities in metabolism.

**methyl donors.** A set of nutrients including folate, $B_{12}$, $B_6$ and choline that participate in important biological processes such as the manufacture of neurotransmitters, detoxification of harmful compounds like homocysteine, or the activation or silencing of our genes.

**methylation.** The act of adding a one-carbon molecule called a methyl group to another substance such as our DNA.

**microbiome.** The collective population of microorganisms (bacteria, viruses, fungi) that inhabit a certain defined location, such as the human intestine.

**microbiome disrupting chemicals (MDCs).** A group of substances that disturb the normal healthy balance of bacteria that reside in our intestines. May refer to items contained in our food such as antibiotics, pesticide residues, artificial sweeteners, emulsifiers, thickeners, and stabilizers.

**microcytic anemia**. A state of low numbers of red blood cells in our blood that are smaller than normal size. Typically, the result of prolonged iron deficiency.

**milk fat globule membrane (MFGM)**. The delivery vehicle for fats in the breast milk that contain a spectrum of proteins and fats bound together in a biological molecule created in the human breast. MFGM has been found to have biological significance.

**mitochondria**. The "powerhouses" of our cells used to create the energy molecule ATP used in most biological processes in our bodies. The end result of metabolizing our food is the production of ATP by our mitochondria.

**MTHFR**. An abbreviation for *methylenetetrahydrofolate reductase*. An important enzyme in our body that converts the biologically inactive form of dietary folate into the active form methyltetrahydro-folate. A significant number of people are found to have alterations of this enzyme, potentially making them more susceptible to having a child with birth defects and developing cardiovascular disease, stroke, and certain brain disorders.

**mucosal microbiome**. The part of the intestinal microbiome that resides in the mucus layer immediately next to the intestine. It may differ from the stool microbiome, which refers to the bacteria detected in a stool sample from the person being studied.

**myelin sheath**. The insulation around a nerve cell that allows nerve conduction and prevents short circuiting.

# N

**necrotizing enterocolitis (NEC)**. A very serious inflammatory condition of the (premature) infant's intestines that can be fatal or require surgery to remove large parts of the baby's intestine.

**neurodevelopment**. The process of growth and maturation of the human brain and nervous system that is most rapid over the first thousand days of a child's life.

**neurodevelopmental disorders**. Any number of conditions that disturb the normal process of neurodevelopment, leaving the child delayed in one or several domains of cognitive, social, or motor functioning. Autism is a common example.

**neurogenesis**. The creation of new neurons, which is most rapid during the first thousand days of life.

**neuron**. A nerve cell in the brain or peripheral nervous system.

**neuronal plasticity**. The ability of the brain to adapt and change its configuration in response to new stimuli and new knowledge.

**neurotransmitters**. Small molecules produced in our brain and nervous system that are the mode of communication between brain cells and nerve cells. Common neurotransmitters include dopamine, serotonin, and acetylcholine.

**neurotrophins**. Nutrients or hormones that support the growth and function of neurons in the brain.

**NAFLD**. An acronym for *non-alcoholic fatty liver disease*. A pathological condition when the liver stores too much fat (triglyceride), causing it to become inflamed. Closely related to insulin resistance and metabolic syndrome.

**non-celiac gluten sensitivity (NCGS).** A condition where the ingestion of gluten-containing foods causes gastrointestinal and other symptoms without the intestinal damage seen in celiac disease.

**non-heme iron.** The type of iron found in plant foods that is less efficiently absorbed as compared to heme-iron.

**non-IgE mediated food allergy.** Allergic food reactions that do not involve the antibody immunoglobulin E (IgE) and are not anaphylactic. May involve other components of the immune system such as T-cells.

**non-immune mediated.** Food reactions that do not involve the immune system and may be more related to an inability to digest and absorb certain foods, or a chemical irritation that results from ingestion of certain foods. Lactose intolerance is a non-immune mediated food reaction.

**natural resources defense council (NRDC).** A large environmental watchdog organization that strives to protect our access to clean air, water, and environment.

# O

**obesogens.** Chemicals in the environment that predispose one to developing obesity and may be epigenetic modifiers and turn on genes for obesity.

**oligoantigenic diet.** Also referred to as the "few foods diet," which eliminates most common allergens such as wheat, dairy, soy, eggs, corn, and nuts and relies on a small select group of less allergenic foods to test for potential adverse reactions to common foods in our diet.

**oligosaccharides.** Special carbohydrate molecules that are not digested by humans, but rather provide food for our microbiome and may be referred to as prebiotics.

**omega-3.** Polyunsaturated fats that have anti-inflammatory properties and are important for brain structure and function. EPA and DHA are the biologically active omega-3 fats.

**omega-6.** Polyunsaturated fats that are needed for cellular structure and function but are often excessive in the modern diet and potentially pro-inflammatory. ARA is the biologically active omega-6 fat.

**omnivorous.** Eating a variety of foods, including meat, grains, and vegetables.

**oxidative stress.** Refers to a situation where the body's production of free radicals through various metabolic processes exceeds the body's ability to neutralize or "quench" the free radicals. This creates oxidative stress and begins to damage the cells and tissues of our body.

**oxidized oils.** Damaged dietary fats that have been exposed to prolonged heat and oxygen, changing their chemical properties, and creating the potential for them to form *free radicals* and create *oxidative stress* in the human body.

**pediatric feeding disorders (PFD).** Any number of maladaptive feeding behaviors leading to a decreased ability to consume a healthy, age-appropriate diet.

**pelvic floor dysfunction.** An abnormal functioning of the nerves and muscles of the pelvis that may be a common cause of pelvic pain and constipation.

**phytates.** Naturally occurring compounds that are found in plant foods that may have some health benefits but can block absorption of nutrients such as iron and zinc.

**phytochemicals/phytonutrients.** Beneficial plant compounds that are not officially classified as vitamins but have protective roles when consumed by humans. May act as antioxidants and beneficial epigenetic modifiers and play a role in feeding the microbiome.

**polyunsaturated fatty acids (PUFAs).** Fats that contain several double bonds (as opposed to saturated fats with no double bonds) thereby changing their chemical properties. May include omega-3 and omega-6 PUFAs.

**prebiotics.** Substances that feed the microbiome, typically soluble fiber, oligosaccharides, and resistant starches.

**precision medicine.** A new paradigm that does away with the one-size-fits-all mentality of classic Western medicine and uses evolving science such as metabolomics, nutrigenomics, and microbiome analysis to determine the best treatment or prevention method for that individual.

**prediabetes.** A state of insulin resistance and rising fasting blood sugars that is the final step prior to development of diabetes. Reversible with diet and lifestyle modification.

**preeclampsia.** A potentially dangerous condition during pregnancy with the development of high blood pressure and protein in the urine.

**pregnancy induced hypertension.** Development of high blood pressure during pregnancy.

**preterm delivery.** Delivering a baby prior to 37 weeks of gestation. Early preterm birth prior to 32 weeks is associated with a number of medical complications for the baby. Even late-preterm birth from 34-37 weeks can carry some risks to the child.

**probiotics.** Beneficial bacteria that when consumed in significant numbers by humans, convey a health benefit.

**R**

**radiofrequency (RF) emissions.** Radiation that can include the spectrum from radio waves to microwaves and emitted by devices such as microwave ovens and cellular phones. Referred to as non-ionizing radiation, it is controversial whether prolonged or excessive exposure in children could be detrimental to their health.

**RDA.** Acronym for *recommended dietary allowances* originally set by the US Institute of Medicine (IOM) to recommend adequate nutrient intake levels to prevent deficiency.

**resistant starch.** Dietary carbohydrates that are not digested by humans but may provide fuel for the microbiome.

**reverse osmosis (RO) filtration.** Use of a semi-permeable membrane to remove 99% of dissolved solids, metals, and impurities from drinking water.

**S**

**saturated fat.** The type of fat containing no double bonds, typically found in animal products but also in palm, coconut, and olive oil.

**short chain fatty acids (SCFA).** Produced when beneficial bacteria ferment dietary fiber and resistant starch. SCFA may play important roles in the human body.

**small intestinal bacterial overgrowth (SIBO).** A state of excessive numbers of the wrong kinds of bacteria residing in the upper intestine, potentially causing a host of symptoms including those consistent with irritable bowel syndrome (IBS).

**speech-language pathologist (SLP).** A specialized therapist trained in treating disorders of speech and eating.

**Standard American Diet (SAD).** Generally refers to the diet that is calorie rich and nutrient poor. It consists largely of highly processed foods while lacking real whole foods. Consumption of the SAD is associated with most modern diseases like cancer, heart disease, and diabetes but may be associated with depression and other brain disorders as well.

**subclinical nutrient deficiency.** A more subtle inadequate intake of a vitamin, mineral, or other nutrient that does not present with classic deficiency symptoms but still results in ill health or suboptimal development.

**synapse.** The junction or gap between two nerve cells that requires neurotransmitters to transmit nerve signals.

**synaptogenesis.** The creation of new connections between existing nerve cells (neurons) in the brain. Synaptogenesis is how learning occurs, and the reinforcement of connections between neurons is thought to be how new information is stored in the brain.

**T**

**TOFI.** An acronym for Thin Outside, Fat Inside. A common condition where people store their fat around their vital organs rather than their bellies and thighs.

**toxicant.** Any toxic agent that can be damaging to the body.

**toxin.** A toxic agent produced by a living organism. (This term is often used instead of the more correct term toxicant to refer to any substance toxic to the human body.)

**trans fat.** An artificially produced fatty acid used in food processing, which is also referred to as partially hydrogenated fat. It has been used heavily in the food supply over the past 40 years, but recently associated with increased risks of cancer, heart disease, and the development of Alzheimer's.

**triglycerides.** The most common transportation and storage form of fats/lipids in the body. Elevated triglycerides in the blood can be harmful and associated with metabolic syndrome and risk of cardiovascular disease.

**type 1 diabetes (T1DM).** An autoimmune disease, typically of childhood, where the immune system attacks and destroys the insulin producing cells of the pancreas. The child then becomes dependent on injected insulin.

**type 2 diabetes (T2DM).** Previously referred to as adult-onset diabetes, is not autoimmune in nature and is the result of prolonged insulin resistance leading to pancreatic exhaustion and elevations in blood glucose and metabolic abnormalities. Often but not always associated with obesity.

## U-Z

**ultra-processed food.** Food-like substances that represent an increasing proportion of the Western diet and are made from substances extracted from real foods such as starches and sugars, often containing many additives and chemicals. Often little to no amount of the original food is left in the product.

**whey.** A common protein found in animal milk and the largest protein component of human breastmilk.

**World Health Organization (WHO).** An international agency that works to improve the health of people globally, often focused on protecting the health of those people in developing nations across the globe.

**zonulin.** A protein discovered in the early 2000s that causes an increase in the permeability of the intestinal barrier and can lead to "leaky gut" if excessive.

www.ingramcontent.com/pod-product-compliance
Lightning Source LLC
Chambersburg PA
CBHW050852150626
46549CB00013B/1429